PRACTICAL SMALL ANIMAL ULTRASONOGRAPHY. ABDOMEN

Plaza Antonio Beltrán Martínez n.° 1, planta 8 - letra I
(Centro empresarial El Trovador)
50002 Zaragoza - Spain

First printing: February 2022

ISBN: 978-84-18339-60-8
DL: Z 66-2022

Design, layout and printing:
Grupo Asís Biomedia, SL
www.grupoasis.com
info@grupoasis.com

edra is an imprint of Grupo Asís

Warning:

Veterinary science is constantly evolving, as are pharmacology and the other sciences. Inevitably, it is therefore the responsibility of the veterinary surgeon to determine and verify the dosage, the method of administration, the duration of treatment and any possible contraindications to the treatments given to each individual patient, based on his or her professional experience. Neither the publisher nor the author can be held liable for any damage or harm caused to people, animals or properties resulting from the correct or incorrect application of the information contained in this book.

Practical SMALL ANIMAL ultrasonography

2nd EDITION

Abdomen

Panagiotis Mantis

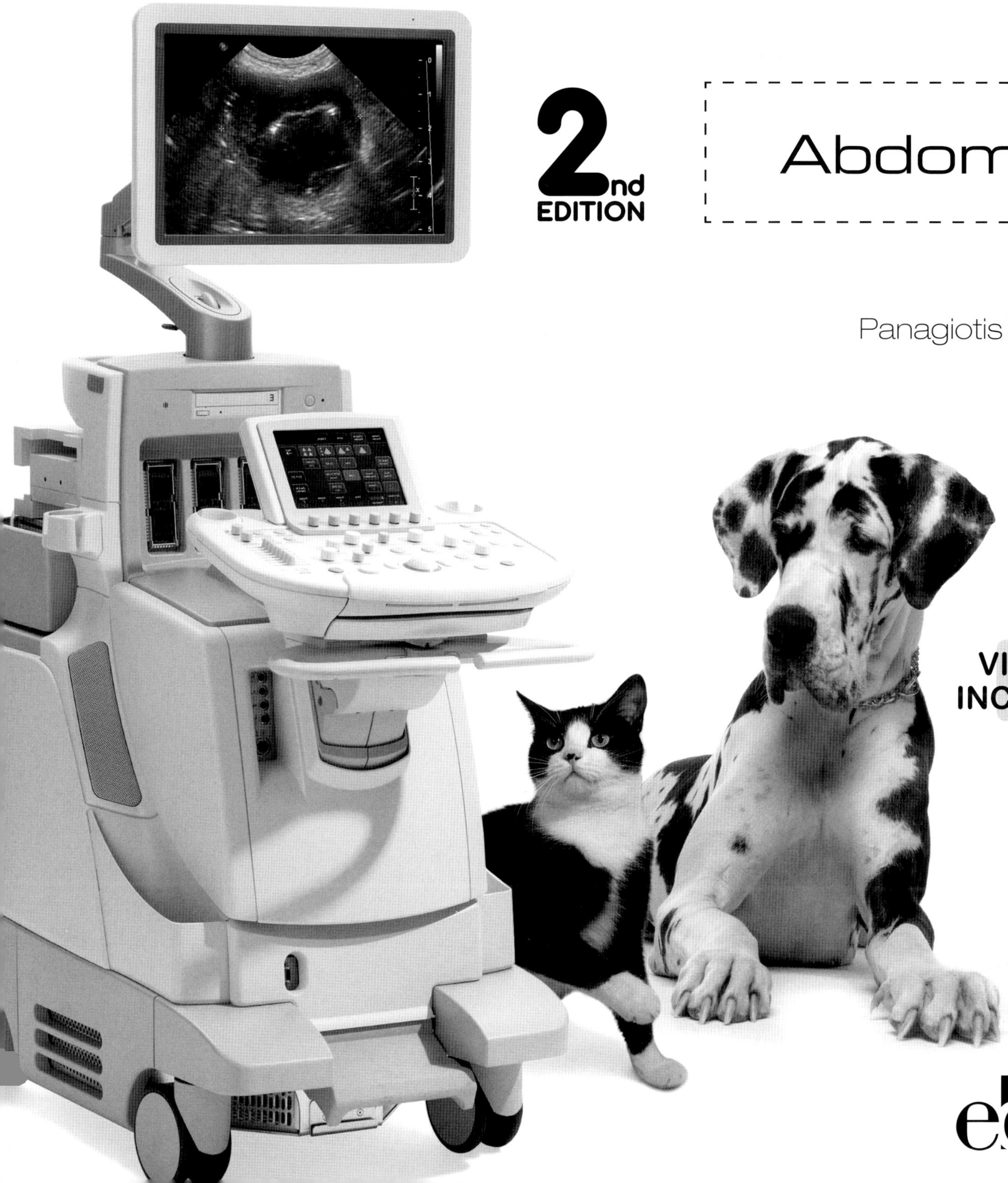

VIDEOS INCLUDED

edra

Acknowledgements

I would like to express my gratitude to the many people who contributed to the production of this book. First, to my editor for her patience with me while preparing and delivering the chapters and for keeping me in the straight and narrow.

A big thank to my colleagues at Dick White Referrals for their help in proofreading the chapters and to my current and previous diagnostic imaging residents for helping to create images displaying the positioning and technique.

Special thanks to Mrs Paula Mann for organising the video recordings and Mr Brian Cox for recording, directing, and editing the video clips that appear in this and the previous edition.

Again, I want to thank my wife Vaia and my children who continuously encouraged and supported me during this time preparing the second edition, despite the amount of time that this work has taken me away from them.

Finally, I would like to thank and ask their forgiveness to all those people who have helped me over the years and whose names I have not mentioned.

The author

Panagiotis Mantis

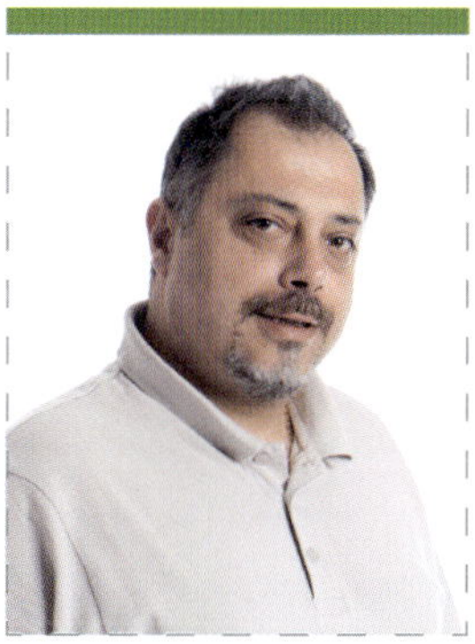

Panagiotis (Pete) Mantis graduated from the Faculty of Veterinary Medicine of the Aristotle University of Thessaloniki, Greece in 1994. He completed his Diagnostic Imaging Residency at the Royal Veterinary College and then worked in first opinion practices and referral hospitals in London before moving for a year to the Swedish Agricultural University in Uppsala. In 2000, he returned to the Royal Veterinary College. He became Senior Lecturer in Radiology and remained at RVC until joining Dick White Referrals in 2017 where he is currently the Head of Diagnostic Imaging.

Pete is a European and RCVS Specialist in Veterinary Diagnostic Imaging, Fellow of the Higher Education Academy and Fellow of the Royal College of Veterinary Surgeons. He is a regular author, speaker and CPD tutor on small animal radiology, ultrasonography, computed tomography, and magnetic resonance imaging. Pete has lectured extensively nationally and internationally and is involved in innovative and very popular online and conventional CPD courses.

Foreword

The needs of those new to ultrasonography and of those who though quite practiced are keen to benchmark and reaffirm their current practice remain. For this reason, it is a pleasure to see the second edition of this successful practical book. This new edition has managed to retain the strength of the previous edition and add new material in the form for example of a chapter on common artifacts and of multiple new illustrations, new examples and new and upgraded images.

The author Dr. Panagiotis Mantis and I have worked together during overlapping periods in our careers at the Royal Veterinary College, London and at the Swedish University of Agricultural Sciences. Since then, over the years we have worked together on many practical ultrasound training courses for veterinary practitioners, covering material at various levels. At the very outset and as time progressed, I could see how Panagiotis has an almost magical ability to place himself in the mind of the person he assists. In so doing, he takes the learner in ultrasound imaging from a place of frustration and confusion to a place of comfort and assurance. As I write this foreword from my office in Copenhagen, I think of the Philosopher Søren Kierkegaard from this city and often cited here, who wrote that the teacher must learn from the learner; must place themself in the student's position in order to take them forward to new places. This teaching philosophy is turned into practical reality in this book. What you have in your hand is a clear, concise and basic practical aid, because the author has the depth of knowledge and experience to make it so.

The first edition of this practical text was published in 2016. In the period since then diagnostic ultrasound has grown in importance, particularly in the investigation of abdominal disease and the time when ultrasound is first encountered has shifted. Currently the initial encounter with veterinary ultrasonography will for many, come as early as the undergraduate courses at veterinary school. The period since the last edition has also seen improvements in image quality, which assist in organ and lesion recognition and increase confidence in those findings, but also have stretched the demands and expectations put on the sonographer.

To mirror these developments this second edition brings the teaching material contained within, up to date and relevant. As you the reader use this book, you will find it holds true to basics and will provide guidance in addressing questions that are of relevance to you, your patients and your clients.

Fintan J. McEvoy
MVB PhD DVSc DVR DipECVDI
Professor of Veterinary Radiology
University of Copenhagen
December, 2021

Preface

This second edition aims to update and improve the first edition and build on it. I hope it will continue to provide veterinary surgeons and veterinary ultrasonographers with straightforward guidance in performing and interpreting ultrasonographic examinations of the dog and cat.

Practical demonstration of the technique is provided by the inclusion of online video clips, with additional comprehensive instructions provided for each abdominal organ. I have included descriptions of normal ultrasonographic appearance along with variations from normal and commonly encountered abnormalities along with examples of commonly encountered artifacts.

The technique should appeal to most examiners and can be performed in first opinion practice. It can be easily adapted for those that prefer to scan the animals on their backs or use their left hand.

I would recommend reading each chapter, watch the technique clips and practice the technique.

I hope you will find this edition useful.

Cambridge, December 1st, 2021
Panagiotis Mantis

Table of contents

1

CHAPTER

MACHINE SET-UP

The typical ultrasound keyboard is full of buttons (Fig. 1) and trying to deal with it can be an intimidating experience. The good news is that you do not have to use all of these buttons of the keyboard. Regularly, once the machine is set up, you will only use a small number of the available buttons repeatedly to perform the ultrasonographic examination.

Before using the machine

Nowadays, most machines come with the screen properly calibrated to start using it. If not, or the image is not to your liking, follow these steps:

1. First, set the contrast of the screen to 90–100 %.

2. Then, set up the brightness using a greyscale bar. The machine probably has one on the side of the image. Alternatively, you can find many greyscale bars on the Internet.

3. Start by setting the brightness to the maximum and then reduce gradually until the darkest level in the greyscale bar is black. The top of the bar should be white, but not extremely bright. If too bright, adjust the contrast to correct it.

Machine buttons and knobs

The most common imaging controls used on a daily basis are detailed below and labelled accordingly in Figures 1 and 2.

1. **Patient details button.** Always input the details of the patient since this is going to be recorded in every image. As a minimum, it is recommended that the animal's name, owner's last name and case number should be entered. The date and time are usually entered by the machine automatically, therefore you just need to make sure that the machine's date and time are set correctly.

2. **Exam presets button.** It allows you to choose the exam presets (for abdominal ultrasound examination use the abdominal preset) that the manufacturer has inserted. In some machines the choice of exam preset is accessed together with the patient details using a single button. These presets are very helpful though some modifications are sometimes required to suit your needs. Go through all the presets and pick the one you prefer to use. Modify the settings to suit you and save the preset as your personal favourite for the abdominal examination.

> If presets do not exist, then it will be necessary to set them. This task requires more experience to be accomplished, so the manufacturer of the machine or supplier's application support team should be the first port of call to get some advice on how to proceed. Radiologists and ultrasonographers can also help you with the settings.

Figure 1. Keyboard of a portable ultrasound machine. The buttons and knobs commonly used are indicated.

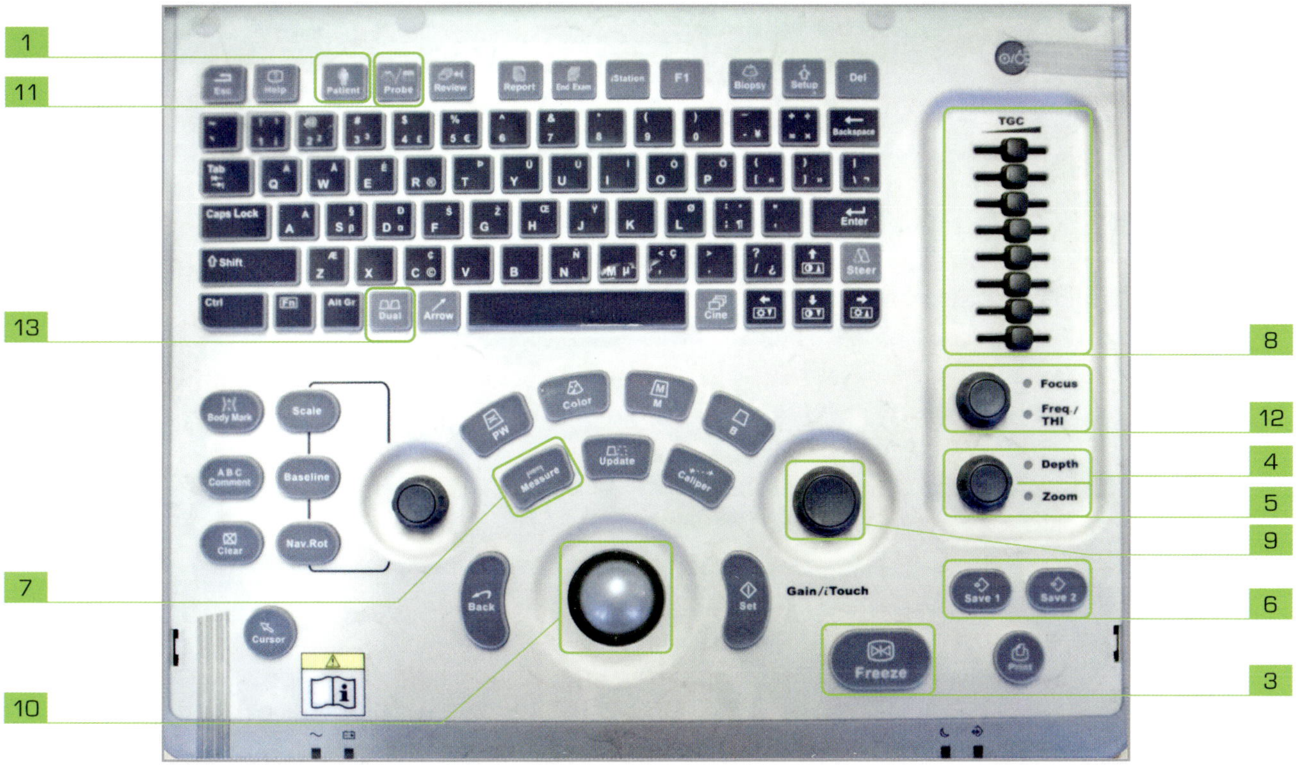

1 Patient details button	6 Save buttons	10 Focal zone control button or knob
2 Exam presets button	7 Measure button	11 Probe selection button
3 Freeze button	8 Time gain compensation (TGC) series of slide buttons	12 Frequency selection button or knob
4 Depth button	9 Overall gain knob	13 Dual-display button
5 Zoom button		14 Auto-optimisation button

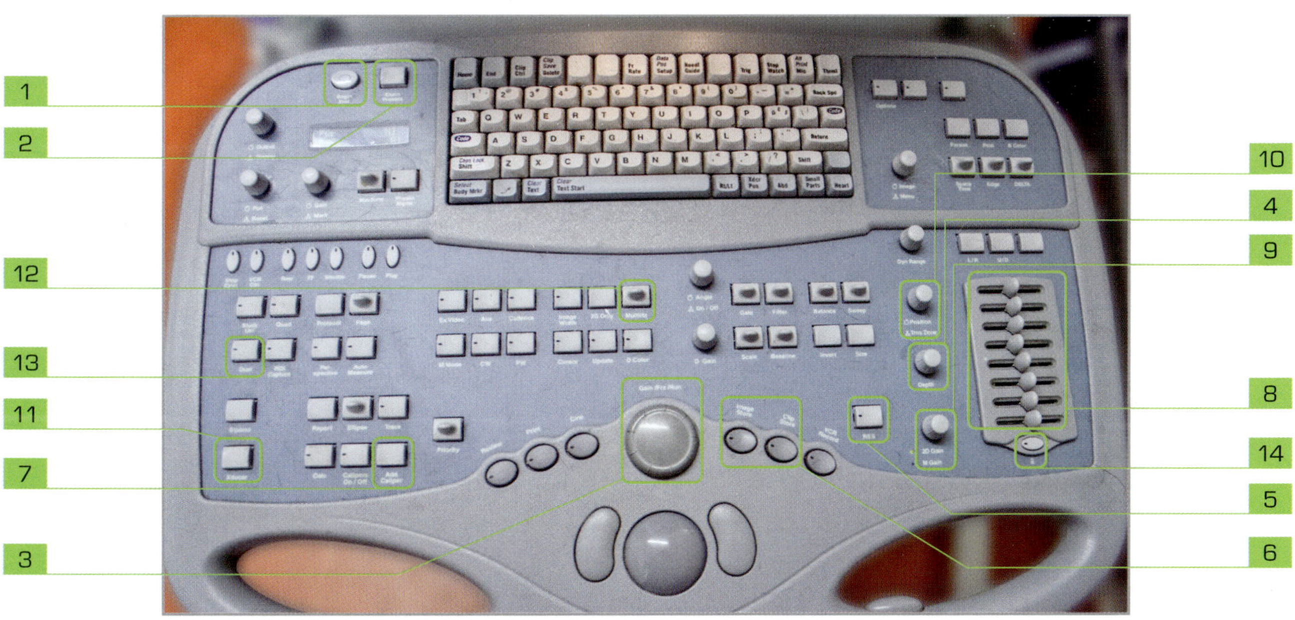

Figure 2. Keyboard of a high-specification ultrasound machine. The buttons and knobs most commonly used are indicated.

3. **Freeze button.** It freezes the images. In some machines the last few hundred frames are saved and this allows the ultrasonographer to go back and choose the best image, since it is commonly not the last one. This is a useful feature but not absolutely necessary.

4. **Depth button.** Depending on the machine, there may be buttons to press or knobs to rotate to increase or decrease the depth during an abdominal examination. It is recommended that any organ being imaged occupies approximately 75 % of the depth visible on the screen for general abdominal examination.

5. **Zoom button.** Some machines will zoom whatever is visible at the centre of the screen and some will allow the operator to choose the area to zoom. It is a very helpful button when examining small structures like the adrenals. It is not usually employed to identify the organ but to create a bigger image of a small organ or area of an organ to examine and save.

6. **Save buttons.** Usually there is one button to save images and another one to save clips. The "clip store" button can usually be adjusted in relation to the length of a clip up to a certain limit.

7. **Measure button.** It is pressed to perform linear measurements using the callipers. There is also a calculations or measurements button that allows the examiner to perform other calculations such as volumes or perimeters. It is a good idea to get into the habit of measuring the diameter or the length-width-height of the lesions. This way it will be possible to compare the lesions to see if they have progressed or regressed when an animal is re-examined.

8. **Time gain compensation (TGC) series of slide buttons.** These buttons adjust the image in specific areas (near-, mid- and far-field). You can set them up using a live image containing a large organ such as the liver. Use your whole hand to slide the buttons so they have an angle from top left to bottom right (greater amplification of the bottom echoes which are weaker) until you see that the liver (or the live image you are using) looks uniform in brightness (Fig. 3). Some machines (usually portable) have two separate knobs instead of a series of slide buttons, one for the near-field and another one for the far-field. These knobs are set up in a similar fashion.

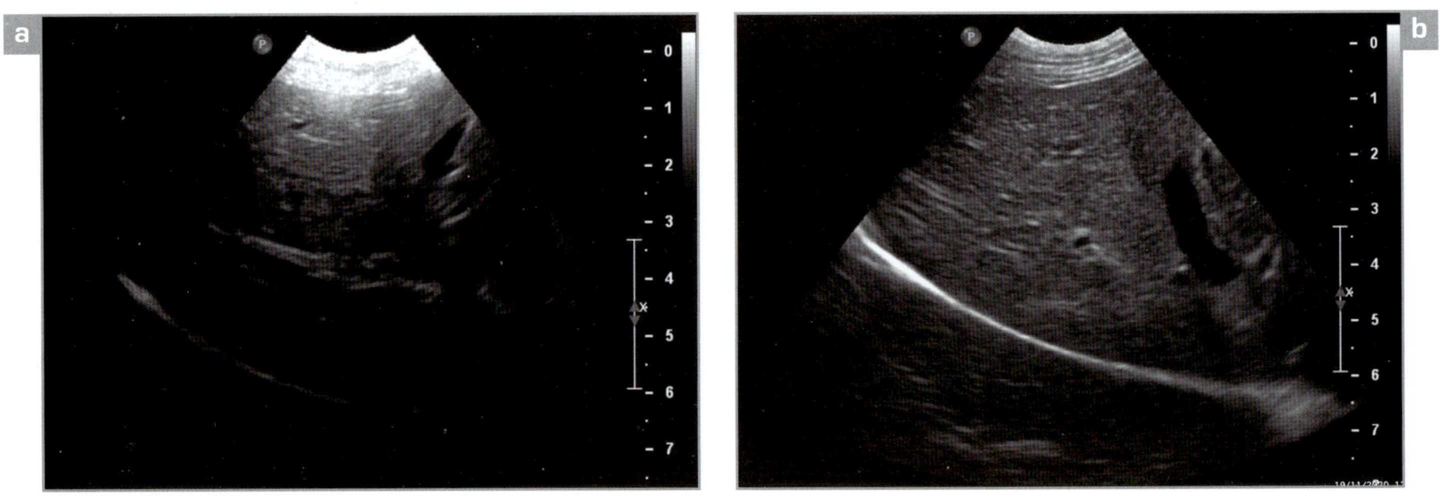

Figure 3. (a) Image from the normal liver of a dog prior to TGC setting. (b) Image of the liver from the same dog after TGC setting. All other settings remained the same. Note that of the liver appears uniform in brightness at all depths after TGC setting.

9. **Overall gain knob.** It amplifies or reduces the amplitude of all returning echoes regardless of the depth at which they were originated and thus increases or decreases the brightness of the image. This button will only be used from time to time during the examination.

10. **Focal zone control button or knob.** Usually, there is one button (or knob) to change the depth of the focal zone and another button (or knob) to modify the number of focal zones (to a maximum that varies depending on the machine). The focal zone is the area in which you get the highest resolution and it can be fixed or, more commonly in newer machines, adjusted to a certain depth. Although more than one focal zone can be set, one or two focal zones are enough for a general abdominal examination. As you increase the number of focal zones, the frame rate decreases and the image is updated more slowly. For a general abdominal examination, the focal zone is set to maximum depth and moved more superficially if a more superficial organ is examined. Then it is set back to maximum depth to continue the examination. The position of the focal zone is indicated on the screen.

11. **Probe selection button.** This button allows you to choose one of the transducers that are connected to the machine. In some machines, the preset is selected from this button after a specific probe is chosen.

12. **Frequency selection button or knob.** In multi-frequency transducers (common in the newer machines) this button (or knob) allows you to increase or decrease the frequency of the transducer employed. Some machines display the actual frequency employed (in MHz) while other machines (commonly portable) offer three choices: Res (resolution, for the highest frequency), Pen (penetration, for the lowest frequency) and Gen (general, for the mid-frequency of the transducer), so the operator needs to know the frequency range of the transducer in advance.

> Always use the highest frequency allowing the organs to be assessed at the required depth.

13. **Dual-display button.** Some machines have a dual-display button that splits the screen into two and allows the examiner to save an image on the left and a separate image on the right in order to compare organs side-by-side, e.g. to compare the liver with the spleen.

14. **Auto-optimisation button.** Some machines have a button that, when pressed, optimises the gain and overall contrast of the image. If available, it can be a good starting point once the preset and frequency have been selected.

15. **Image width.** The ultrasonographer can increase or decrease the image width when using a sector probe. We can increase or decrease the angle of viewing as required e.g. to include the whole kidney in the image. Some machines have this setting in the menu and others have it as a knob. This did not apply to linear probes. However, the trapezoidal image that can be created with the latest linear array transducers increases the width of the far field partially overcoming this limitation of the linear transducers. We usually use a sector image with an angle of 75–80 degrees for general scanning, when employing a sector probe for the examination.

Of course, you will have to consult the manual in order to identify the exact location and appearance of these buttons and knobs in your machine. You may also find other controls such as dynamic range, grey maps, line density, persistence, reject, tissue harmonic imaging, speckle reduction and spatial compound imaging. Most of these controls are set up with the presets. Tissue harmonic imaging and spatial compound imaging are more advanced modalities and beyond the scope of this book. If required, you can learn more about them from the recommended further reading list at the end of this book.

A few quick notes

- A dynamic range allows the operator to set how the echo intensity is displayed as shades of grey:
  - A wide range will provide a smoother image since more shades of grey are displayed. This is preferred for abdominal ultrasound.
  - A narrow range will provide a more black-and-white image (higher contrast) as fewer shades of grey are displayed. This is preferred for echocardiography.

- A grey-scale map determines how dark or white each level of grey is displayed. Generally, grey-scale maps that display more shades of grey are preferred for abdominal ultrasound. Some ultrasound machines provide also colorised grey-scale maps. These are not commonly used. They may assist in increasing lesion visibility in some instances.

- Line density sets the number of scan lines in the image:
  - A high line density improves resolution and reduces the frame rate.
  - A low line density increases the frame rate and reduces resolution.

- Persistence is also known as "frame averaging". Increasing this parameter raises the number of frames that are averaged to provide the visible image. With high persistence the image update is reduced and the image appears smoother, i.e. with less noise. Since on abdominal ultrasound a fast image update is not paramount, it is usually set higher, while in echocardiography it is set low.

- Reject is a filter that limits the lower level of echo that is displayed, thus eliminating weaker, potentially artefactual, signals.

- In tissue harmonic imaging (THI) mode the transducer does not only "listen" for returning echoes in the fundamental frequency (the frequency it sends), but also "listens" for echoes in multiples of the lowest fundamental frequency emitted (harmonic frequencies). The images generated with this mode have higher resolution because they contain fewer artifacts. Harmonic imaging is generally useful when scanning larger patients and not very useful for superficial scanning. In the author's experience, THI can have a positive effect on the image in some patients or areas examined; however, in a different area of the same patient or a different patient THI can be detrimental to the image.

- Speckle reduction eliminates weak signals that are not representative, while it enhances strong signals providing an improved image.

- Spatial compound imaging (SCI) combines images from multiple scan lines and scan angles into one single image. SCI improves image contrast. There are usually various choices that the examiner can select with SCI. The usefulness of SCI in veterinary ultrasound practice is still debated.

- When the sound is reflected from moving structures, like blood cells, the reflected sound has a different frequency to the frequency of sound that was emitted, the Doppler shift. The Doppler shift can be displayed in different ways. Doppler ultrasonography is used to detect the presence, speed, direction and character of the blood flow within the vessels. There are 4 types of Doppler ultrasound: pulsed wave (PW) and continuous wave (CW) Doppler (termed spectral Doppler) and colour flow Doppler and power Doppler. Duplex Doppler ultrasonography is termed the simultaneous display of pulsed or continuous wave Doppler and B-mode images. Triplex Doppler is the combination of B-mode and colour and PW or CW Doppler display. For more details on Doppler, check the recommended further reading.

Technique

1. Sit with the screen and keyboard in front of you and the patient on your right (or the patient on your left if you are left handed). The animal can be positioned in right lateral recumbency with the head of the animal towards the machine and its limbs towards you (Fig. 4a) if you are right-handed (and for some left-handed examiners) or the animal can be positioned on its back with the head of the animal towards the machine for right (Fig. 4b) and left (Fig. 4c) handed examiners. The author prefers to position the animal in rigth lateral recumbency because he is rigth-handed. Having the animal on the site is also easier, since it usually requires one assistant to hold the animal, especially if more assistants are not available. Similar steps can be followed with the animal on the back.

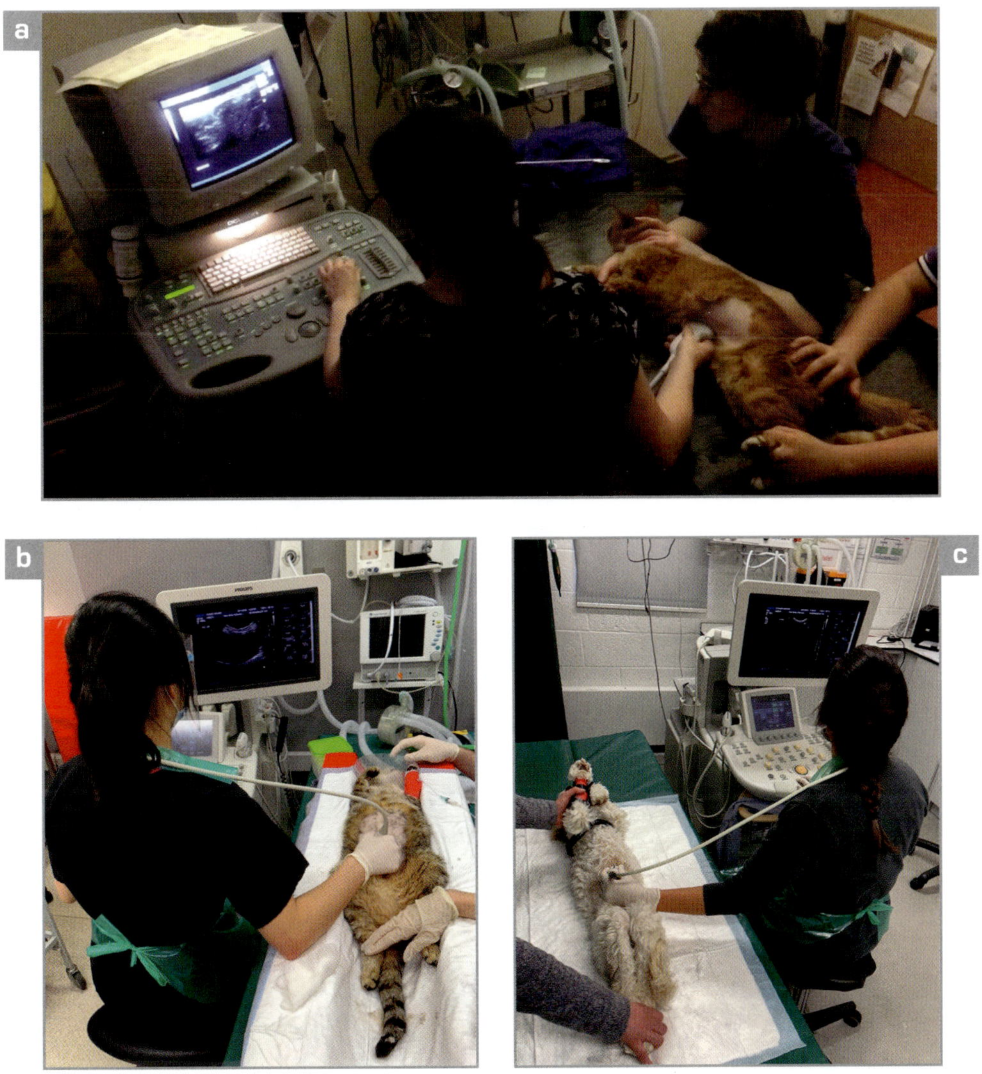

Figure 4. Positioning to start an abdominal ultrasound. **(a)** The animal is in right lateral recumbency and to the right of the examiner. The machine is in front of the examiner. The examiner holds the tarnsducer with the right hand and manages the keyboard with the left hand. **(b)** The animal is on its back (dorsal recumbency) and to the right of the examiner. The machine is in front of the examiner. This way, the right hand can be used to hold the transducer and the left hand to click the buttons and turn the knobs on the keyboard. **(c)** More helpful for left handed examiners. The animal is on its back (dorsal recumbency) and the machine is on the left of the examiner. The examiner can hold the transuder with the left hand and manage the keyboard with the rigth hand.

2. Press the "patient" button and set the patient details.

3. Select probe: Curvilineral or microconvex probe for dogs and cats. Consider linear probe for small dogs and cats and superficial structures.

4. Set the abdominal preset of choice.

5. Set an appropriate depth for liver (depending on the size of the animal).

6. Position and prepare the animal (Fig. 4 and 5).

7. Position the transducer to visualise the liver on the screen (see the Liver chapter for technique) (Fig. 6).

8. Select the appropriate frequency.

9. Set TGC and overall gain so that the liver appears of similar brightness at every depth (see Fig. 3).

10. Set focal zone number to one or two and the position to the deepest point possible.

11. You are now ready to start.

The TGC does not usually require any change throughout the ultrasound scan, but the overall gain, depth and frequency do.

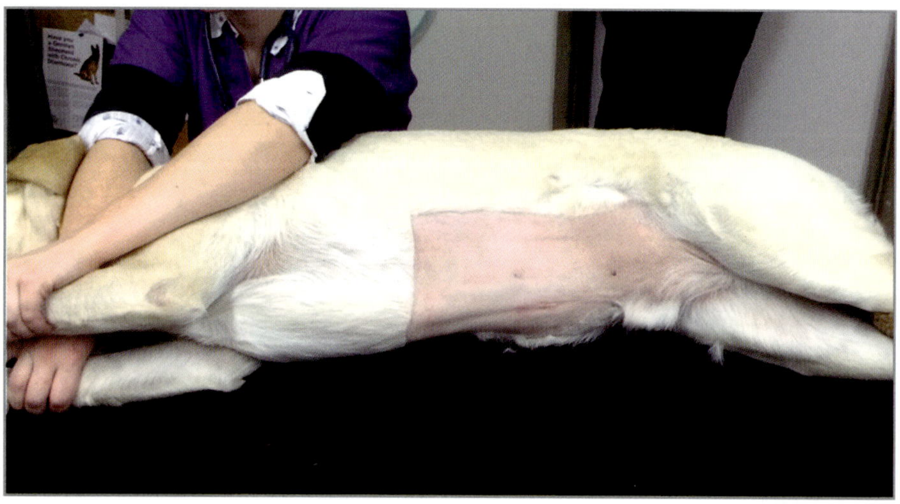

Figure 5. For a general abdominal ultrasound, wide clipping from the xiphoid process cranially to the pelvic inlet caudally, and latero-laterally half way up the side, should be performed. With experience, the clipped area can be reduced in extent.

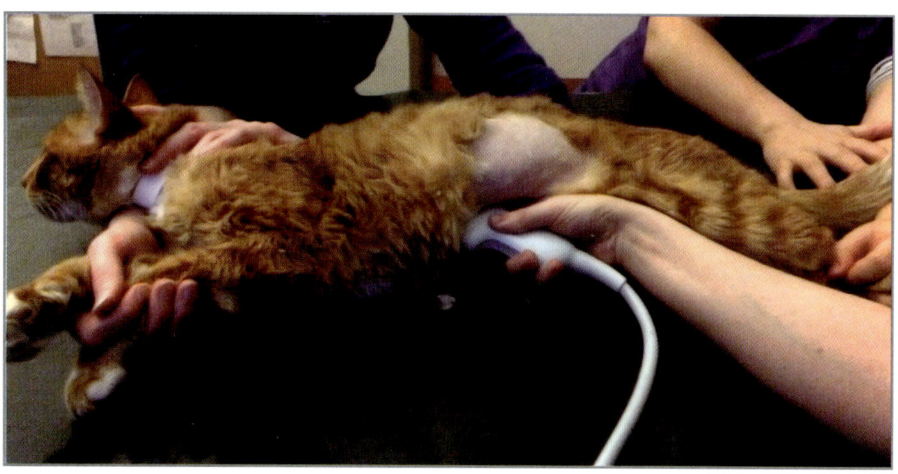

Figure 6. Position to acquire an image of the liver adequate to set up the machine. The transducer is parallel to the table, behind the xiphoid process and points towards the animal's shoulder. This way, the liver is commonly in the middle of the screen. If not, slight cranio-caudal angling (rocking) of the transducer will bring it to the middle of the screen.

2

CHAPTER

HOLDING THE TRANSDUCER AND TRANSDUCER MOVEMENTS

Holding the transducer

The transducers used in ultrasonography have an indicator (marker) in the form of an embossed or engraved mark. This marker corresponds to a mark that is identified in the top left or right corner of the image on the screen (Fig. 1).

> For abdominal ultrasound, the marker is usually displayed in the top left corner of the screen and this will be assumed for the techniques described in this book.

In order for the operator to use and move the transducer while only looking at the screen, the operator can hold the transducer with a finger on the marker. Usually the thumb or index finger is placed on the marker, depending on how one holds the transducer (Fig. 2). By knowing which finger is on the transducer's marker, the operator understands his or her orientation on the screen without the need to look at his or her hand (Fig. 3).

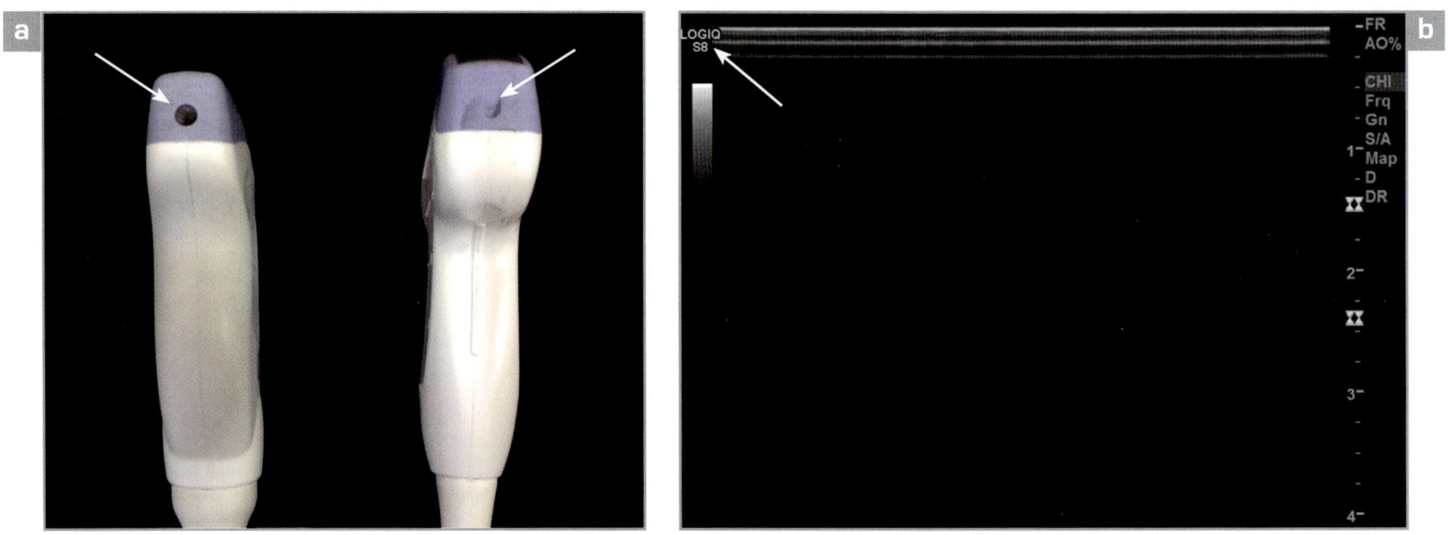

Figure 1. Linear (left) and curvilinear (right) transducers from an ultrasound machine. The marker is visible on the transducer **(a)** and displayed on the screen **(b)**.

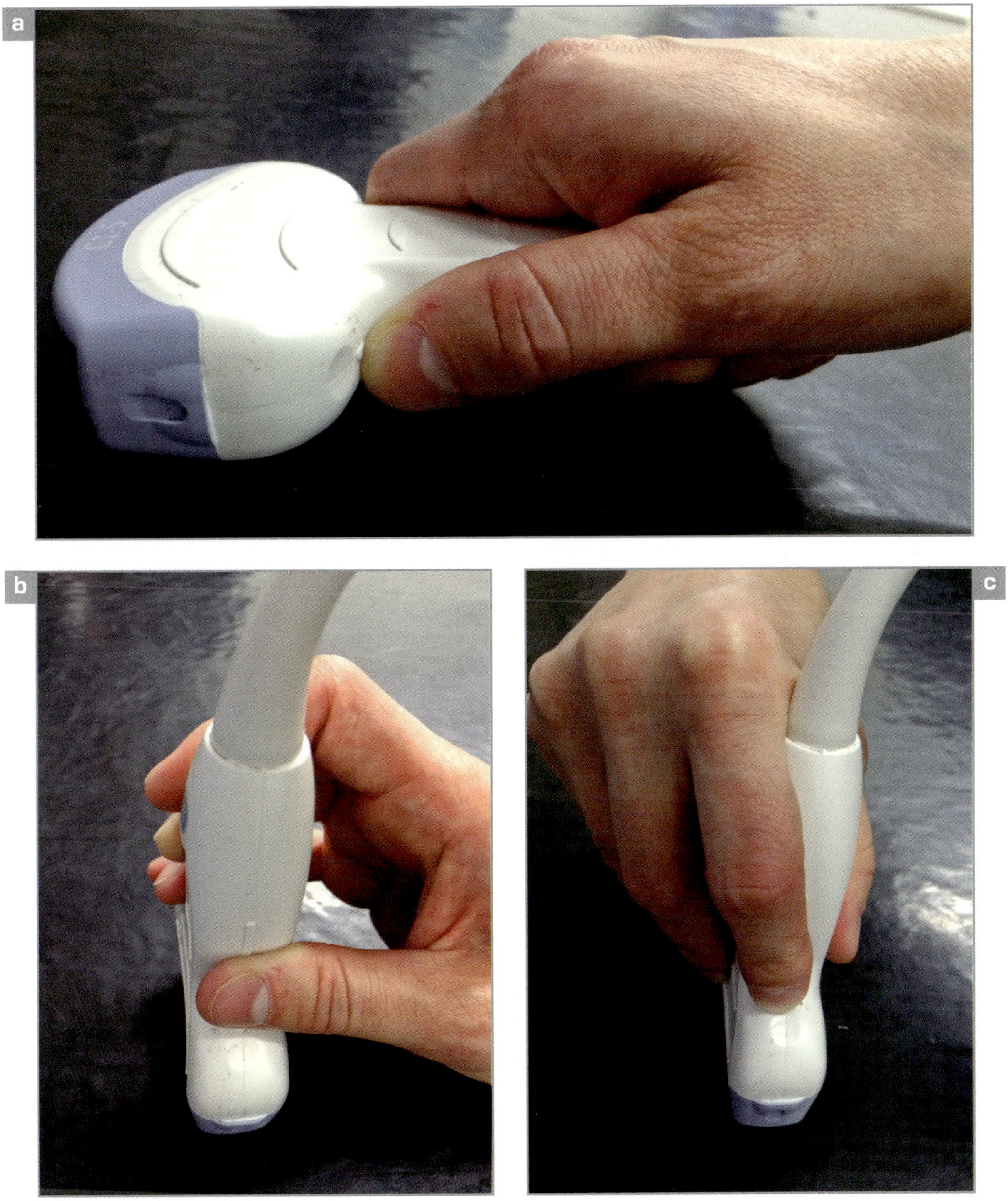

Figure 2. **(a, b)** The operator holds the transducer with the thumb on the marker. **(c)** The operator holds the transducer with the index finger on the marker.

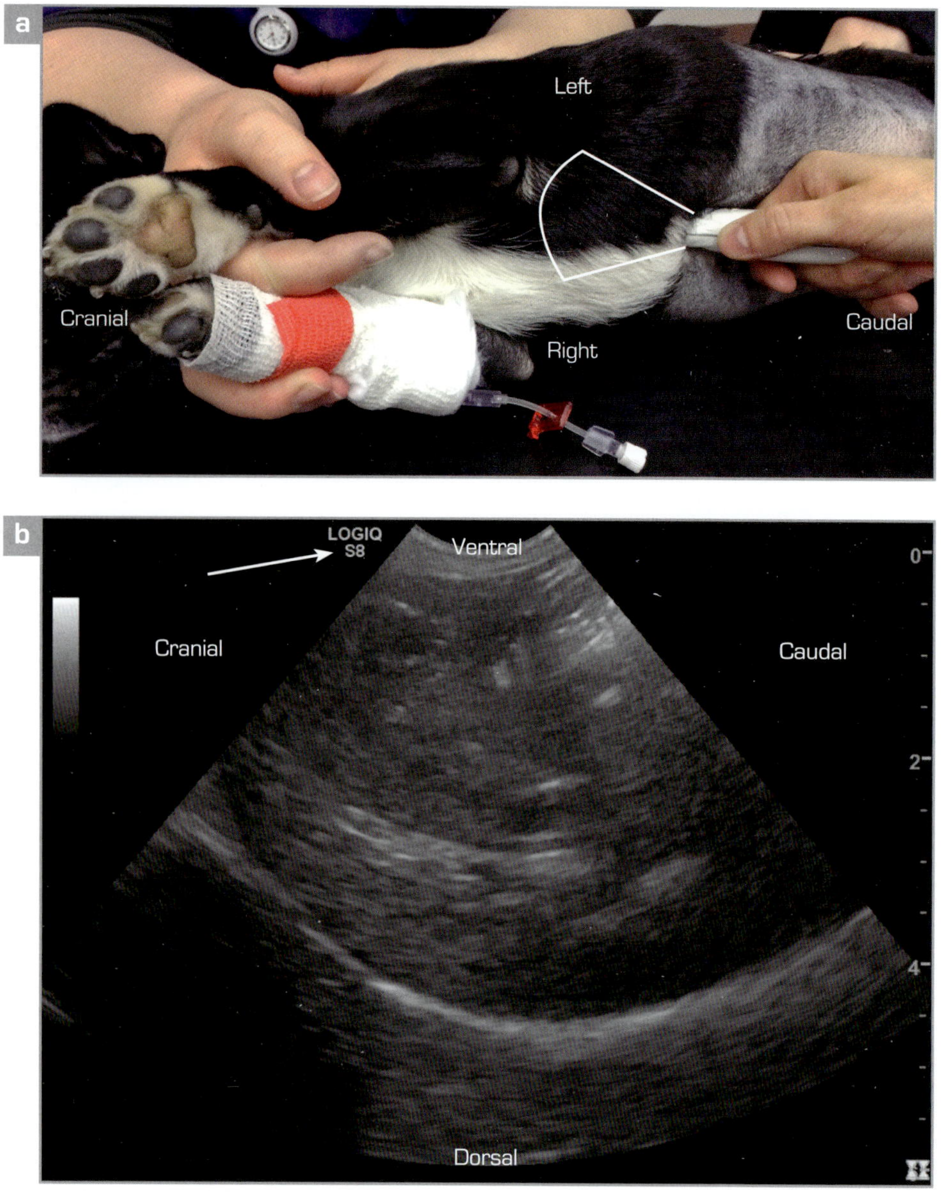

Figure 3. (a) Placement of the transducer for the evaluation of the liver with the marker pointing cranially. **(b)** An ultrasound image acquired with the orientation identified thanks to the knowledge of the location of the marker (arrow) and orientation of the transducer.

Transducer movements

There are five transducer movements:

1. **Sliding:** the transducer is held perpendicular or at an angle to the skin and it is moved cranially, caudally, and/or from side to side (Fig. 4).

2. **Rotation:** the transducer is held perpendicular or at an angle to the skin and is rotated clockwise or anticlockwise as we look at the transducer from its back (Fig. 5).

3. **Pressure:** the transducer is held perpendicular or at an angle to the skin and the abdomen is compressed by applying pressure to the transducer (Fig. 6).

4. **Rocking:** the transducer is held still at one point and is tilted forwards and backwards along the axis of the beam (Fig. 7).

5. **Fanning:** the transducer is held still at one point and is tilted side to side perpendicular to the axis of the beam (Fig. 8).

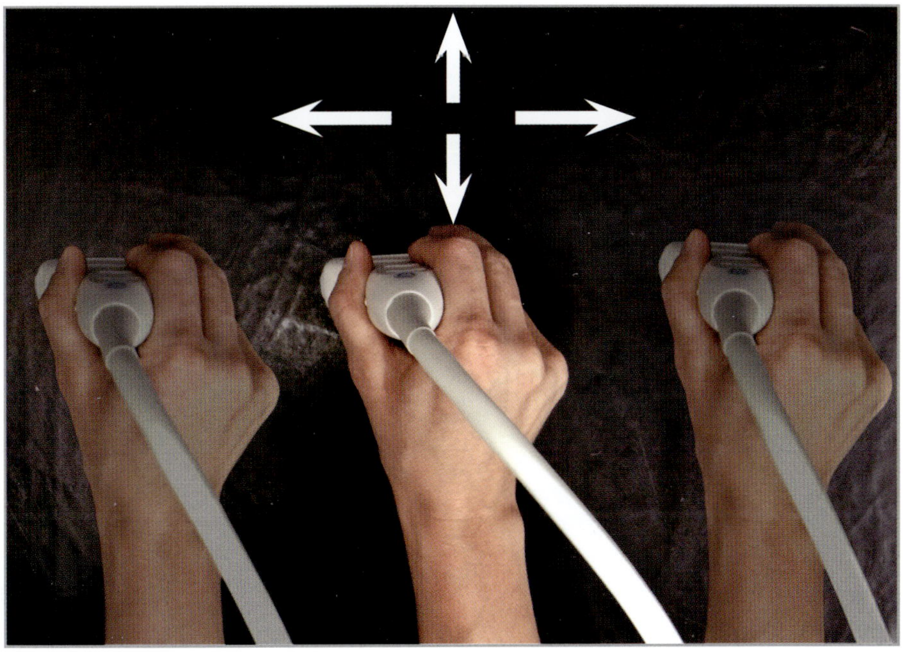

Figure 4. Sliding. The transducer is held perpendicular to the skin and it is moved in a sliding fashion (vertically and horizontally).

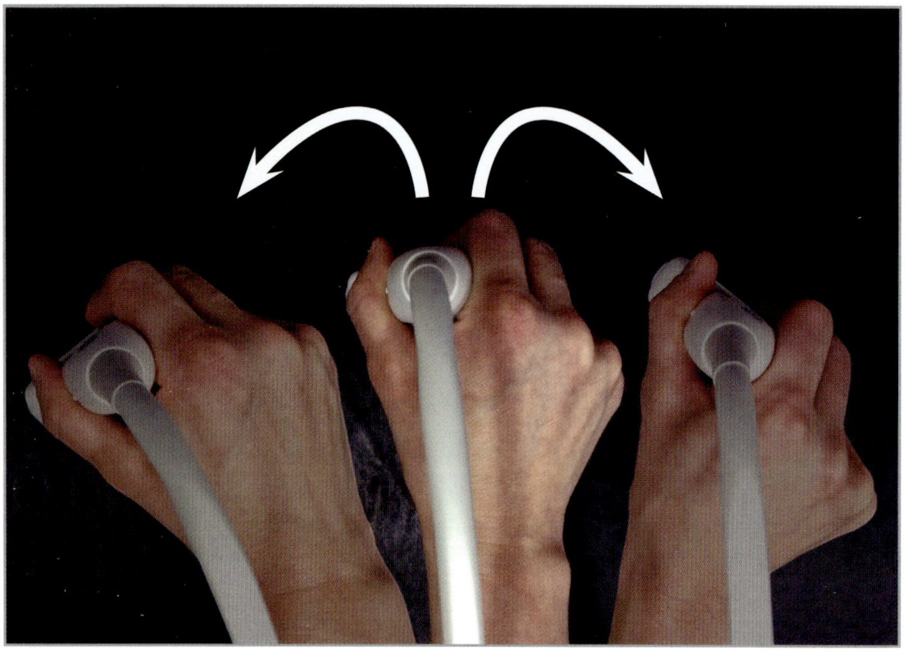

Figure 5. Rotation. The transducer is held perpendicular to the skin (middle image) and is rotated clockwise (right image) and anticlockwise (left image).

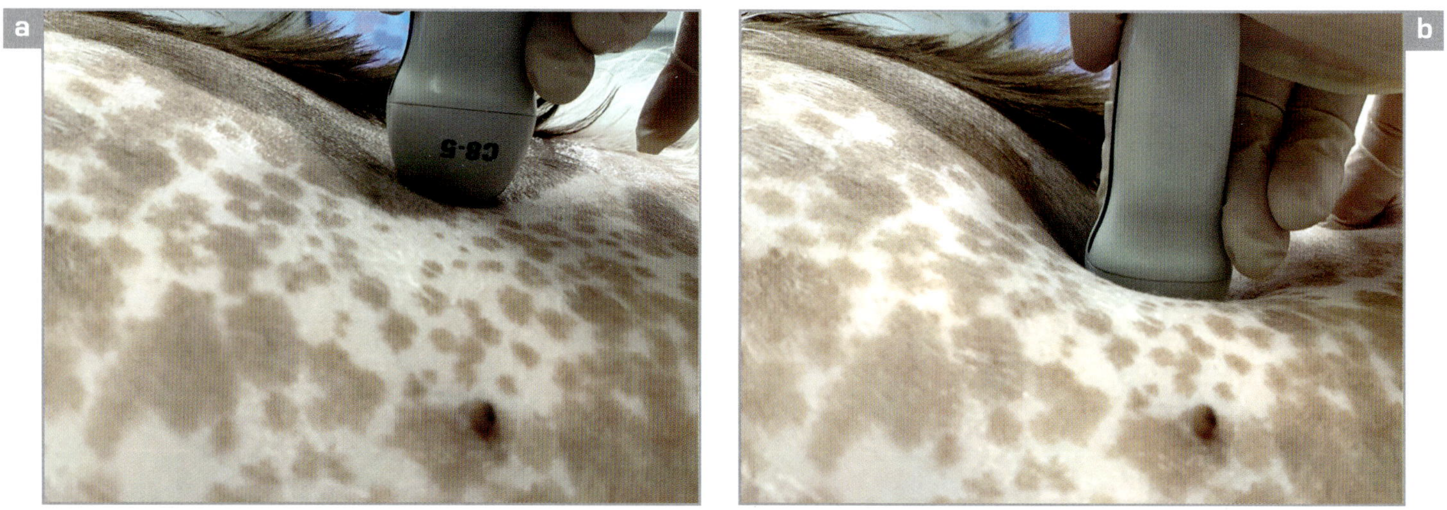

Figure 6. Pressure. The transducer is perpendicular to the skin and the abdomen is compressed by applying pressure to the transducer. **(a)** The transducer touches the skin. **(b)** Pressure is applied to the transducer.

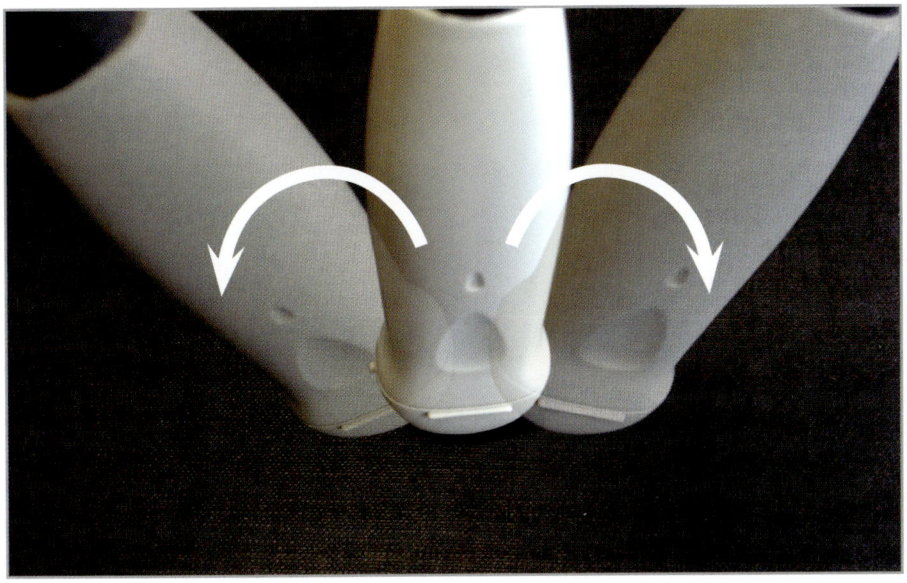

Figure 7. Rocking. The transducer is held still at one point of the abdominal wall and tilted forwards and backwards in a rocking fashion (like a rocking chair).

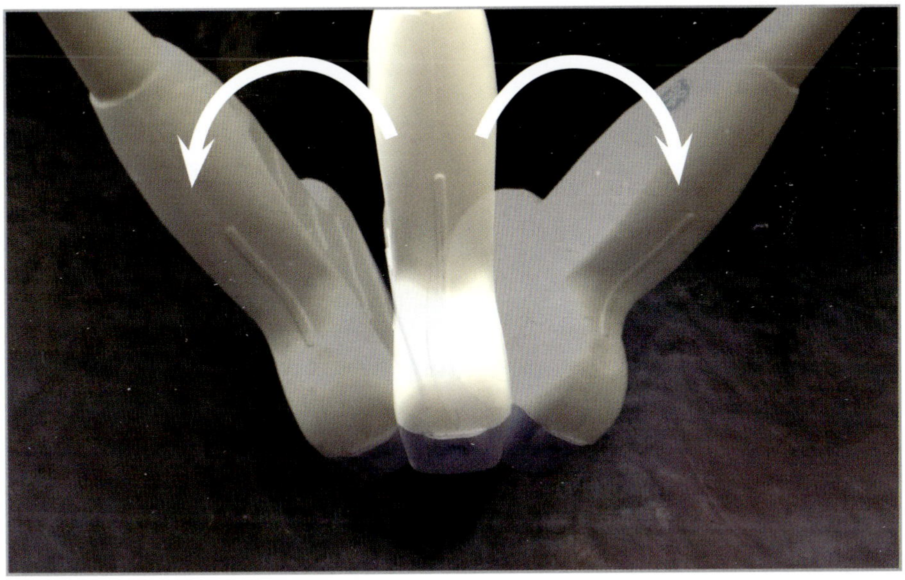

Figure 8. Fanning. The transducer is held still at one point of the abdominal wall and tilted from side to side in a fanning fashion (like a handheld fan).

Exercises

- Hold the transducer in your hand placing your thumb on the marker. Perform the five movements as described above. You do not need an animal to do this.
- Place the transducer on the side of a dog or cat with the marker pointing to the head. Think which side is cranial, caudal, left, right, dorsal and ventral. Keep in mind that where you place the transducer is at the top of the screen (see Fig. 3).

3

CHAPTER

ARTEFACTS

Introduction

Ultrasound artefacts are commonly encountered during an abdominal ultrasonographic examination.

> Artefacts can be confusing and/ or disruptive; however, at times they can help with the understanding and diagnosis of the abnormality seen.

- Ultrasound artefacts can result from equipment computer software assumptions such as:
  - Sound travels in straight lines.
  - Echoes originate only from objects located along the beam axis.
  - The intensity of the returning echoes is directly related to the scattering strength of the imaged structures.
  - The speed of sound is the same through different tissues and is 1540 m/s or 6.5 μsec/cm (13 μsec for a 1 cm return trip).
- Artefacts may also be environmental or induced by equipment or operator. These are usually considered "controllable" since, if the cause is identified and removed (e.g. patient motion, external device interference), the artefacts are not generated.
- By contrast, ultrasonographic artefacts arising from beam-patient interactions are considered of limited control. They can be useful (assist with the understanding of the underlying pathology of the lesion) or useless (interfering or/and confusing).

Selected artefacts seen during the ultrasonographic examination of the abdomen are presented in this chapter. Doppler artefacts are beyond the scope of this book.

Acoustic shadowing

Acoustic shadowing appears as an anechoic area beyond a hyperechoic reflector. It is commonly seen behind bone and other mineralised structures, because they reflect a large percentage of the sound beam and absorb most of the remaining sound. This results in a well-defined acoustic "shadow" beyond the hyperechoic reflector (Fig. 1). This artefact can be seen with calculi and mineralisation (e.g. cases of nephrocalcinosis).

> Keep in mind that a very small calculus or calculi outside the focal zone (see machine set up) may have a faint or no shadow or may have acoustic shadowing with unclear margins.

When there is a soft tissue gas interface, 99 % of the sound is reflected and the result is an acoustic shadow that contains some echoes and that is why it is termed "dirty shadowing" (Fig. 2).

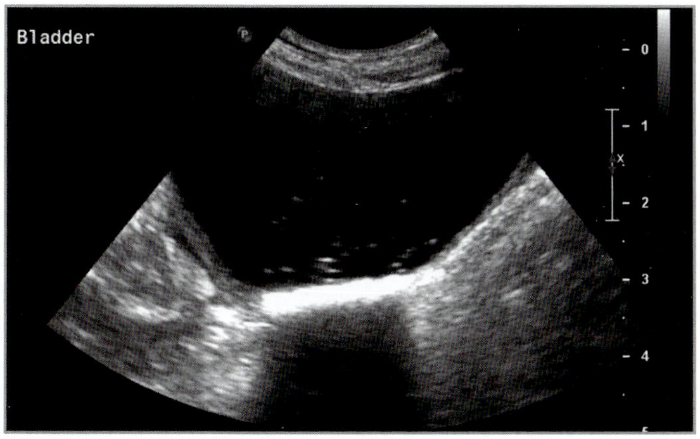

Figure 1. Hyperechoic calculi on the dependent aspect of the urinary bladder of a dog. Observe the acoustic shadow bellow them.

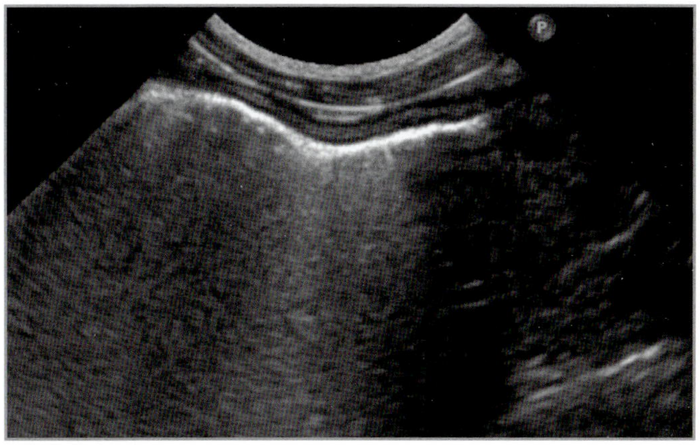

Figure 2. Dirty shadow below intestinal gas.

Acoustic enhancement

Acoustic enhancement is usually seen as increased echogenicity below fluid-filled structures (Fig. 3) or, less commonly, below solid structures that attenuate less sound than the surrounding tissues. It appears so because of the increased amplitude of echoes below (deep to) a low attenuating structure.

> When you see acoustic enhancement below lesions, always consider the possibility of cystic or cavitary lesion.

a

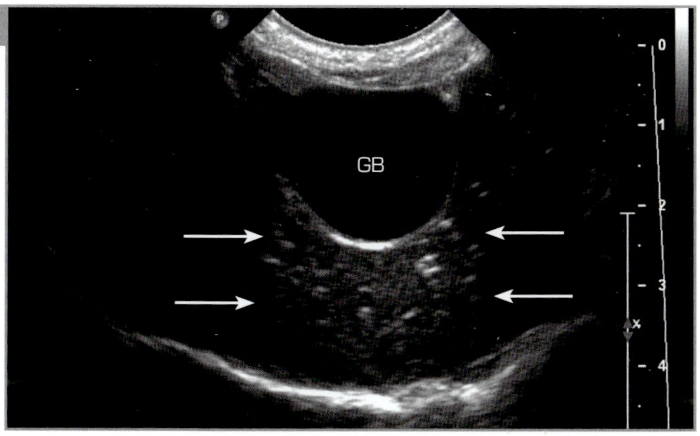

b

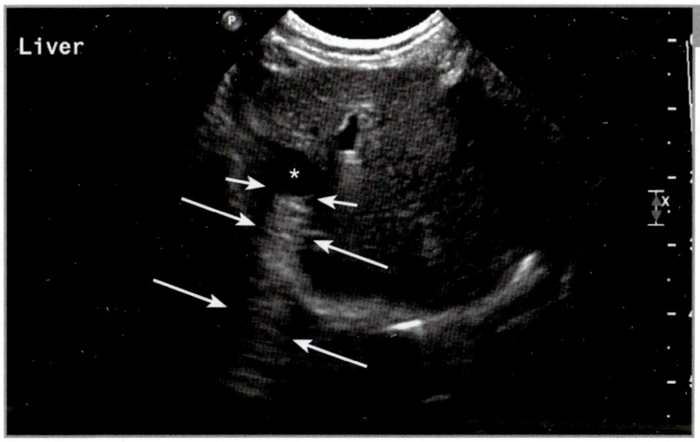

Figure 3. (a) Acoustic enhancement (between arrows) is visible below the gallbladder (GB) of a dog. (b) Cystic lesion (*) in the liver of a dog displaying distal acoustic shadowing (arrows). Edge shadowing can be seen at the lateral edges of the artefact (thin arrows).

Acoustic reflection and refraction (Edge-shadowing)

Edge shadowing (Fig. 3b) appears as an area with no echoes, i. e. as acoustic shadow, that can be seen at the margins of round or oval structures. This is due to interaction of the sound beam with the curved periphery of the structuress such that part of the beam is being reflected while the remainder part of the beam is refracted. The reflected beam does not return to the transducer because the surface of the reflector is not perpendicular to the beam. It is also known as "edge-shadowing".

This artefact can be seen at the gallbladder margins, at the margins of intestines seen end-on and even at hydronephrotic kidneys. Although this artefact can be useful, it can also interfere with the examination of areas where the edge-shadow extends to.

Reverberation artefact

Reverberation artefact (Fig. 4) occurs when a high intensity returning sound beam hits the transducer and is reflected back into the body. This process may repeat so that the sound makes two, three or more return trips between the transducer and patient a second time and this may happen a third or more times. This is misinterpreted as a strong echo originating form a certain depth and then at twice that depth and thrice that depth, etc.

The result is a display of evenly spaced echoes. The number of these echoes depends on the penetrating power of the beam and the transducer sensitivity. The distance between each dispelled echo is the distance between the transducer and the original reflector.

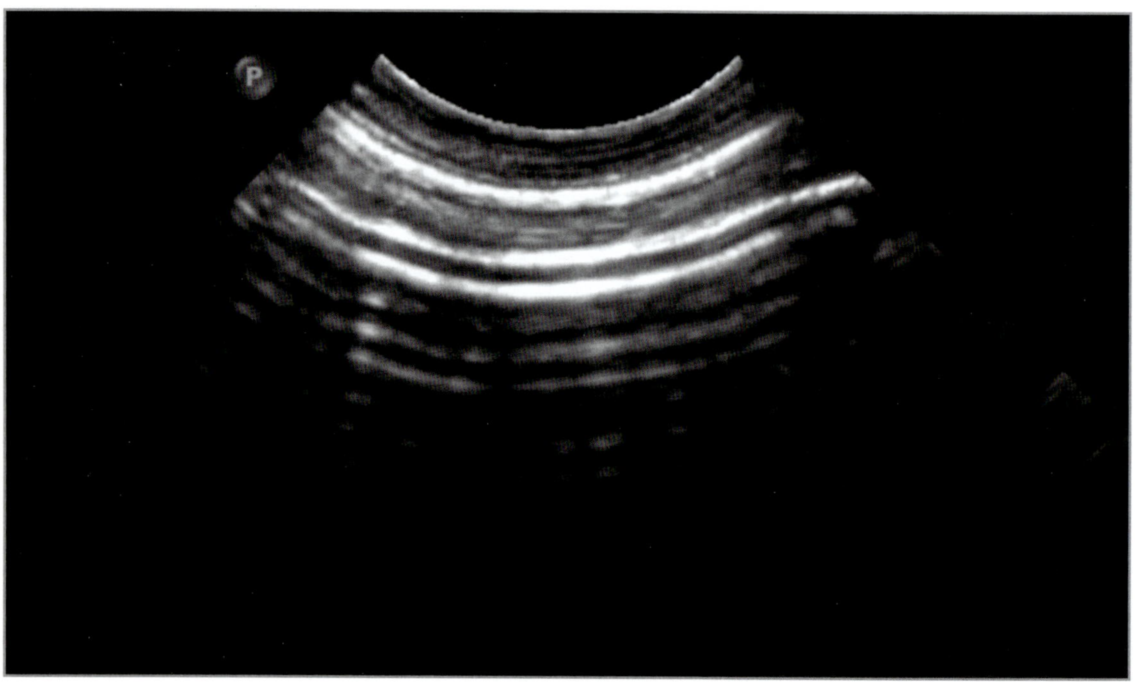

Figure 4. Reverberation artefact due to poor transducer contact.

Ring down artefact

The ring down artefact (Fig. 5) is only associated with gas bubbles. It occurs when an ultrasound pulse encounters a bugle-shaped fluid collection that is between two layers of gas bubbles. The trapped fluid resonates and emits a continuous signal back to the transducer. It is commonly encountered when examining the gastrointestinal tract. Its appearance makes is often confused with the comet tail artefact.

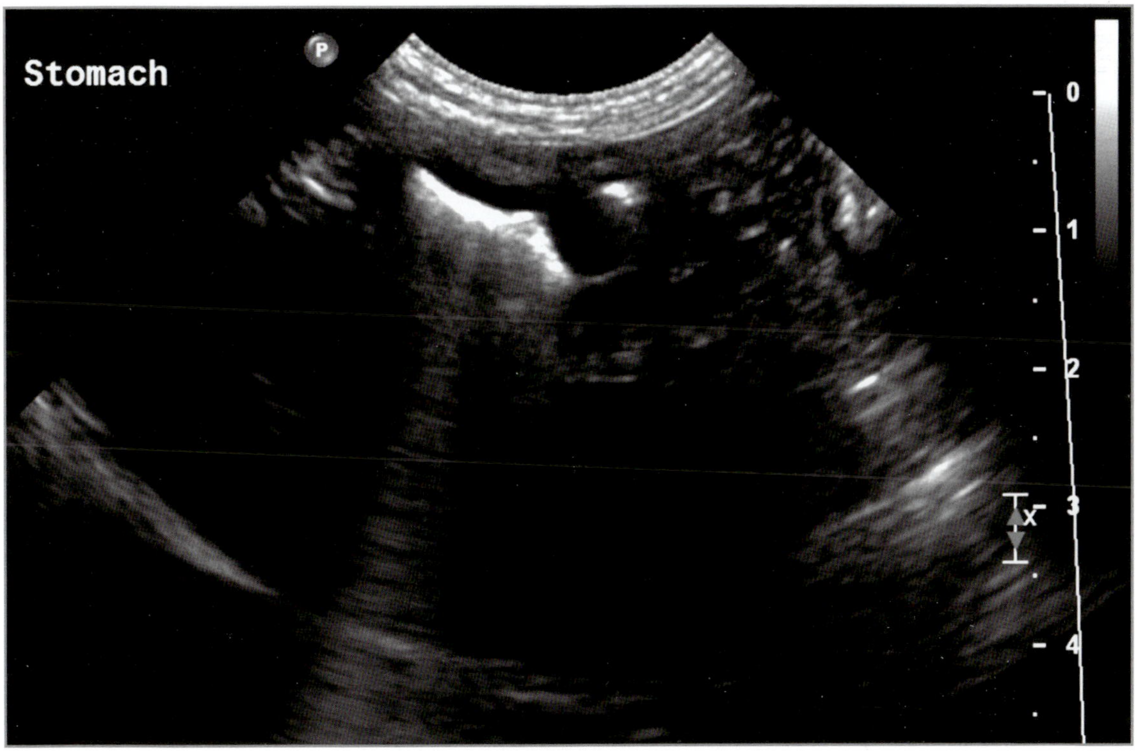

Figure 5. Ring down artefact seen distal to the stomach.

Comet tail artefact

The comet tail artefact is recognised by the closely spaced echoes that has the shape of the tail of a comet (Fig. 6). It is commonly seen below calcific/ crystalline highly reflective objects, and it occurs because of the large acoustic impedance mismatch between these objects and surrounding tissue. It is believed to be a special form of reverberation artifact. It often confused with the ring down artefact, but it is created by a different mechanism.

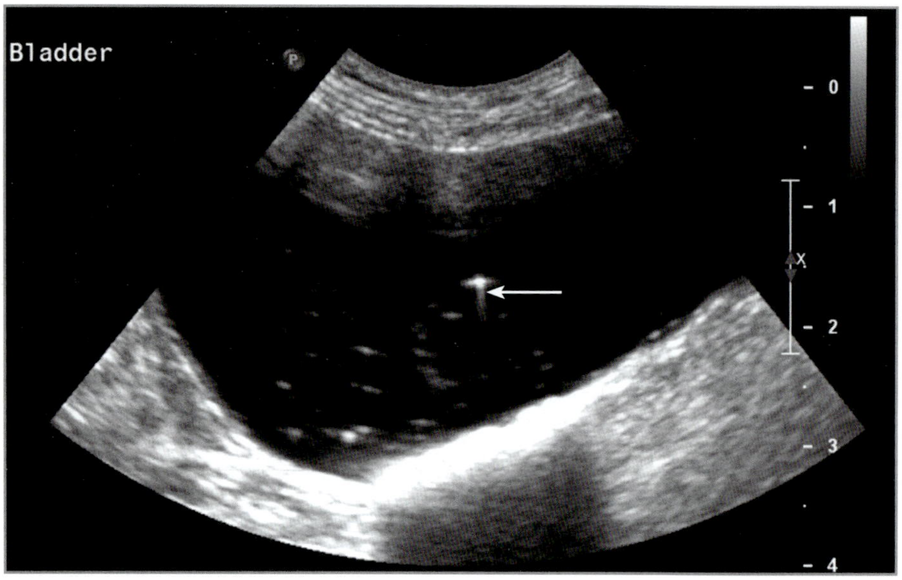

Figure 6. Comet tail artefact in the middle of the urinary bladder (arrow). Observe also the acoustic shadowing below the calculi at the depended aspect of the urinary bladder.

Slice thickness artefact

Slice thickness artefact (Fig. 7), also called section thickness or partial volume artifact, creates echoes in curved fluid filled structures that may be confused for particulate material ("pseudosludge") or can create echoes blood vessels and ducts. The artefact results from all echoes in the width of the imaging pulse being compressed into a thin slice for graphic representation. To distinguish true material in a fluid filled structure from slice thickness, we need to keep in mind that slice thickness artefact has a meniscus while true sediment has a flat interface. Also, this artefact may appear in the non-dependent aspect of the structure.

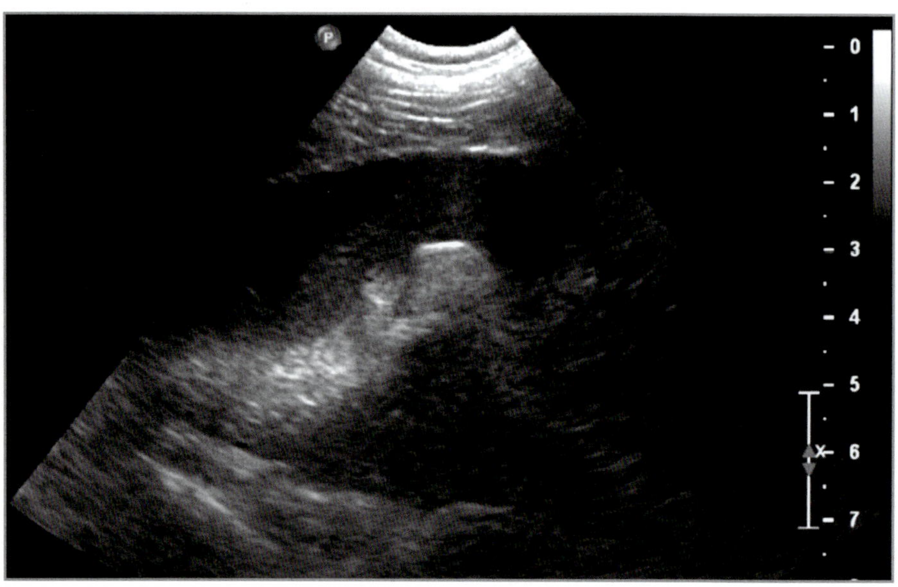

Figure 7. Slice thickness artefact appears as echoes in the urinary bladder.

Mirror image artefact

The mirror image artefact (Fig. 8) shows structures that exists on one side of a strong reflector also appearing on its other side. Commonly seen when examining the liver distal to the lung-diaphragm interface because of the almost total reflection of the sound from the air-filled lung. The sound beam may travel through the liver where it is reflected back to a different part of the liver and then reflected back to the transducer through the diaphragm. The computer assumes that sound is travelling in straight lines only and displays the data as further liver tissue incorrectly located at greater depths.

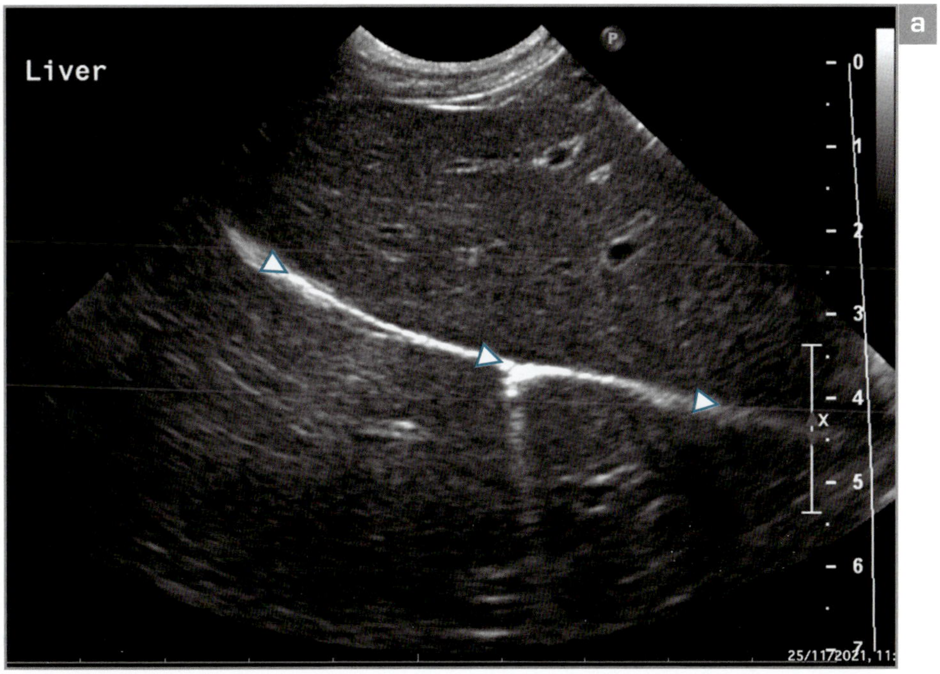

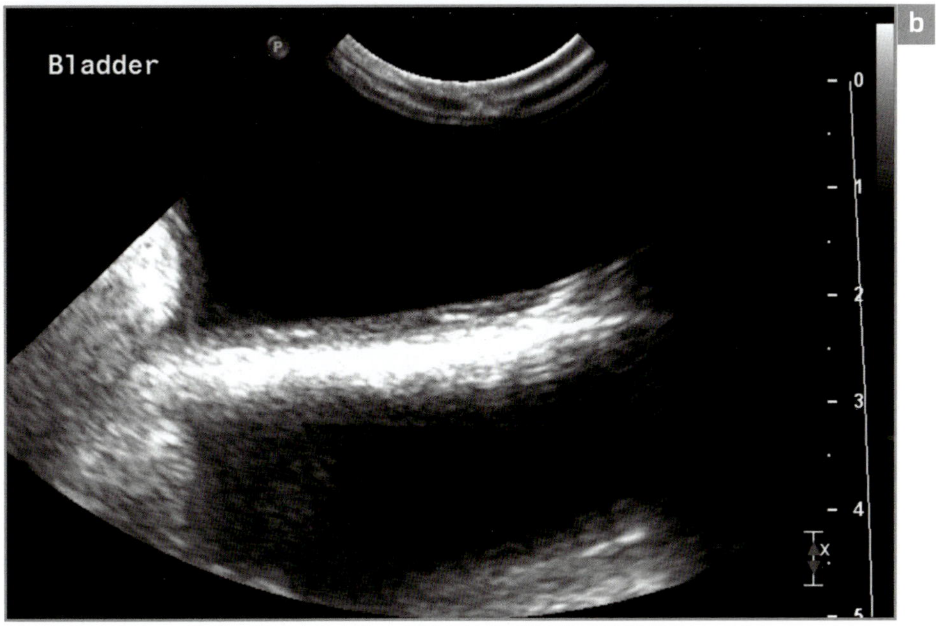

Figure 8. (a) Mirror image artefact with the liver appearing also beyond the lung-diaphragm interface (▷).
(b) Mirror image artifact at the level of the urinary bladder. The very bright straight hyperechoic area is the tabletop. The urinary bladder is visible on top of the image and the mirror image bellow the straight hyperechoic area.

Side lobe artefacts

These artefacts result from secondary beams outside the main beam. Side lobes are weaker than the primary beam. The echoes produced are less intense and they are best seen in anechoic structures like the urinary bladder where they appear as echoes in the anechoic content (Fig. 9). It may resemble in appearance to the slice thickness artefact.

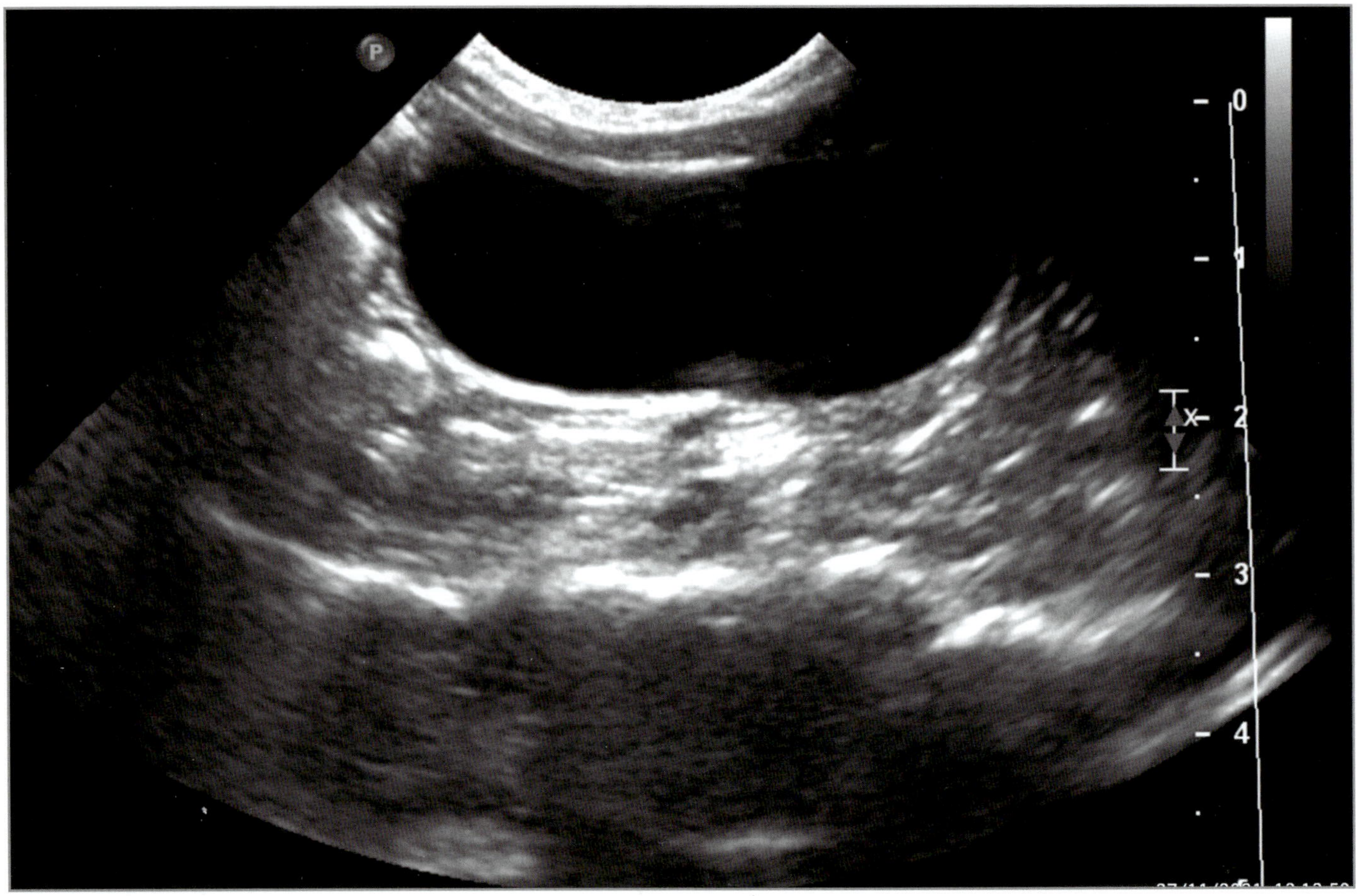

Figure 9. Side lobe artefact appears as echoes in the urinary bladder lumen.

Propagation speed error

This occurs when two tissues in the near field have different propagation velocities. Organs and margins deep to the two tissues may appear irregular or interrupted bellow the tissues (Fig. 10). This is because the computer always assumes that the velocity of the sound is constant at 1540 m/sec. Propagation speed errors displace structures along the path of the beam i.e. axially.

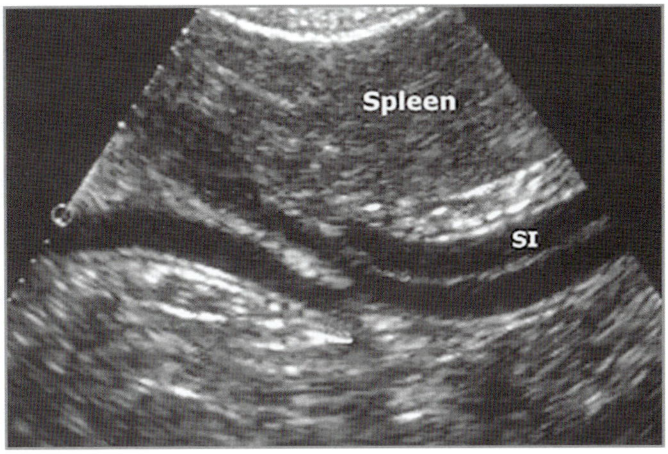

Figure 10. Propagation speed error artefact resulting in a loop of small intestine (SI) appearing interrupted. Courtesy of C.R. Lamb.

Range ambiguity artefact

In sonography one of the software assumptions is that for each pulse echoes are received prior to the emission of the next pulse. Range ambiguity artefact (Fig. 11) results when a pulse is transmitted before the energy of the previous pulse has dissipated. Then the previous pulse may generate echoes from a reflector out of the field of view that will be placed in the field of view. Decreasing the pulse repetition frequency (e.g. increasing depth or widening sector angle) or selecting a lower frequency transducer will reduce or eliminate the artefact.

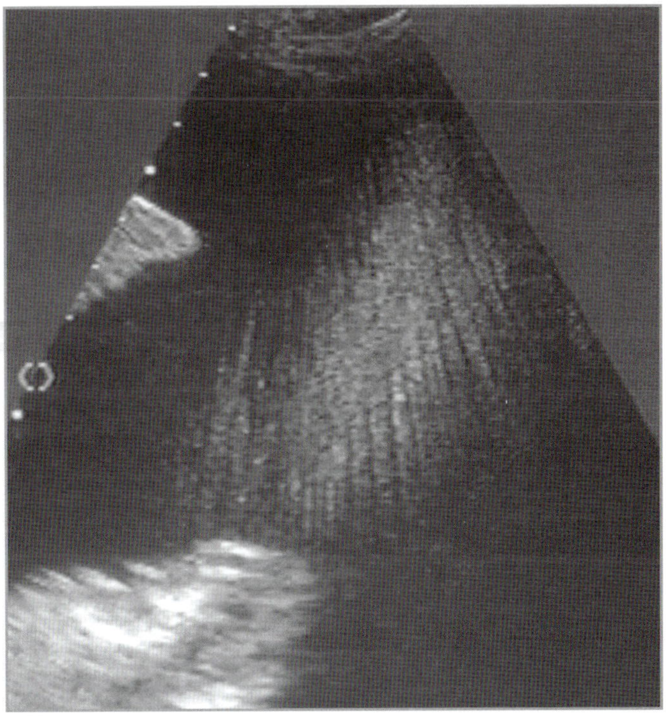

Figure 11. Range ambiguity artifact. Courtesy of C. R. Lamb.

Electronic interference

Electronic interference from electrical equipment or radio frequency signals can be seen on screen even without the transducer touching the patient (Fig. 12). Switching off the interfering equipment or changing examination room, if the external signal cannot be turned off, should resolve this artefact.

> There are more ultrasound artefacts. For more detailed information regarding ultrasound artefacts and their causes look for further information in the recommended further reading

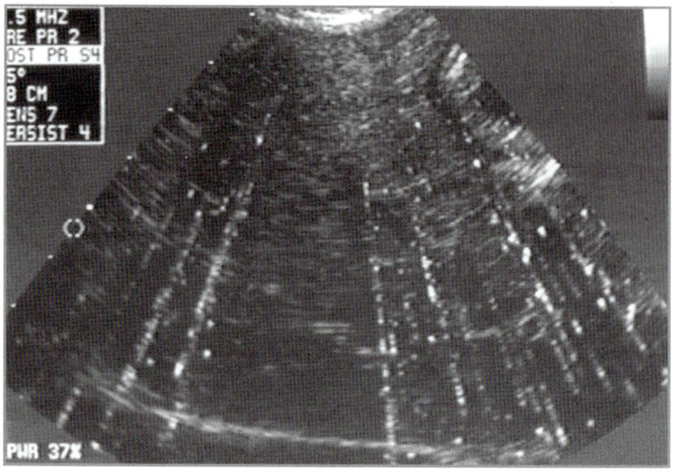

Figure 12. Electronic interference artefact. Courtesy of C. R. Lamb.

4

CHAPTER

LIVER AND GALLBLADDER

Scanning technique

The animal is placed in right lateral recumbency with the head towards the ultrasound machine.

1. Position the transducer parallel to the tabletop just caudal to the xiphoid process with the marker pointing cranially (Fig. 1).

2. Orient the transducer's axis so that it points towards the shoulder joints (Fig. 1).

3. Rock the transducer cranially or caudally to view the liver in the middle of the screen.

4. Fan the transducer to the left and to the right of the animal ensuring that the whole liver is examined (Fig. 2).

5. Rotate the transducer 90° anticlockwise and fan the transducer cranially and caudally ensuring that the whole liver is examined (Fig. 3).

6. The gallbladder will be visible on the right side of the animal (Fig. 4).

7. The liver and gallbladder can be evaluated while moving the transducer.

8. In large dogs, it may be difficult to evaluate the right dorsal liver from this approach. Positioning the dog in left lateral recumbency and placing the transducer intercostally, dorsal and cranial to the right kidney, will allow more detailed examination of this part of the liver.

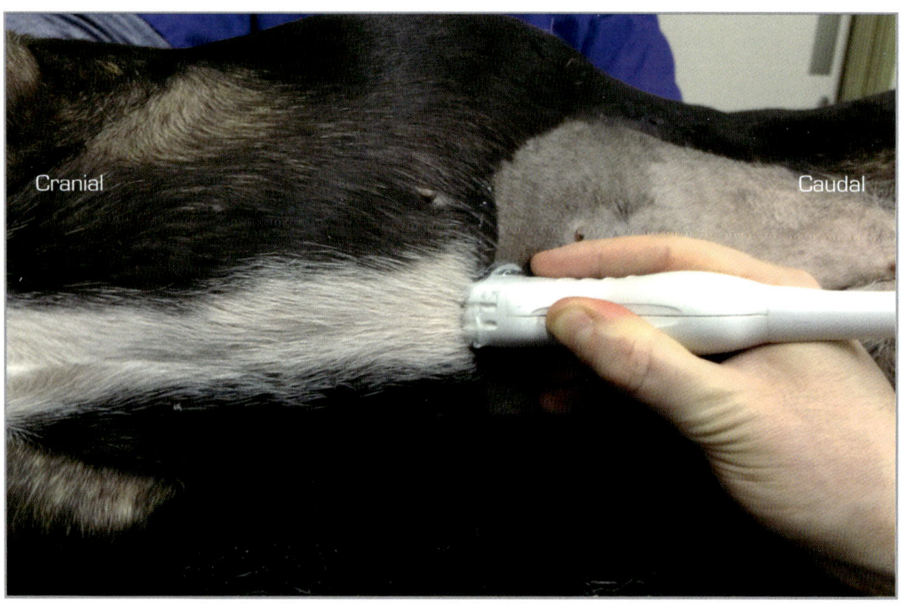

Figure 1. Initial position of the transducer to assess the liver and gallbladder. The transducer is positioned parallel to the tabletop just caudal to the xiphoid process with the marker towards the head of the animal. It is then pointed towards the shoulders.

If it is difficult to examine a dog adequately because it is very deep-chested (i.e. with limited space caudal to the xiphoid), or it has excessive gastrointestinal gas, or its liver is small-sized, then clip the hair on both sides and examine the liver by placing and moving the transducer intercostally through the 10th to 12th intercostal spaces (right and left).

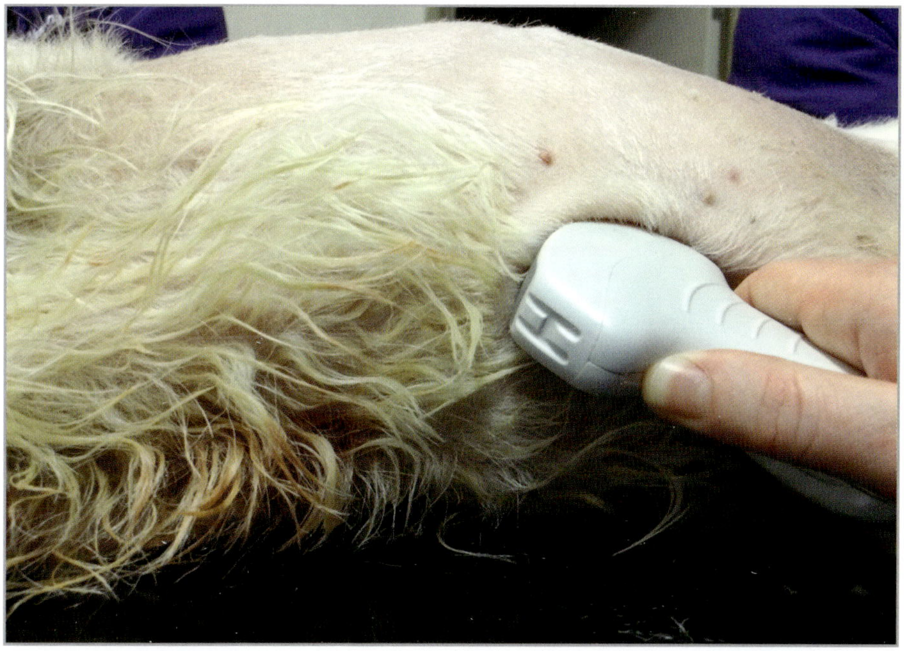

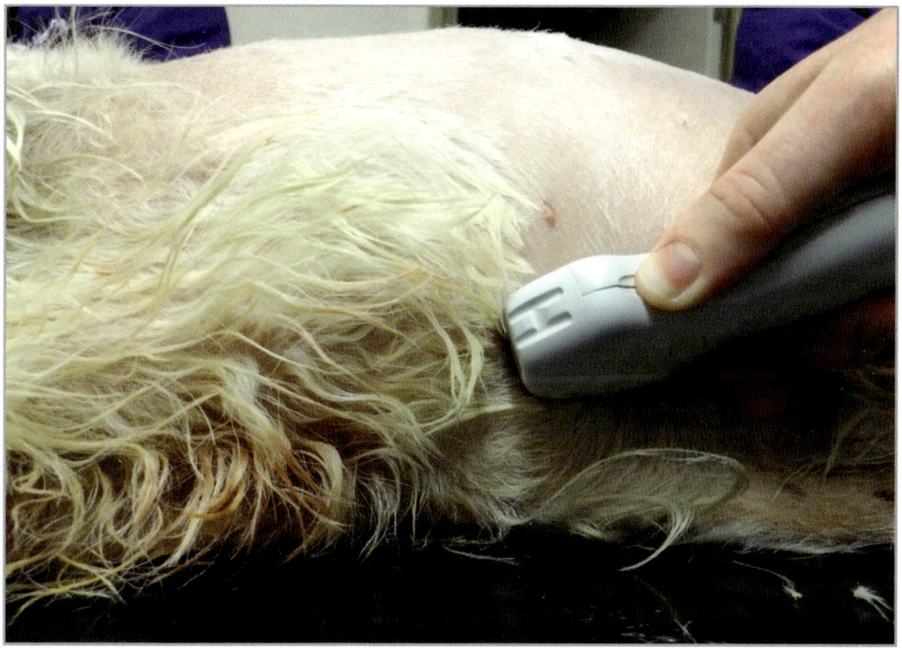

Figure 2. In order to examine the liver in a sagittal orientation, the transducer is fanned to the left and to the right of the animal until the whole liver and the gallbladder are examined.

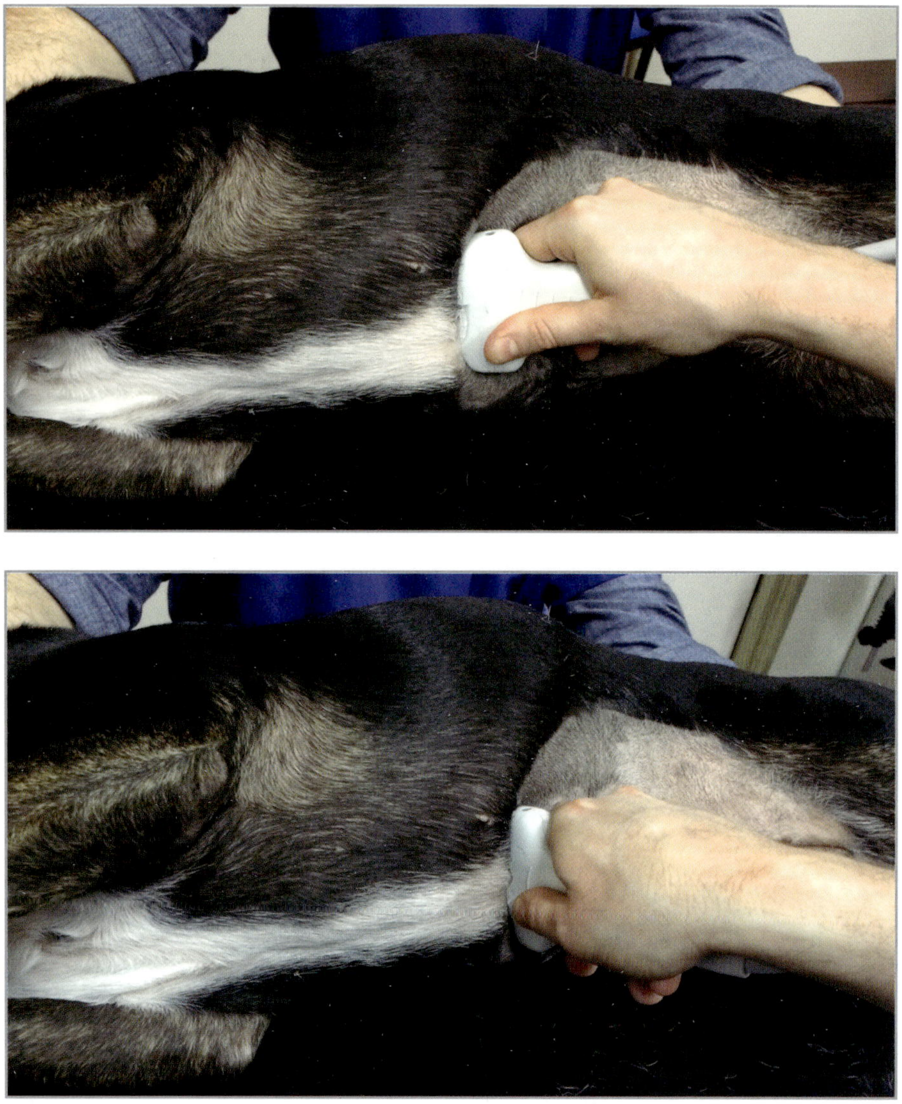

Figure 3. Following the sagittal examination, the liver and gallbladder are examined in a transverse orientation by rotating the transducer 90° anticlockwise and fanning the transducer cranially and caudally until the whole liver and the gallbladder are examined.

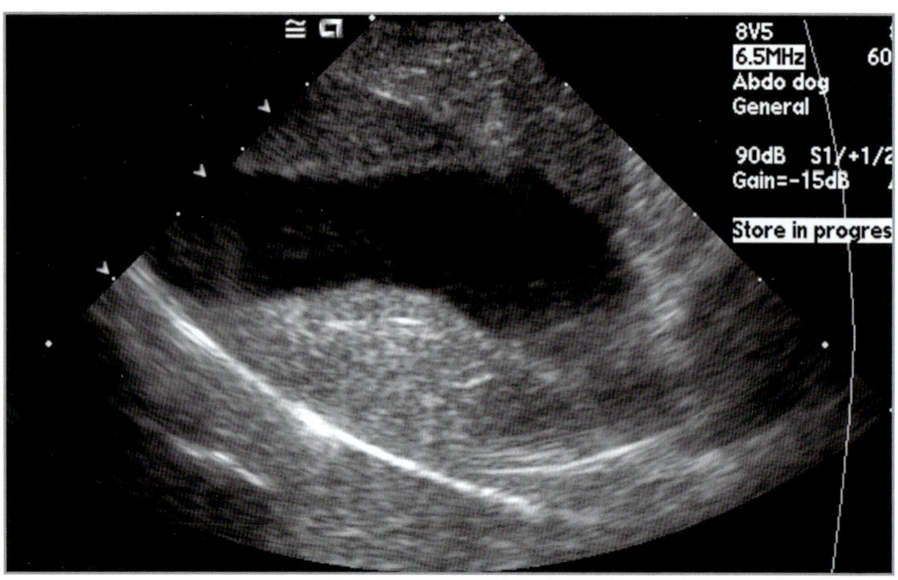

Figure 4. The gallbladder is visible on the right side of the animal as the transducer is fanned towards the right.

Searching for shunt

1. Rotate the animal to left lateral recumbency with the head towards the machine and the limbs away from the examiner (Fig. 5).

2. Place the transducer in a transverse orientation near the spine (at the last intercostal space or behind the last rib) with the marker towards the spine and identify the right kidney (Fig. 5).

3. Slide the transducer cranially, for one or more intercostal spaces, until you see the liver and can identify, from dorsal to ventral, the aorta, caudal vena cava (CVC) and portal vein (Fig. 6).

4. Follow the CVC and portal vein in transverse orientation to search for any evidence of communication. Examine the portal vein branches for evidence of an enlarged vessel that may be the location of the shunt origin.

5. Identify the CVC and rotate the transducer clockwise (the transducer´s marker now points towards the animal's head) to examine the CVC in a longitudinal view. Evaluate it using colour-flow Doppler and pulsed-wave Doppler.

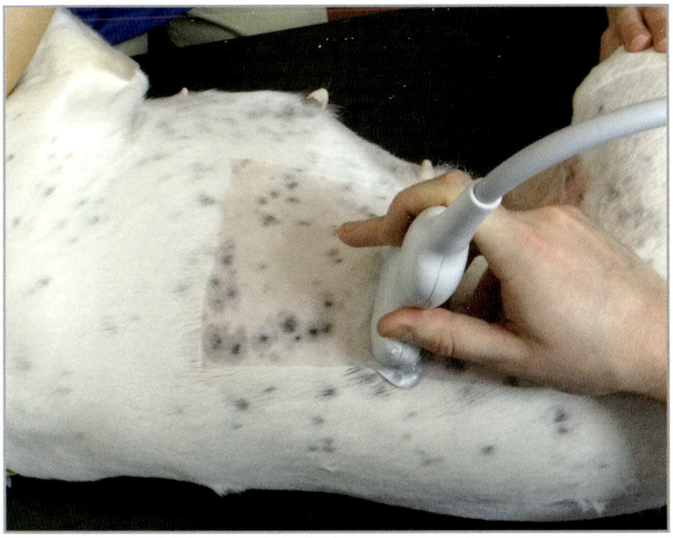

Figure 5. To search for a portosystemic shunt, a right intercostal window is commonly used. The transducer is placed in a transverse orientation near the spine (at the last intercostal space) with the marker towards the spine in order to identify the right kidney. From there, the transducer is moved cranially (one intercostal space at a time) to identify the aorta, caudal vena cava and portal vein.

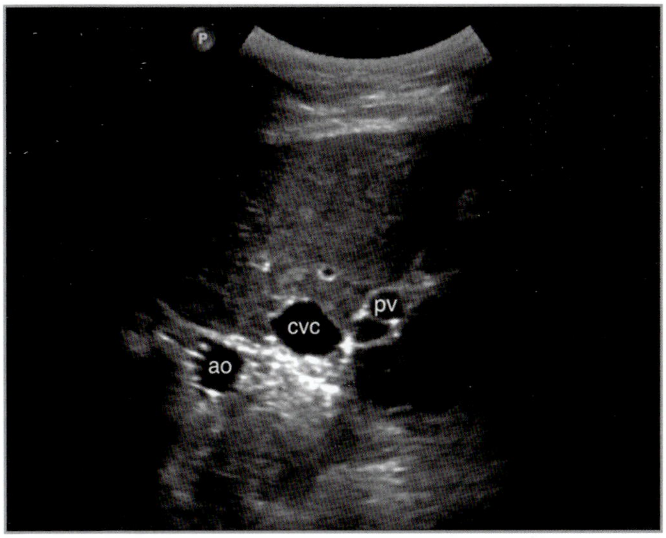

Figure 6. Right dorsal intercostal approach. The transducer is placed cranial to the right kidney. The aorta (ao), caudal vena cava (cvc) and portal vein (pv) can be identified from dorsal (left) to ventral (right).

6. Fan your transducer ventrally to identify the portal vein and assess it. You can also measure the portal blood flow velocity using pulsed-wave Doppler (Fig. 7). Doppler examination is beyond the scope of this book.

7. Fan dorsally to identify the aorta along its long axis. Look for a vessel immediately adjacent to the aorta that can indicate an enlarged azygus vein in case of portoazygus shunt

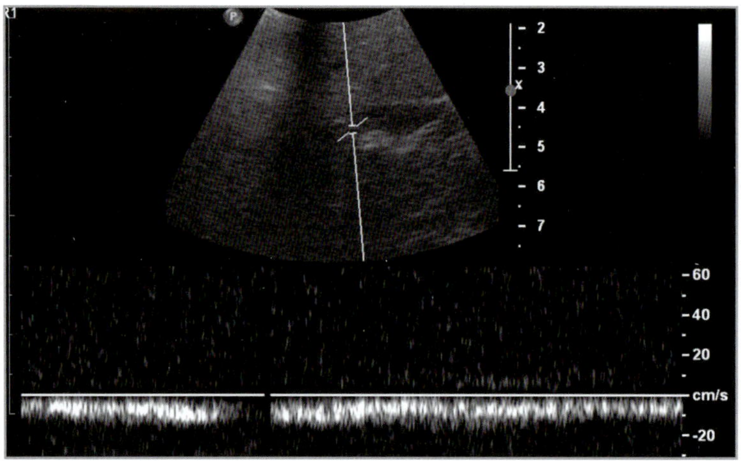

Figure 7. Long-axis view of the portal vein acquired from the right dorsal intercostal approach. The pulsed-wave Doppler spectral tracing of the portal vein is visible having a flat profile, bellow the baseline and not being influenced by the cardiac cycle or respiration.

Normal appearance

Liver

The liver is caudal to the diaphragm, dorsal to the falciform fat and is bounded caudally by the right kidney, stomach and spleen (from right to left). The echogenic line seen cranial to the liver corresponds to the lung-diaphragm interface (Fig. 8). The liver is divided into the left, right, quadrate and caudate lobes. The left and right lobes are, in turn, divided into medial and lateral sublobes. These lobes and sublobes cannot be clearly distinguished in a healthy animal. They are easier to recognise when ascites is present.

The hepatic parenchyma is uniform, moderately echogenic, and has a coarse echotexture. The echogenicity of a normal liver is similar, or slightly increased or decreased, compared with the renal cortex and is less echogenic than the spleen in the dog and the cat when they are visualised at the same depth and with the same gain settings. The normal hepatic parenchyma is less echogenic than the falciform fat (Fig. 9).

Different vessels are visible within the liver. It is easy to distinguish between the portal veins and the hepatic veins. The portal veins have bright walls while the hepatic veins do not; the hepatic veins appear as anechoic tubes (Fig. 9).

The intrahepatic arteries are not normally seen. When visualised, the main hepatic artery is dorsal to the portal vein and common bile duct (CBD). Doppler ultrasonography can help in distinguishing between them.

The left lateral liver margin is normally sharp and the liver does not normally extend well beyond the rib cage limit.

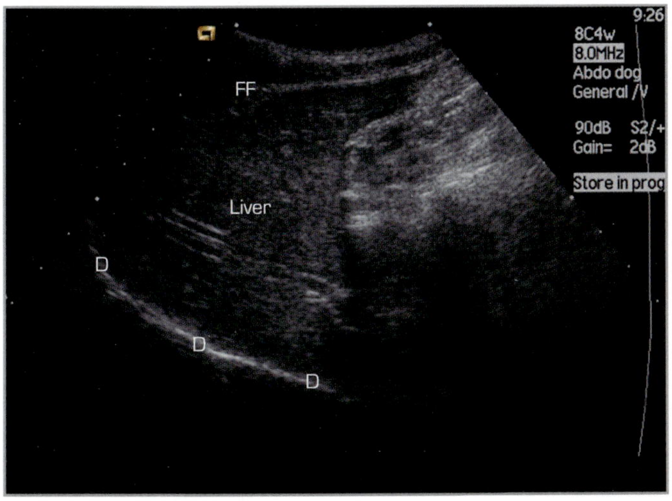

Figure 8. Sagittal view of the liver of a dog. The lung-diaphragm interface (D) is visible cranial to the liver. FF: falciform fat.

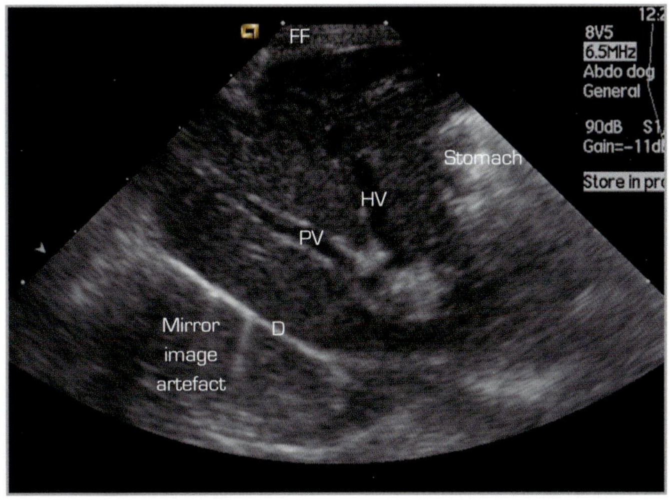

Figure 9. Sagittal view of the liver of a dog. The portal vein (PV) and hepatic vein (HV) are visible and easy to distinguish. Observe also the mirror image artefact. FF: falciform fat; D: lung-diaphragm interface.

Gallbladder

The gallbladder is a round-to-oval anechoic structure to the right of the midline, between the right medial sublobe and quadrate lobe of the liver (see Fig. 4). Its size varies depending on the time elapsed since the last meal before the scan: if the animal has eaten recently it may be empty and difficult to see, whereas if the animal has not eaten for a while it may be large and filled with bile. A small amount of dependent echogenic sediment (sludge) may be present in healthy dogs.

> The normal gallbladder wall has been reported to be up to 3 mm thick in dogs while in cats it has been reported to be less than 1 mm thick.

The CBD can be seen ventral to the main portal vein and has a diameter of less than 3 mm in healthy dogs. In healthy cats, the common bile duct is normally less than 4 mm in diameter (Fig. 10).

In young dogs, it may be difficult to see the gallbladder wall. In older dogs, the gallbladder wall is more visible and slightly "lumpy" in appearance due to mucinous gland hyperplasia, although its thickness may be normal.

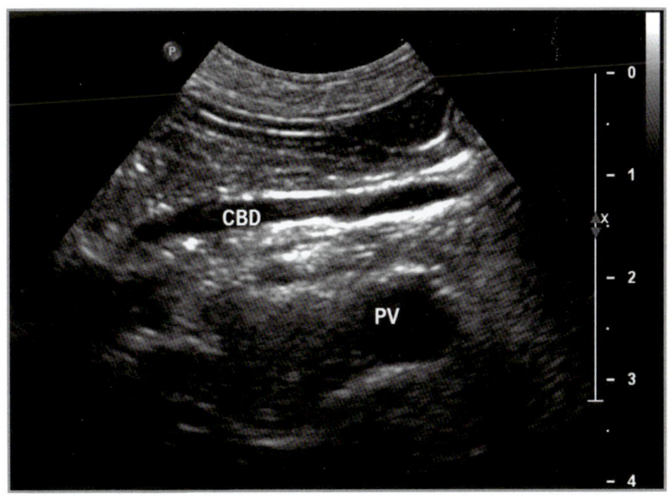

Figure 10. The normal common bile duct (CBD) of a dog visible ventral to the portal vein (PV).

Variations from normal

Liver

Focal and multifocal lesions

The presence of focal and multifocal lesions in the liver (Fig. 11) is not specific to a disease and there is a long list of disorders that may be included in the differential diagnoses for each appearance (Table 1). Most notably, neoplasia and regenerative nodules should be considered in almost any combination of focal and multifocal hepatic lesions. Although other clinical and imaging findings may indicate a particular disease, further tests are usually required to reach a final diagnosis, including ultrasound-guided aspiration and/or biopsy.

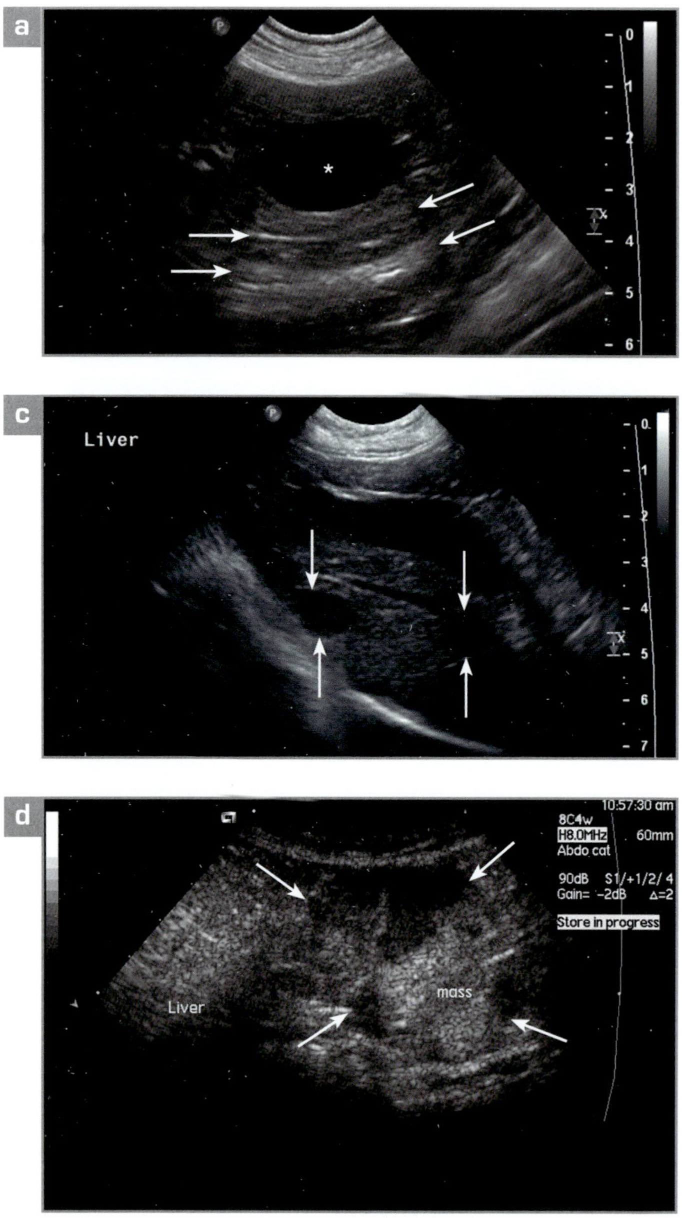

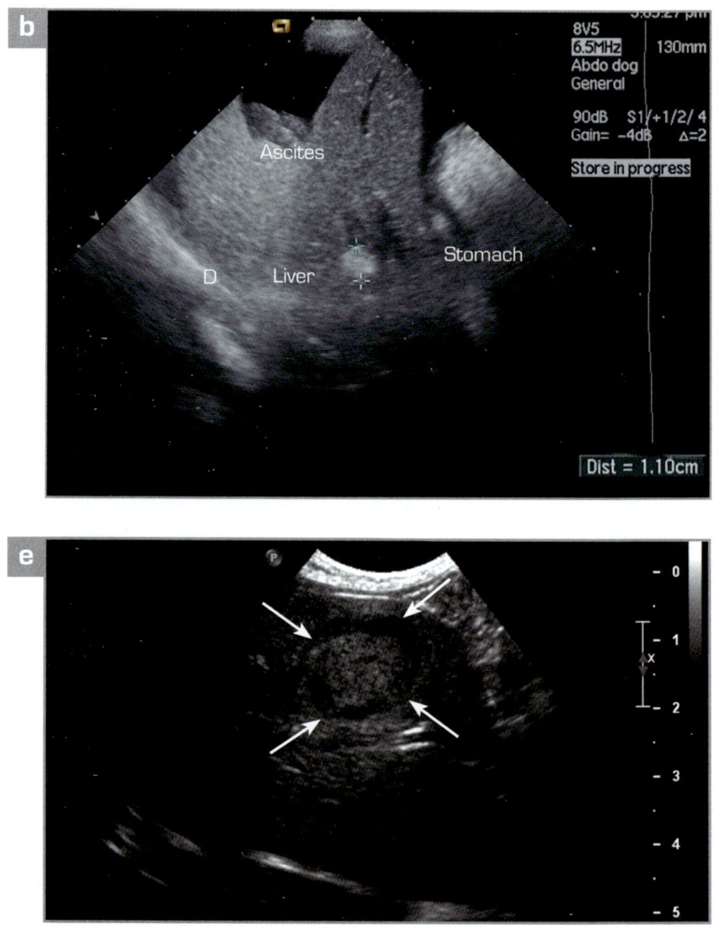

Figure 11. Liver lesions. **(a)** Incidental anechoic cyst in a canine liver. Observe the acoustic enhancement artifact (arrows).
(b) A hyperechoic nodule (between callipers) is visible in the liver. Ascites can also be seen (D: lung- diaphragm interface).
(c) Hypoechoic hepatic nodules (arrows) in a dog with metastatic carcinoma.
(d) Mixed echogenicity liver mass (between arrows).
(e) Target-like liver nodule with hyperechoic centre and hypoechoic periphery (between callipers).

Table 1. Differential diagnosis of focal or multifocal hepatic nodular lesions or masses.

Ultrasound appearance	Most likely differential diagnoses
Anechoic lesions (Fig. 11a)	• Cyst (e.g. polycystic disease) • Biliary cyst • Cystadenoma • *Peliosis hepatis*
Hyperechoic (Fig. 11b)/isoechoic lesions	• Neoplasia (primary, metastatic) • Nodular hyperplasia • Haemorrhage • Abscess • Granuloma • Infarct
Hypoechoic lesions (Fig. 11c)	• Neoplasia (primary, metastatic) • Nodular hyperplasia • Abscess • Granuloma • Infarct • Hepatocutaneous syndrome • Liver lobe torsion (reduced or absent blood flow, usually left medial or lateral liver sublobes)
Mixed echogenicity lesions (Fig. 11d)	• Neoplasia (primary, metastatic) • Nodular hyperplasia • Cyst (infected) • Abscess • Haematoma • Telangiectasia • Liver lobe torsion (reduced or absent blood flow, usually left medial or lateral liver sublobes)
Target-like lesion (Fig. 11e)	• Malignant neoplasia • Nodular hyperplasia • Hepatitis (chronic active or pyogranulomatous) • Cirrhosis (also small, lumpy liver)

Diffuse changes

Diffuse changes result in changes in size, shape and echogenicity. Again, the diffuse appearance is not pathognomonic of a disease.

Uniformly increased echogenicity (Fig. 12) has been reported in vacuolar hepatopathy (including lipidosis), steroid hepatopathy, chronic hepatitis, lymphoma/lymphosarcoma, mast cell tumours and cirrhosis.

A diffusely hypoechoic liver is an uncommon finding and it is usually associated with hepatitis (acute). It has also been reported in infiltrative diseases (e.g. lymphoma), amyloidosis, and leukaemia.

Mixed echogenicity of the liver parenchyma is equally not specific and may be seen in neoplasia (primary, metastatic), hepatocutaneous syndrome and, in general, in any hepatopathy that does not affect the whole liver evenly.

The liver may appear normal on ultrasound in cases of acute hepatitis, infiltrative disease and toxic hepatopathy.

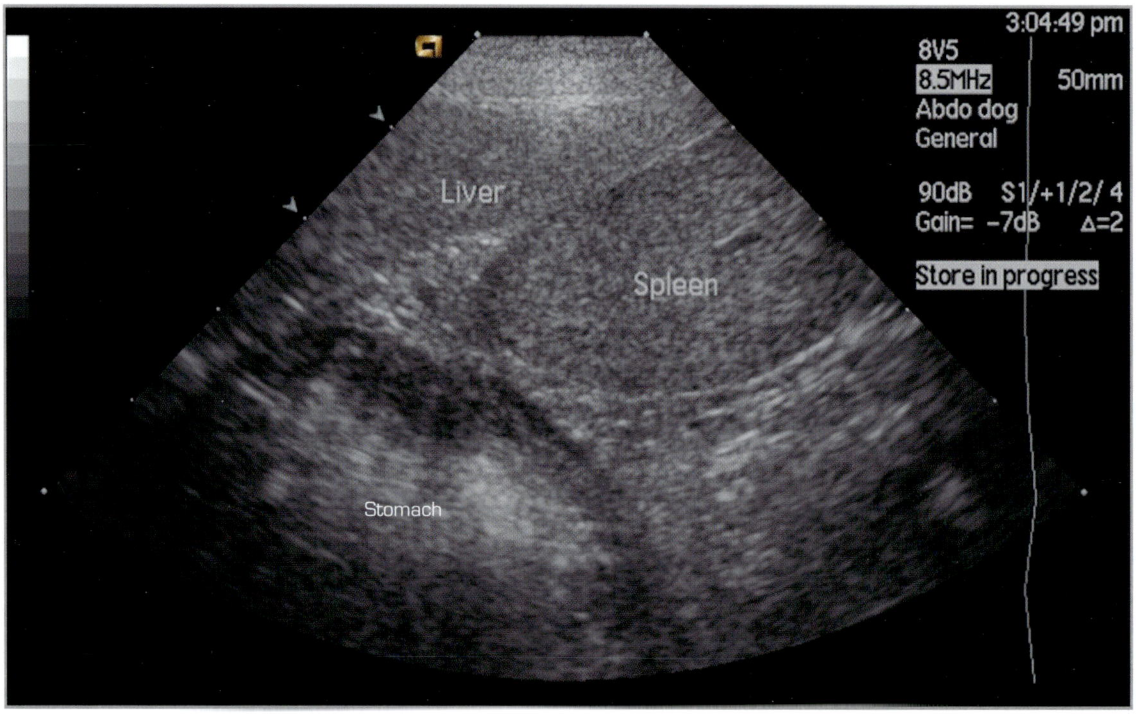

Figure 12. Dog with a hyperechoic liver. The abnormal liver is hyperechoic to the normal spleen.

The assessment of liver size is subjective and secondary signs, such as increased distance between diaphragm and stomach, hepatic extension beyond the rib cage and a rounded caudal liver margin (Fig. 13), are used as signs to diagnose hepatomegaly. Hepatomegaly can be seen with hepatic lipidosis, steroid hepatopathy and neoplasia.

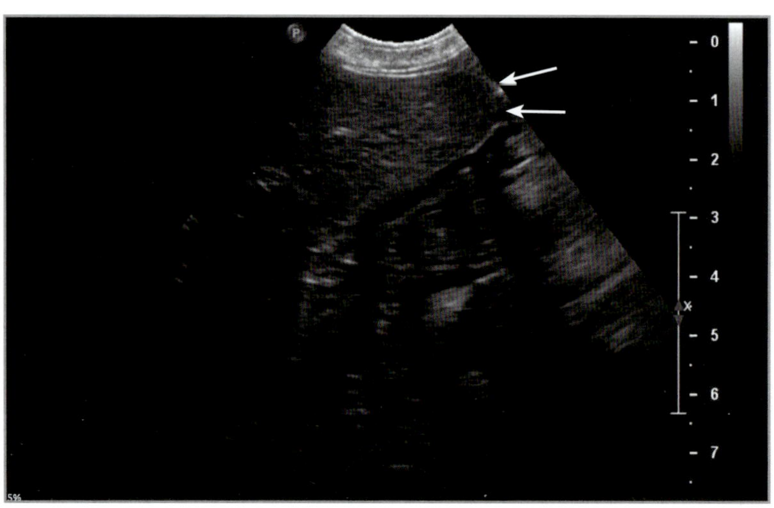

Figure 13. Hyperechoic liver with rounded caudal margin (arrows) extended well beyond the rib cage in a dog with hepatomegaly.

Microhepatica makes the liver difficult to evaluate on ultrasound examination; it is usually seen with chronic hepatitis, cirrhosis and portosystemic shunts. A cirrhotic liver appears as small, hyperechoic and "lumpy" in outline.

Gallbladder

Congenital conditions, such as a bilobed gallbladder and septa in the gallbladder, may be seen even in clinically normal animals. In cats, the gallbladder has more of a "U" shape and, depending on the transducer's orientation, it may appear as a double gallbladder. Rotation of the transducer should clarify whether the appearance of a double gallbladder is a true double gallbladder or the folded shape of the gallbladder itself.

A thickened gallbladder wall shows a "layered" appearance (Fig. 14). Care should be taken not to confuse this appearance with that of a thickened gallbladder wall in animals with ascites due to the fluid around the gallbladder. A thick gallbladder wall is a non-specific finding that can be seen with primary gallbladder disease or be secondary to a systemic disease.

Sediment (sludge) is commonly seen in the gallbladder of clinically normal animals.

Choleliths (Fig. 15) and choledochal calculi have the same appearance as any other calculi, i.e. hyperechoic and with shadowing. Differentiation from mineralised polyps is required. This can be done by turning the animal and observing that the calculi have dropped to the dependent aspect, while in the case of polyps the structures will remain in the same location.

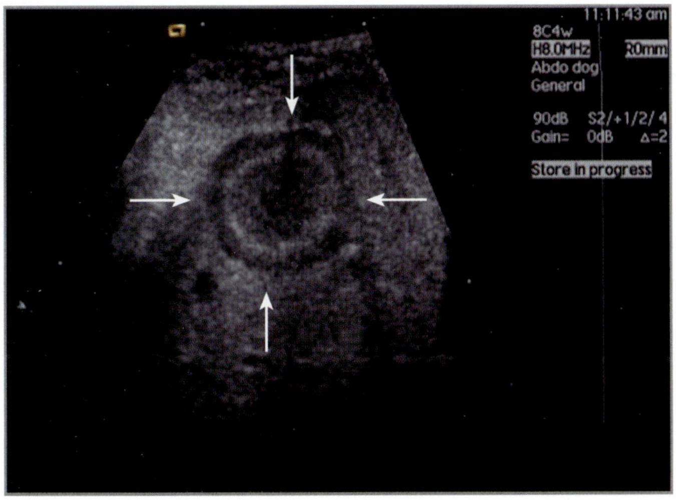

Figure 14. Cholecystitis in a dog. The gallbladder (arrows) has a "layered" wall appearance and contains more echogenic bile.

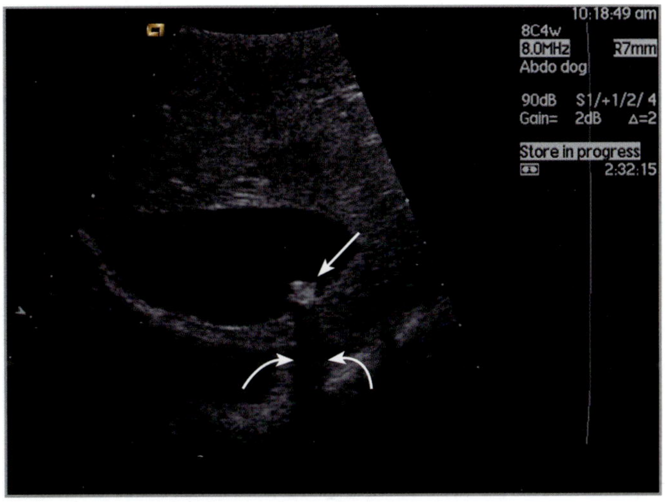

Figure 15. Cholelithiasis in a dog. The calculus (straight arrow) is hyperechoic with distal acoustic shadowing (curved arrows) and it is visible on the dependent aspect of the gallbladder.

Emphysematous cholecystitis (Fig. 16) appears as a thickened gallbladder wall containing bright foci and reverberation artefacts in the non-dependent aspect of the lumen as well as within the wall.

Gallbladder polyps (Fig. 17) appear as echogenic projections from the gallbladder wall to the lumen, sometimes resembling cauliflower. Gallbladder polyps are commonly an incidental finding that remain asymptomatic unless they cause obstruction. They can also be seen in chronic inflammation.

Gallbladder mucocoeles in dogs are of unknown aetiology. In these cases, the bile is more echogenic and has a "kiwi" (Fig. 18) or asteroid pattern. Though other patterns may also be seen, gallbladder distention is commonly present.

With gallbladder rupture, there is presence of fluid around the gallbladder, extending into the peritoneum. Hyperechoic fat can also be seen surrounding the gallbladder, which appears small in size and difficult to see while the area of the rupture may not be identified.

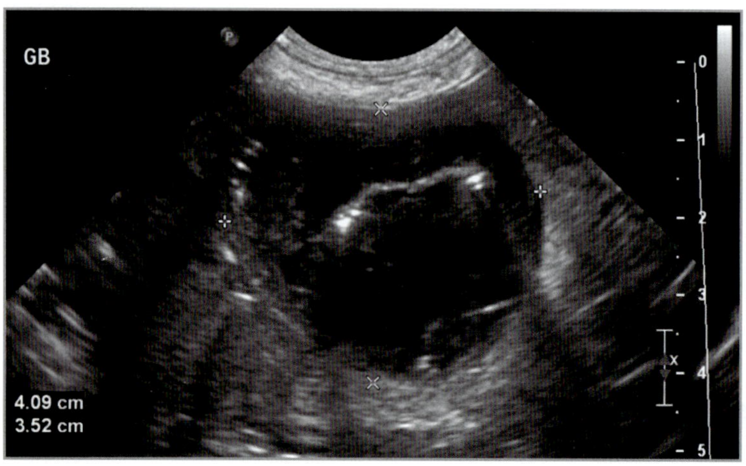

Figure 16. Emphysematous cholecystitis in a dog. Gallbladder between calipers.

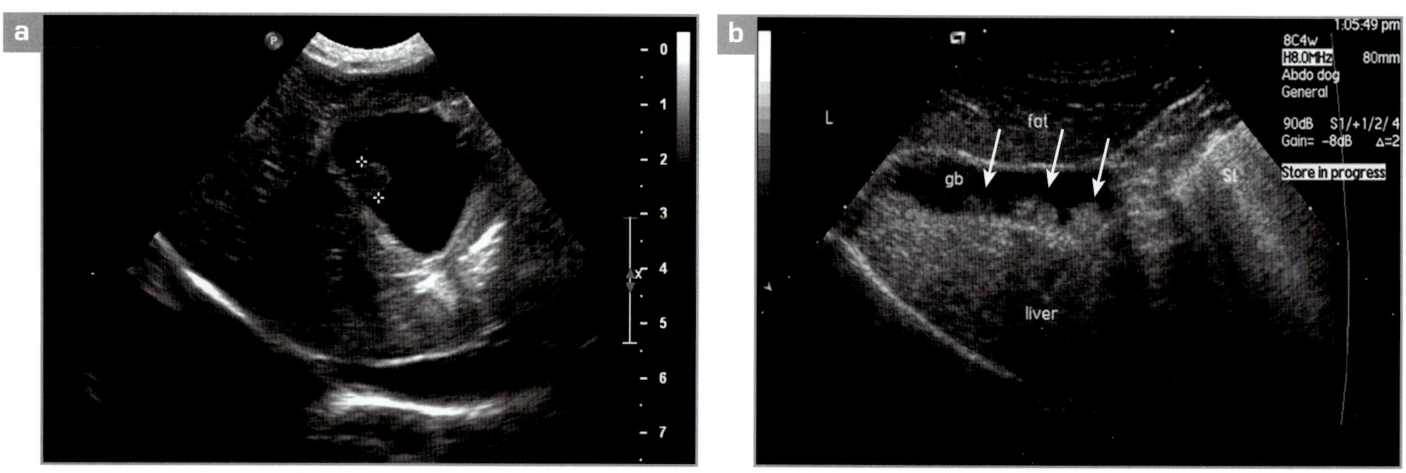

Figure 17. (a) Single polyp (between callipers) in the gallbladder of a dog. **(b)** Three polypoid projections (arrows) from the gall bladder wall of another dog consistent with polyps. gb; gallbladder.

CBD obstruction causes dilatation of the common bile duct (Fig. 19) and subsequent dilatation of the gallbladder within 24 hours, although the intrahepatic ducts may take more than a week to dilate. Dilated intrahepatic ducts (Fig. 20) appear similar to portal veins on ultrasound and colour-flow Doppler may be necessary to differentiate between them.

The CVC and hepatic veins may be dilated secondary to right-sided heart failure, thrombi and space-occupying lesions.

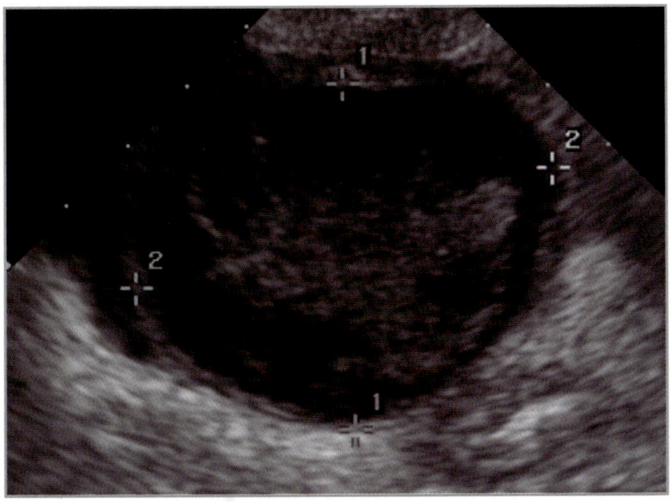

Figure 18. Gallbladder mucocoele in a dog (between callipers). The bile is more echogenic than normal and has a "kiwi" appearance.

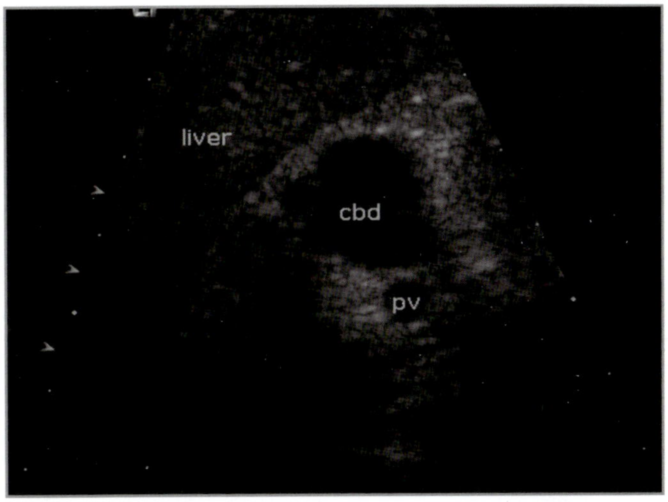

Figure 19. Common bile duct (Cbd) dilatation in a cat with pancreatitis. pv: portal vein

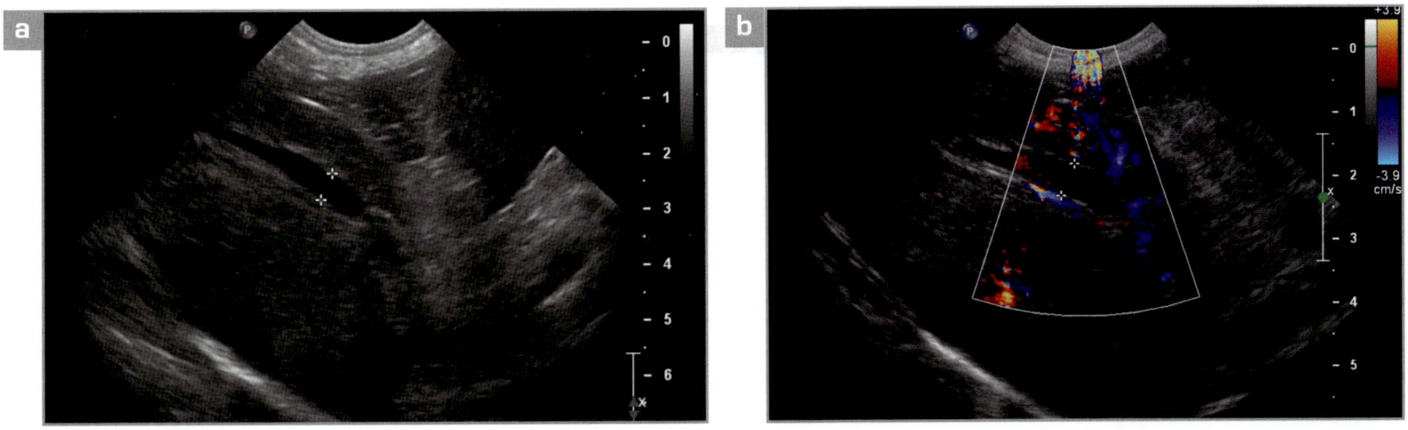

Figure 20. (a) Dilated intrahepatic duct in a dog. (b) Colour-flow Doppler shows the lack of signal from the dilated duct.

Portosystemic vascular anomalies

Portosystemic shunts can be identified by ultrasound. Ultrasound is more sensitive for extrahepatic shunts than for intrahepatic shunts. Hyperechoic kidneys and urolithiasis are common secondary findings associated with shunts. On the scan, an anomalous vessel is seen draining into the CVC (Fig. 21a), hepatic vein, splenic vein or azygos vein (Fig. 21b).

Portosystemic shunts can be single or multiple, congenital or acquired, and intrahepatic or extrahepatic. Congenital extrahepatic shunts are typically seen in small-sized dogs and cats (Fig. 21), while congenital intrahepatic shunts occur more commonly in large dog breeds (Fig. 22). In older dogs and cats, multiple acquired shunts secondary to chronic liver disease are relatively frequent, although these patients can also have congenital shunts that have not been diagnosed previously.

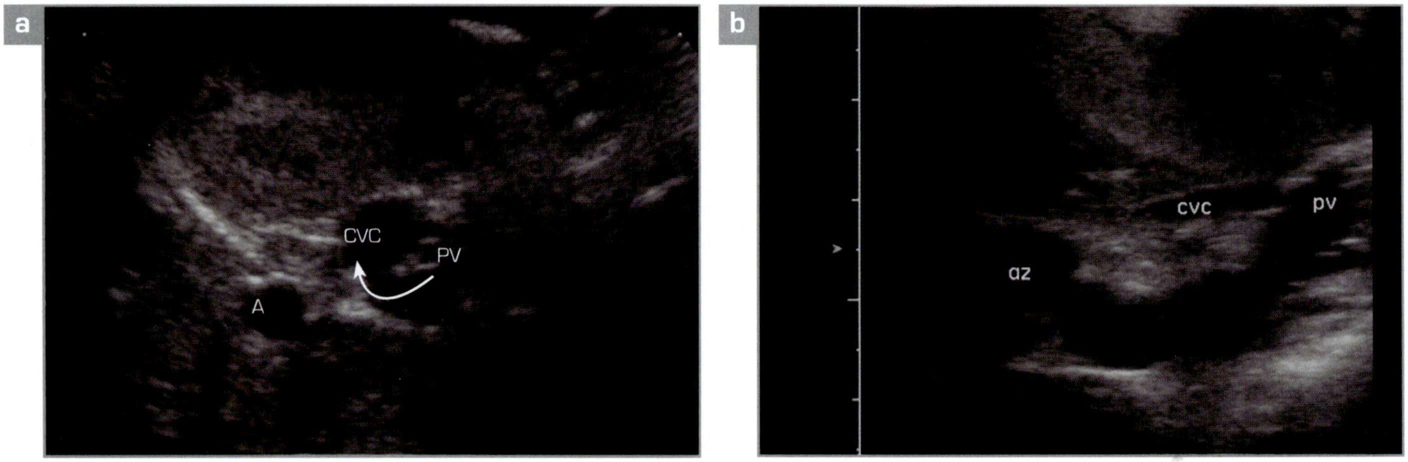

Figure 21. (a) Transverse view using a right intercostal approach in a dog with a single extrahepatic shunt. The shunt (arrow) is visible connecting the portal vein (PV) with the caudal vena cava (CVC). A: aorta. **(b)** Right intercostal oblique view in a dog with a portoazygos shunt. A vessel can be seen connecting the portal vein (pv) with a vessel next to the aorta, which is the dilated azygos vein (az). cvc: caudal vena cava.

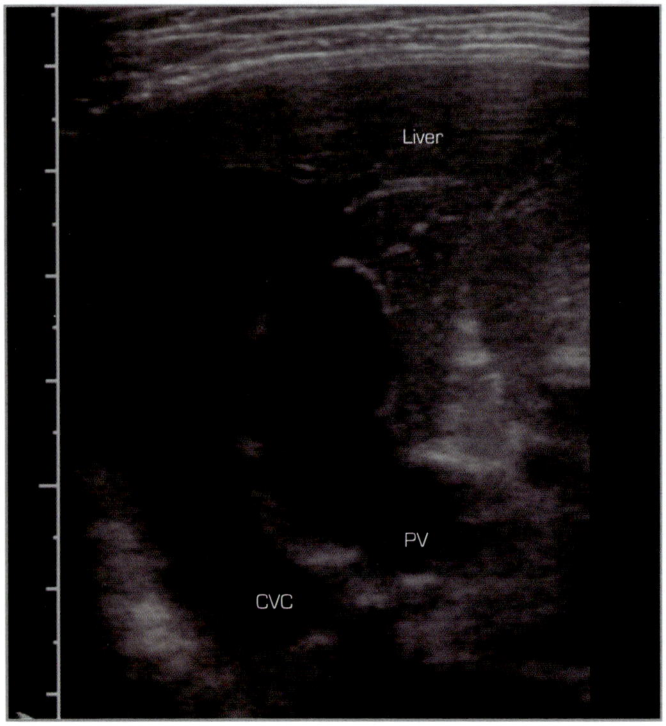

Figure 22. Oblique view using a right intercostal approach. An intrahepatic vessel appears to connect the portal vein (PV) with the caudal vena cava (CVC) consistent with a right divisional intrahepatic portosystemic shunt.

5

CHAPTER

SPLEEN

Scanning technique

The animal is positioned in right lateral recumbency with the head towards the ultrasound machine.

The head of the spleen is located caudal to the stomach in the craniodorsal portion of the left side of the abdomen, adjacent to the abdominal wall and between the gastric fundus and the left kidney. The position of the tail of the spleen is more variable. That is the reason why we look for the head of the spleen initially and then evaluate the remaining spleen by following it caudally.

> While the head of the spleen is usually located between the gastric fundus and the left kidney in the left abdominal cavity, its tail varies in position.

Due to its superficial location, a 7.5 MHz (dogs), 10 MHz (cats) or higher-frequency transducer is commonly used when examining the spleen, applying minimal, if any, pressure. Although it is not usually necessary, a standoff pad can be used to visualise the part of the spleen in the near field.

1. From the liver, with the marker of the transducer pointing towards the head of the animal, slide the transducer onto the left abdominal wall along the last rib, feeling the rib cranial to the transducer, until you identify the spleen on the screen (Fig. 1a).

> It is very important not to apply excessive pressure on the abdominal wall while searching for the spleen.

2. Once you see the spleen, you are either near the cranial margin or just caudal to it. If the latter, then slide the transducer cranially to the last intercostal space to identify the cranial margin of the spleen.

3. Fan the transducer dorsally to see the part of the spleen under the rib cage and then fan it ventrally before you return to the starting position.

> When fanning the transducer dorsally towards the cranial aspect of the spleen, make sure you fan it dorsally enough to see the whole head of the spleen, as it is visible coming from the top to the bottom of the screen.

4. Slide the transducer a centimetre or two caudoventrally and repeat the fanning dorsally and ventrally.

5. Repeat this until the caudal margin of the spleen appears on the screen (Fig. 1b).

6. Then, rotate the transducer 90° clockwise and slide it cranially following the spleen to reassess it in a transverse orientation (Fig. 2).

7. As you move the transducer, evaluate the appearance, echogenicity, echotexture and margination of the spleen along with the location, appearance and direction of the splenic veins.

8. If the spleen is small it may be completely in the rib cage. If you cannot identify the spleen with the previous technique, and you have checked that there is no history of previous splenectomy, slide the transducer along the last intercostal space (and possibly the intercostal space more cranial) to identify a smaller spleen.

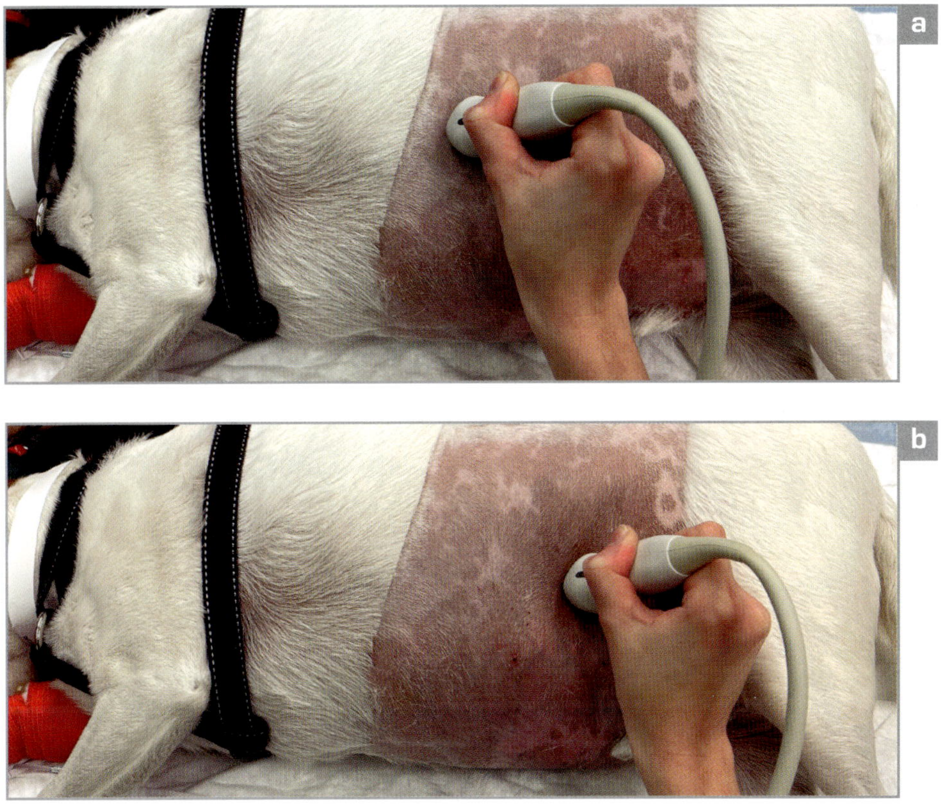

Figure 1. (a) The spleen is located following the last rib up from the liver. **(b)** Fan the transducer up and down to examine the spleen and then slide it caudally to continue the examination until reaching its caudal edge.

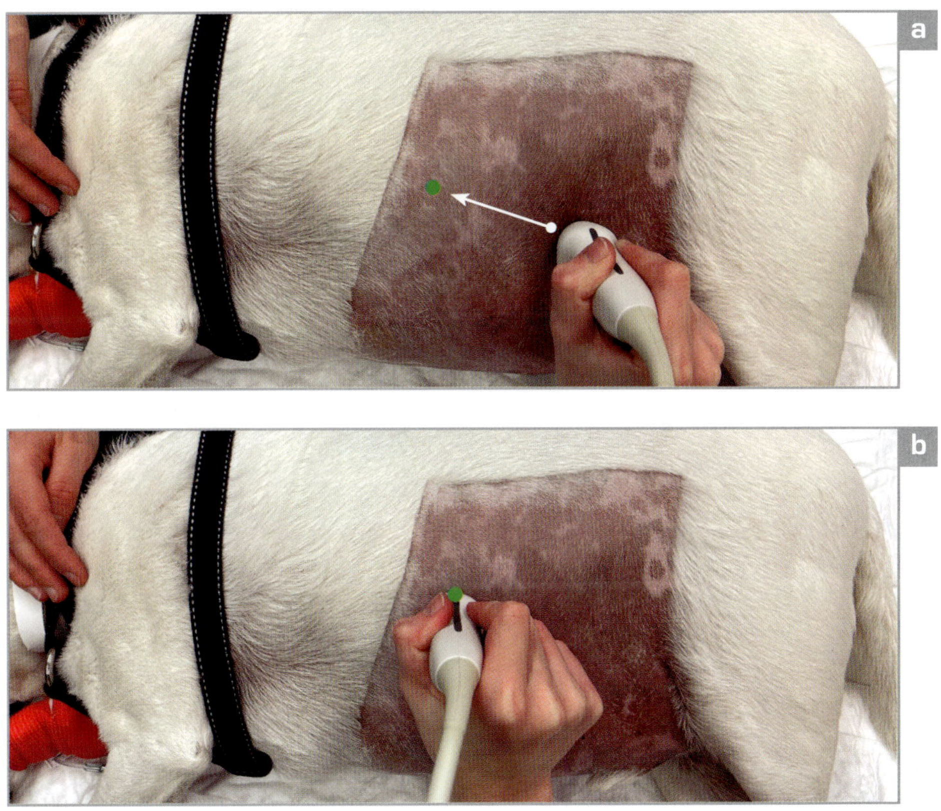

Figure 2. (a) Once you reach the tail of the spleen and its caudal edge is visible, rotate the transducer 90° clockwise. **(b)** Follow the spleen by sliding the transducer cranially until the cranial edge.

Normal appearance

The spleen commonly lies within a centimetre from the skin. In cats, it is very thin, only up to approximately 1 cm thick. It is long and tongue-shaped in its long axis, with a more triangular appearance in short-axis views.

The splenic capsule is thin and distinctly hyperechoic to the splenic parenchyma when the ultrasound beam hits it perpendicularly. The splenic parenchyma is uniformly hyperechoic with a finely granular echotexture (Fig. 3). The spleen is more echogenic than the liver and renal cortex.

The splenic veins can be seen entering the splenic hilum as anechoic tubular structures (Fig. 3a). They are not normally identified within the spleen unless the organ is congested, which is fairly common. The splenic arteries are not usually seen in routine splenic ultrasonographic examinations and require Doppler ultrasonography to be properly evaluated.

a

b

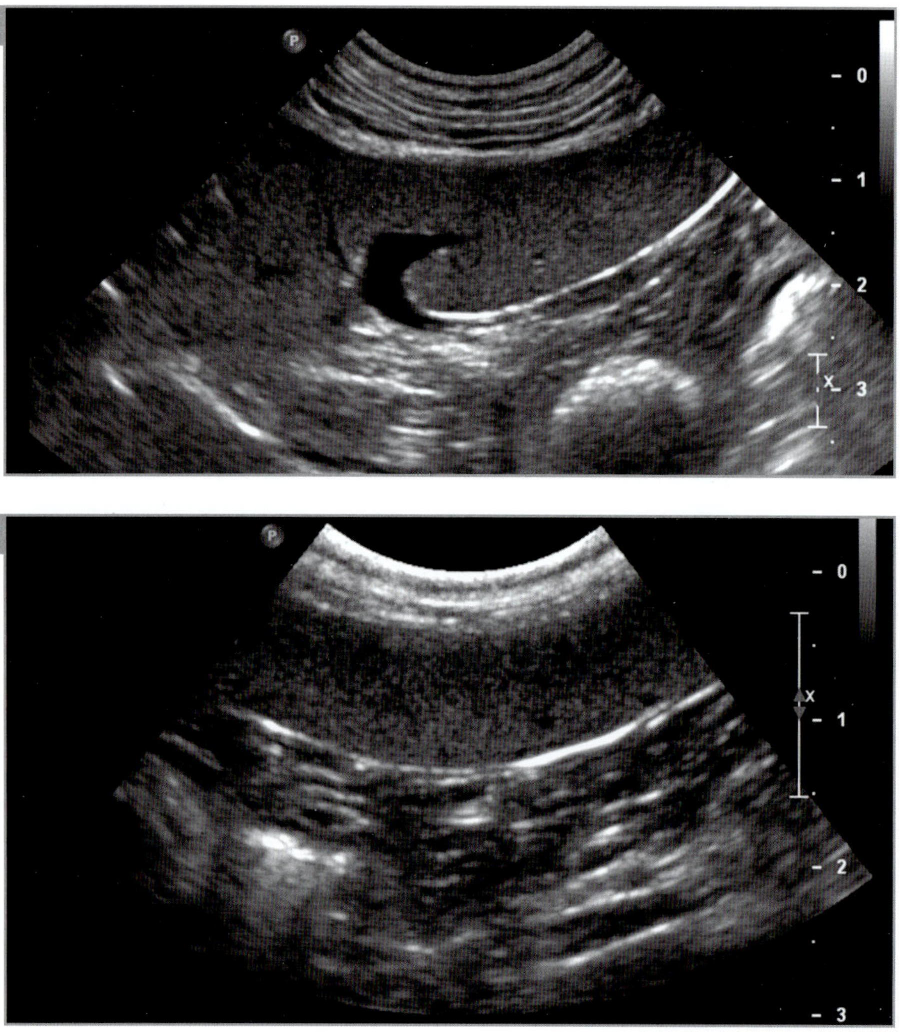

Figure 3. Normal spleen in a dog (a) and in a cat (b). The spleen is uniformly hyperechoic and has a distinct hyperechoic capsule.

Variations from normal

Focal and multifocal lesions

Splenic nodules are a non-specific finding. They can vary from small nodules to large masses and may indicate a number of diseases (Table 1).

Table 1. Differential diagnosis of focal or multifocal splenic nodular lesions or masses.

Ultrasound appearance	Most likely differential diagnoses
Anechoic (Fig. 4), hypoechoic (Fig. 5), isoechoic lesions (Fig. 6)	• Neoplasia (primary, metastatic) Multiple small hypoechoic nodules are suggestive of lymphoma. • Nodular hyperplasia • Haematoma • Extramedullary haematopoiesis • Infarct • Necrosis • Abscess • Granuloma • Cyst
Hyperechoic lesions (Fig. 7)	• Myelolipomas (incidental) • Neoplasia (primary, metastatic) • Nodular hyperplasia • Haemorrhage in the parenchyma • Infarct • Necrosis • Abscess • Mineralised granuloma • Gas bubbles
Mixed echogenicity lesions (Fig. 8)	• Neoplasia (primary, metastatic) • Nodular hyperplasia • Haematoma • Abscess • Telangiectasia
Target-like lesions (Fig. 9)	• Malignant neoplasia (Fig. 9) • Nodular hyperplasia

> Some nodules can be isoechoic to the spleen and the only way to identify them is to observe the margin of the spleen and/or the direction of the splenic veins (Fig. 5).

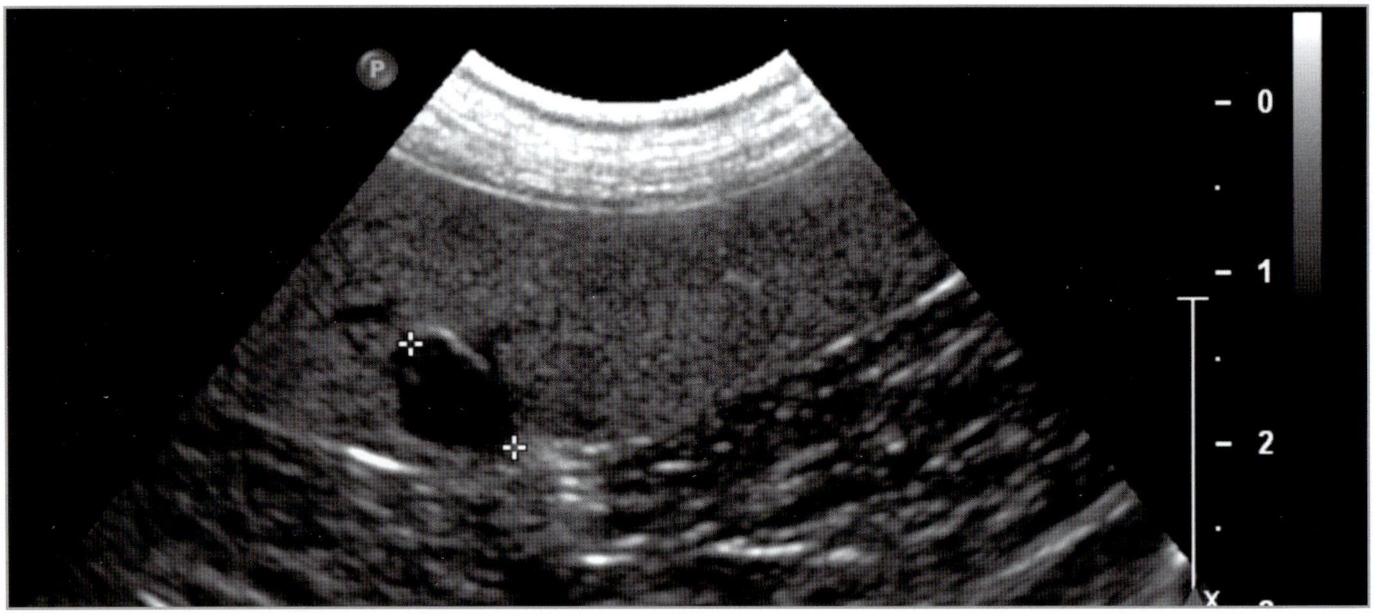

Figure 4. Anechoic nodule in the spleen of a 6-year-old Pug. The fine needle aspirates were consistent with lymphoma. Observe the lack of acoustic enhancement.

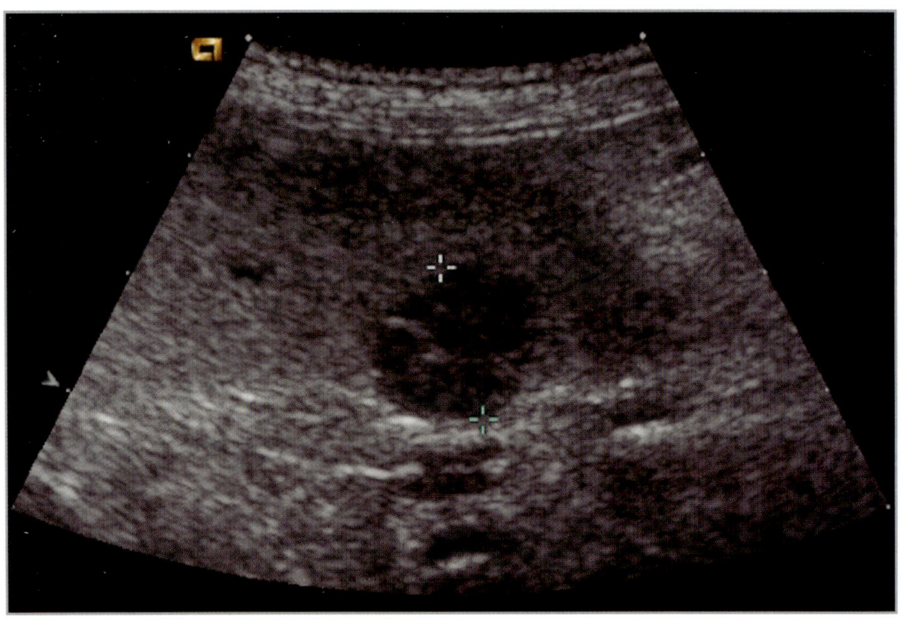

Figure 5. Hypoechoic nodule (between callipers) in the tail of the spleen of a dog.

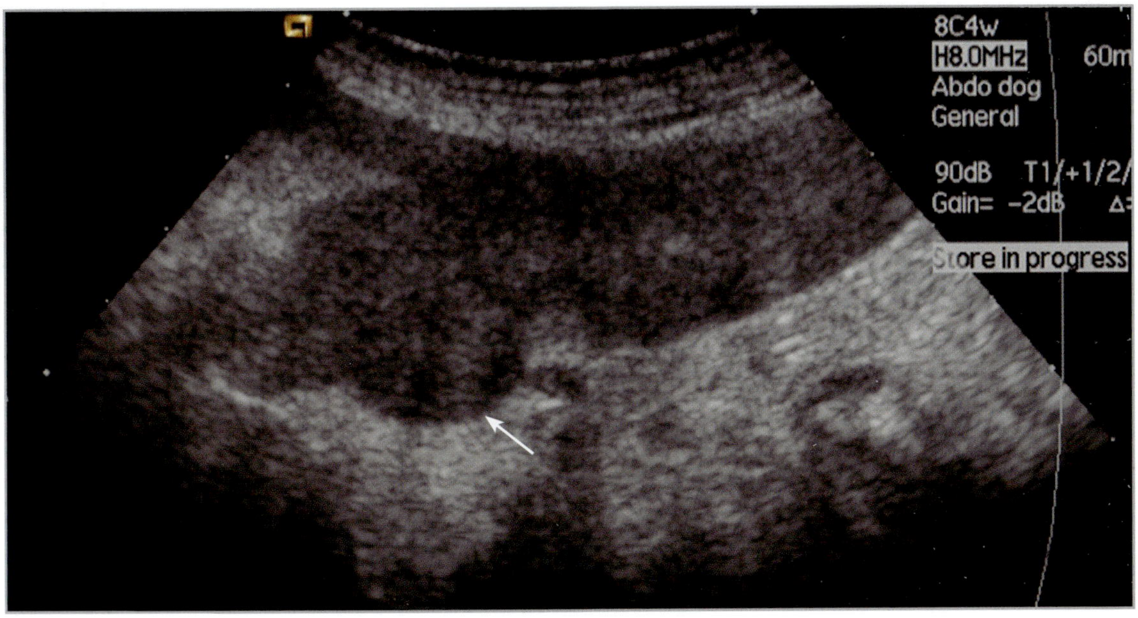

Figure 6. Isoechoic nodule in the spleen (arrow), bulging from the surface of the spleen.

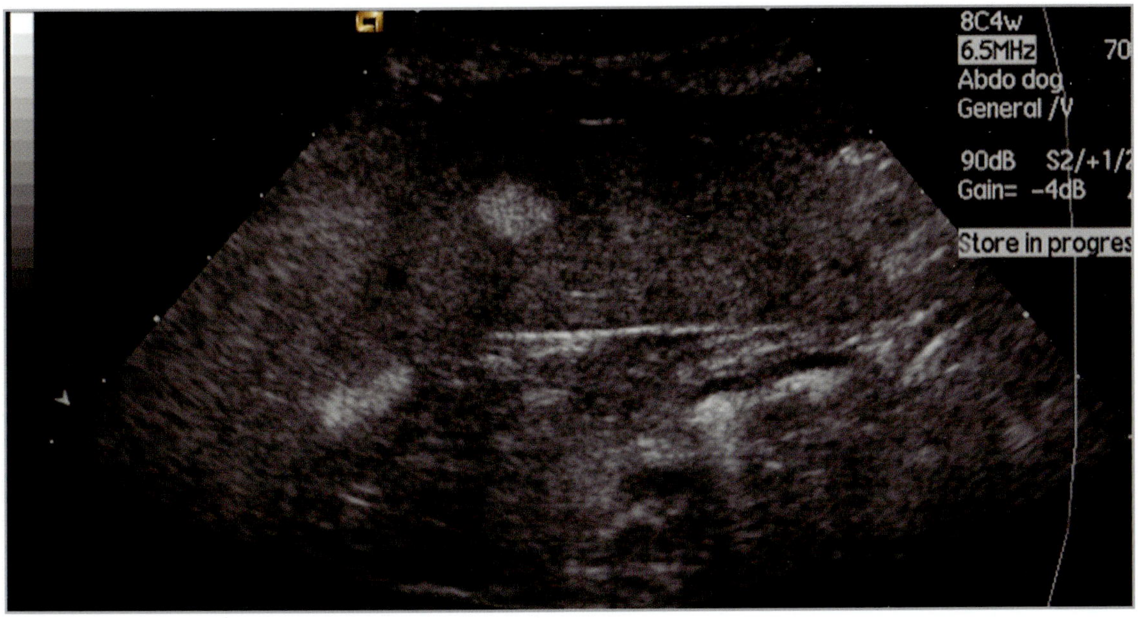

Figure 7. Hyperechoic nodule in a canine spleen. Hyperechoic nodules in the spleen often represent myelolipomas, a common incidental finding.

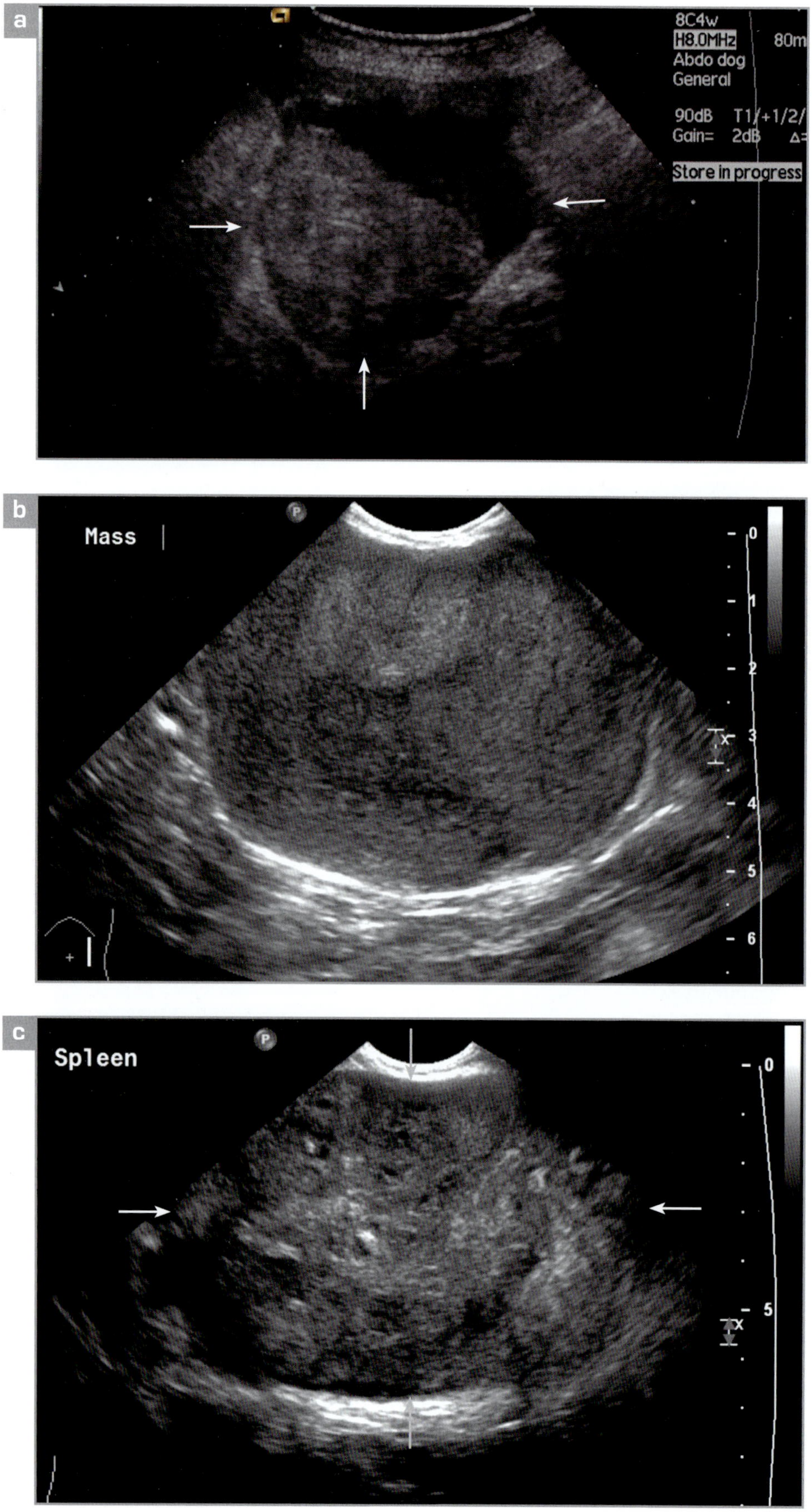

Figure 8. (a) Cavitary mass in the spleen of a dog (arrows). This mass was a haematoma. Note that haemangiosarcomas, for example, can have a similar appearance. (b) Splenic haematoma appearing as a mildly mixed echogenicity mass. (c) Mixed echogenciity mass (arrows) with small cystic areas, confirmed as splenic haemangiosarcoma, in a 10-year-old female miniature Schnauzer.

Splenic masses may have any echotexture and may or may not contain cavities (Fig. 8). The ultrasonographic appearance is not specific to certain conditions and these masses can represent malignant or benign conditions. Rupture of splenic masses resulting in haemoabdomen can be seen with malignant lesions (e.g. splenic haemangiosarcoma); however, it can also be seen with benign lesions. On the other hand, target-like lesions with a hypoechoic periphery and hyperechoic or isoechoic centre have been associated with malignancy, i.e. metastatic lesions (Fig. 9). Nevertheless, these target-like lesions can also be seen with benign processes i.e. hypeplastic nodules.

Splenic vein thrombosis (Fig. 10) may appear as echogenic material in the splenic veins. With splenic infarction (Fig. 11) , the affected areas appear hypoechoic and relatively well marginated with decreased or absent blood flow on colour-Doppler or power-Doppler examination.

Fibrosis, dystrophic or metastatic mineralisations, gas (e.g. from gas forming bacteria) and foreign bodies create focal, hyperechoic lesions with distal acoustic shadowing. If the mineralised foci are small the distal acoustic shadowing may not be seen (Fig. 12).

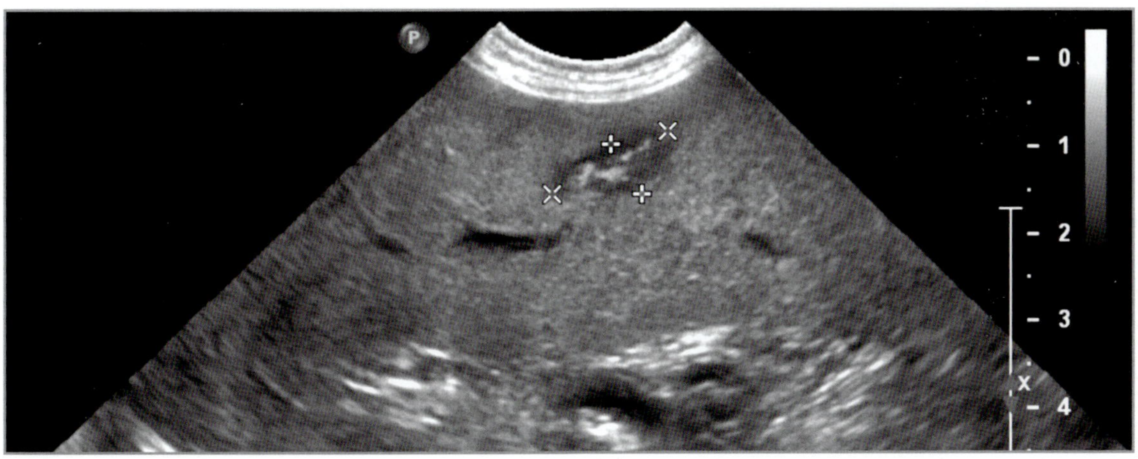

Figure 9. Target-like lesion in the spleen (between callipers) in a 10-year old crossbred dog. Observe the hypoechoic periphery and hyperechoic centre. Fine needle aspirates from the lesion were compatible with plasma cell neoplasm.

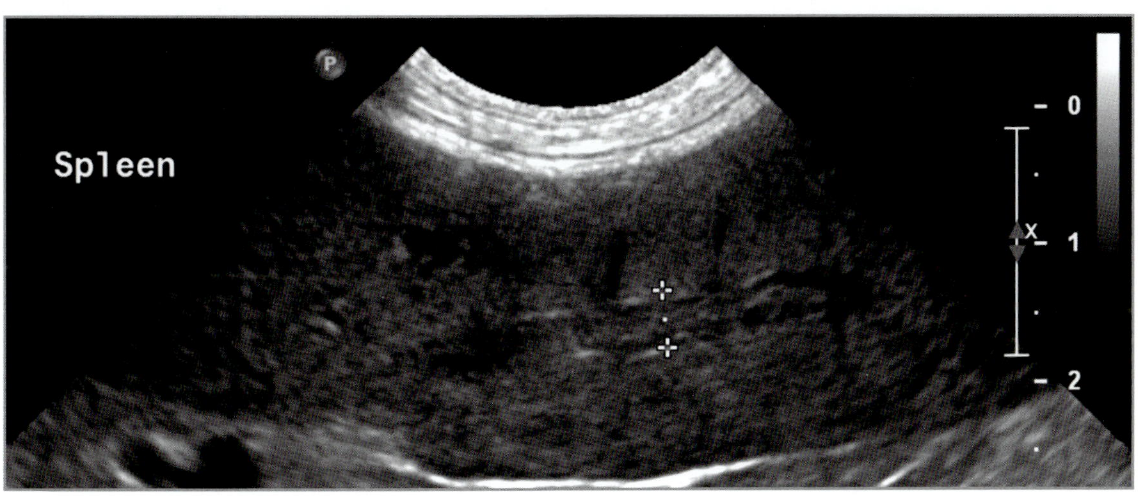

Figure 10. Splenic vein with thrombosis. Observe the echogenic material in the splenic vein (between callipers).

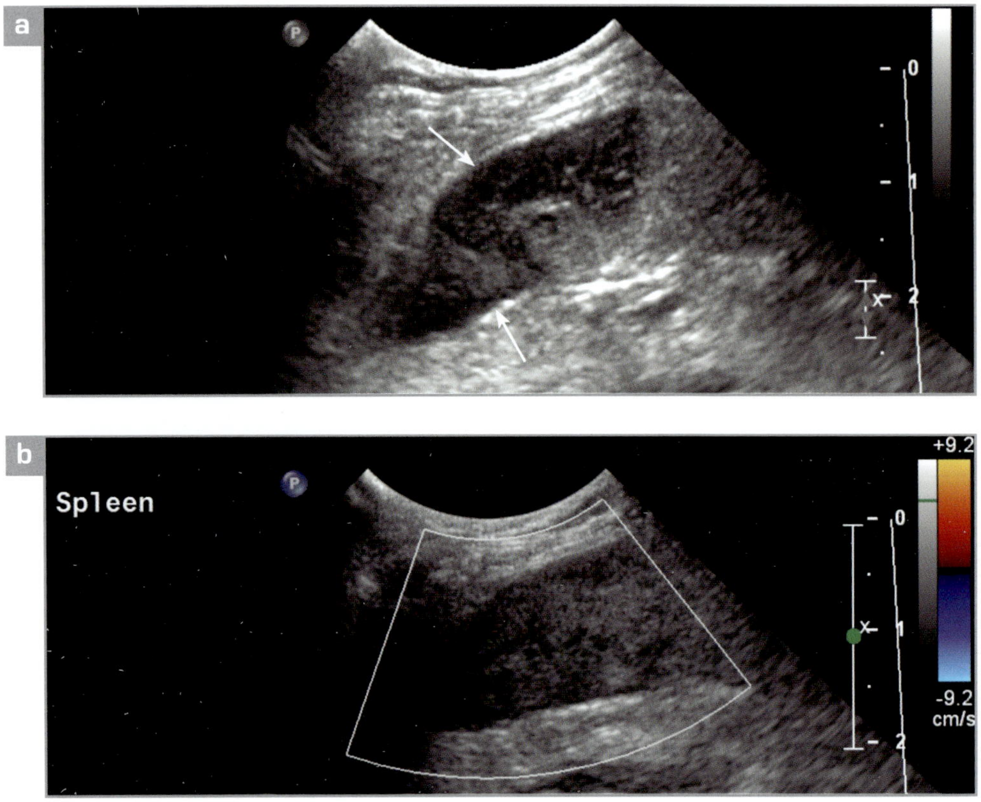

Figure 11. Splenic infract in a dog. **(a)** A hypoechoic and relatively well marginated area is visible in the periphery of the spleen, **(b)** with absent blood flow on colour-Doppler.

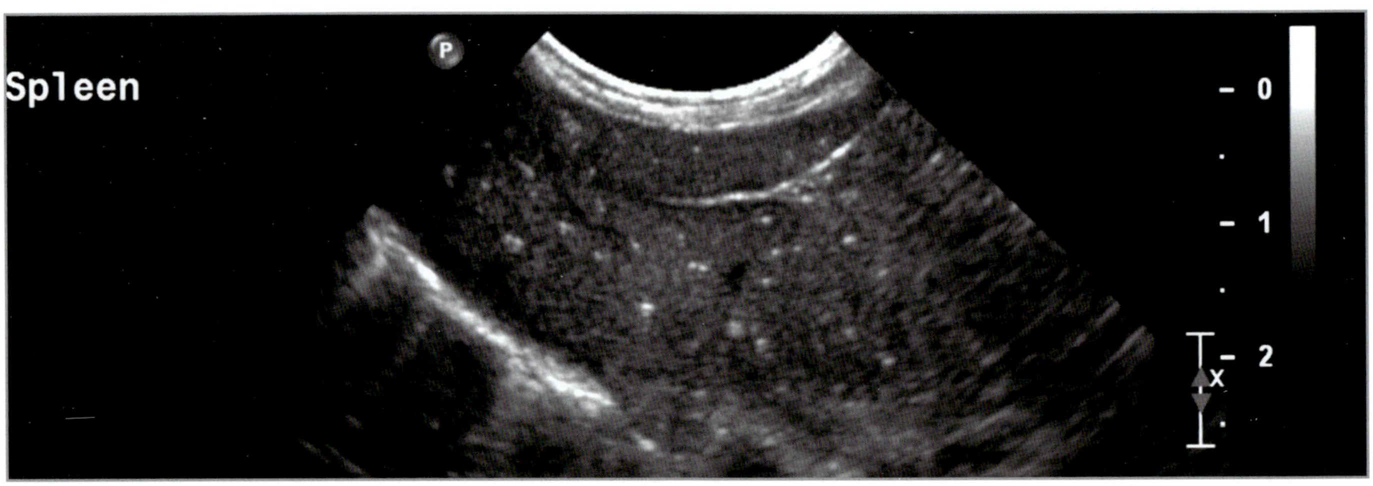

Figure 12. Sagital image of the spleen with hyperechoic foci throughout the parenchyma in an 8-year old female Chihuahua with hyperadrenocorticism.

Diffuse changes

When the spleen is enlarged, the margins appear more rounded, and the organ extends further caudally (occasionally up to the level of the urinary bladder).

Common causes of splenomegaly with normal echogenicity include sedation (e.g. with acepromazine) or general anaesthesia and they should be considered along with other clinical reasons of splenomegaly such as extramedullary haematopoiesis, lymphoid hyperplasia, neoplasia and chronic or haemolytic anaemias. In cats with splenomegaly, the spleen commonly folds on itself. Some dog breeds, like German Shepherd dogs, tend to have large and folded spleens.

With splenic torsion, the spleen is enlarged and hypoechoic, having what is commonly referred to as a "starry sky" appearance (Fig. 13). This appearance can also be seen with extensive venous thrombosis. Other causes of splenomegaly include infectious diseases, extramedullary haematopoiesis and malignant infiltration (Fig. 14).

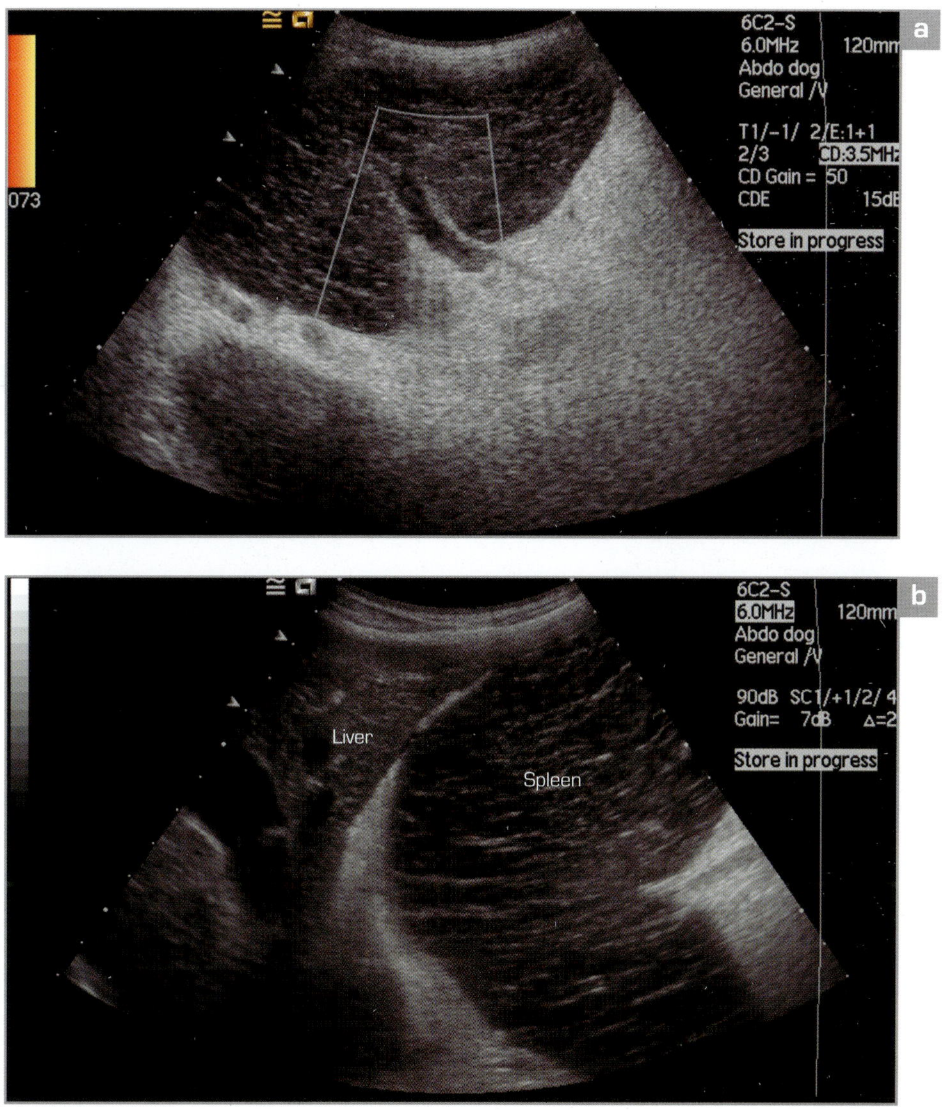

Figure 13. Splenic torsion. (a) The spleen is hypoechoic with hyperechoic foci. No flow is detected in the splenic vein with power Doppler. The surrounding mesentery is markedly hyperechoic. (b) The spleen is hypoechoic to the liver.

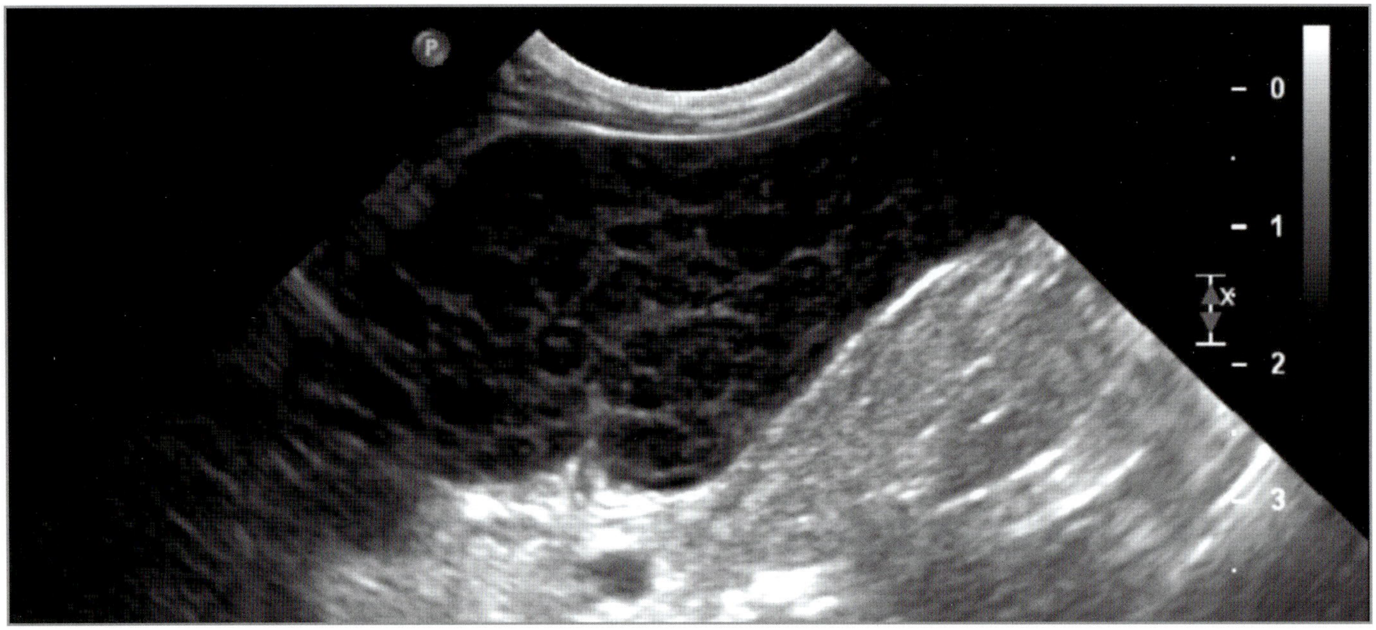

Figure 14. Sagital iimage of spleen of a 17-year old Border-Collie diagnosed with lymphoma. The spleen has a honeycomb appearance.

> The assessment of splenic size is subjective and there are no accurate measurements to determine it.

A small spleen may be very difficult to identify and it can be seen in animals with significant blood loss or in shock. It can also be seen with advancing age secondary to lyphoid atrophy. A small spleen will also have a more triangular shape even in its long axis and appear more hypoechoic than normal.

> Just in case, when you have difficulty locating the spleen always make sure there was no previous splenectomy.

Accessory spleen(s) can be seen. They can be congental or acquired. They have the same echogenicity and echotecture with the spleen but usually smaller size (Fig. 15). Accessory spleens may be difficult to differentiate from peritoneall masses.

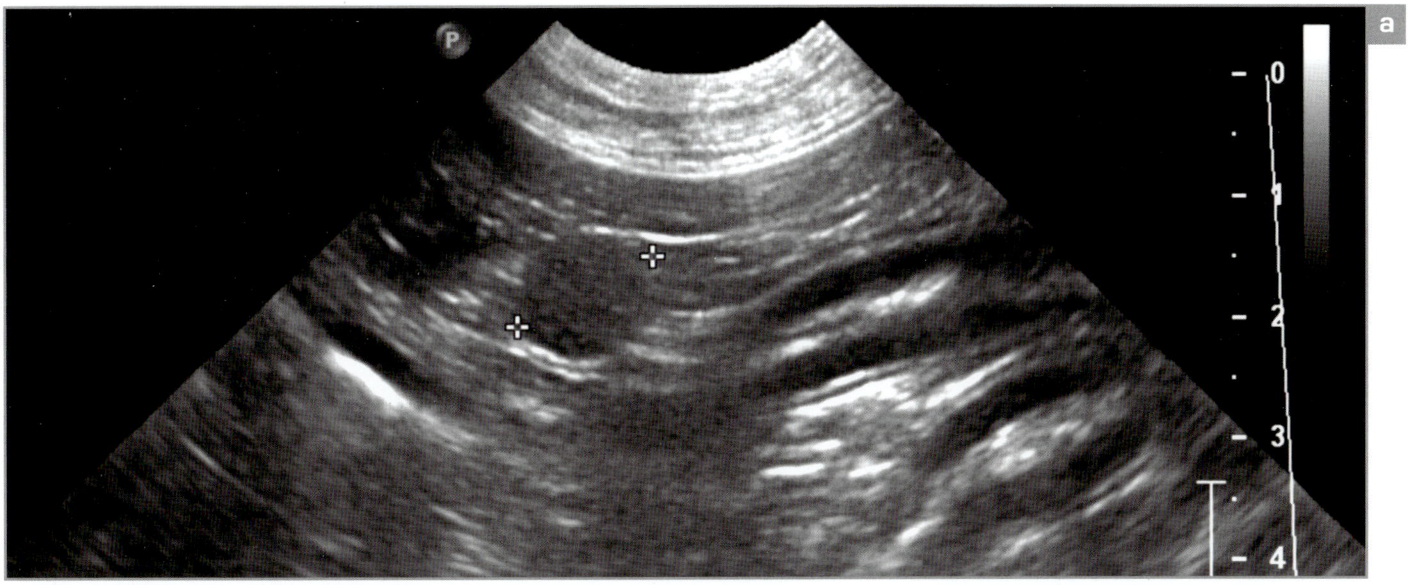

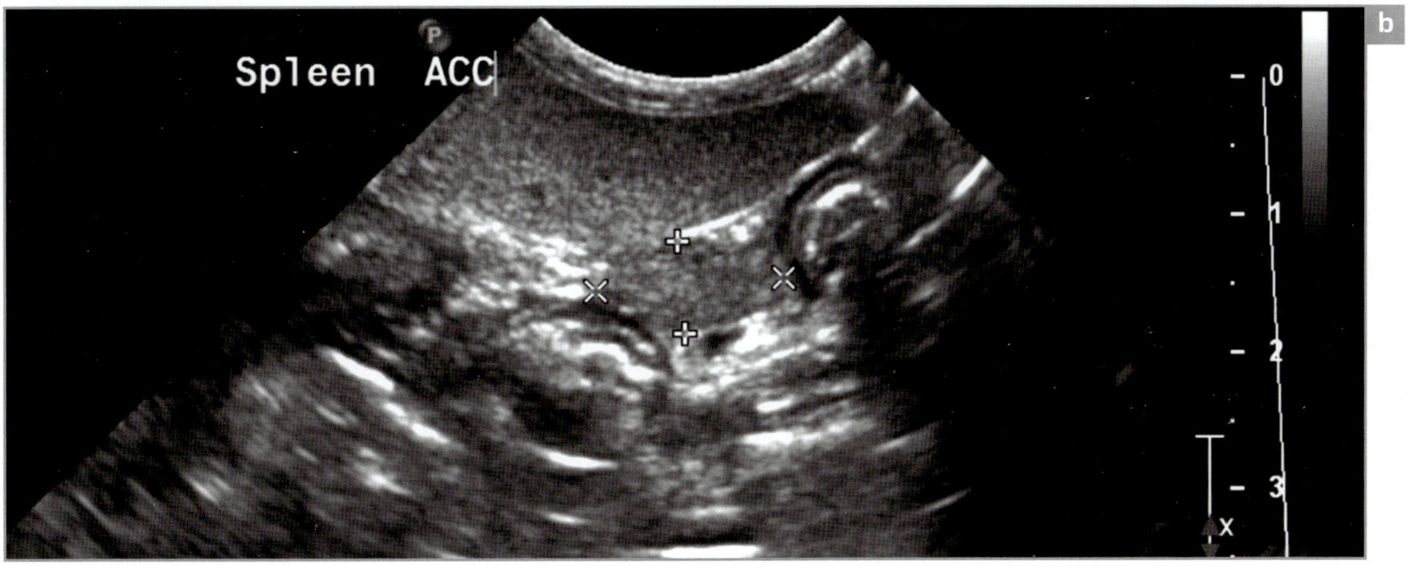

Figure 15. Accesory spleen in (a) 8-year-old male Dalmatian and in (b) a 15-year-old male neutered Maine Coon.

6

CHAPTER

GASTROINTESTINAL TRACT

Scanning technique

The animal is positioned in right lateral recumbency with the head pointing towards the ultrasound machine and the limbs towards the examiner.

The stomach is located just caudal to the liver as the transducer is moved along the last rib towards the spleen. Most of the gastrointestinal tract can be evaluated in right lateral recumbency. Sometimes, the animal also needs to be positioned in left lateral recumbency in order to examine the pyloric region of the stomach and part of the small intestine. This is particularly relevant in large-sized dogs, where due to increased animal size and increasing scanning depth, complete evaluation from one side is not possible.

Most of the gastrointestinal tract can be examined using a 7-8 MHz transducer. In small dogs, and especially in cats, a 10 MHz (or higher) transducer is commonly employed. In large dogs, sometimes a 6, 5 or 4 MHz transducer may be useful due to the increased scan depth that is required.

Stomach

1. From the liver, with the marker of the transducer pointing to the head of the animal, slide the transducer towards the left of the animal along the last rib, feeling the rib cranial to the transducer. The stomach can be identified just caudal to the liver.

2. The first image is along the short axis of the stomach (Fig. 1).

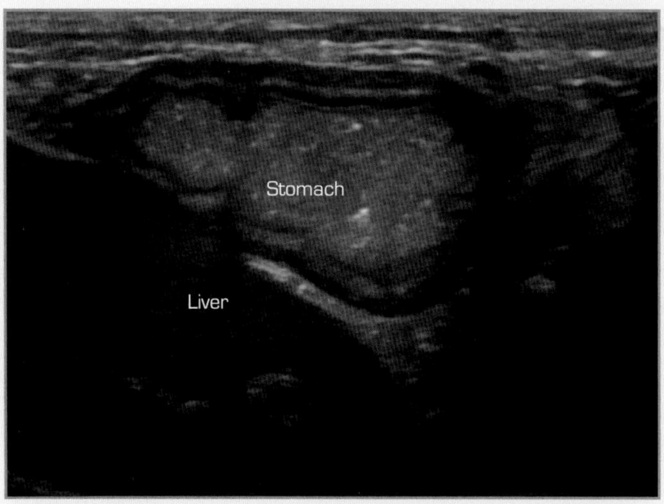

Figure 1. View along the short axis of the stomach. Some rugal folds are visible.

3. Fan and slightly slide the transducer dorsally towards the spine to evaluate the body and fundus of the stomach (Fig. 2a) and then fan and slightly slide the transducer ventrally (Fig. 2b) for the examination of the pyloric region.

4. Rotate the transducer clockwise, approximately 90° or slightly less, until you get a longitudinal view of the stomach in which the stomach appears to run across the screen with the fundus to the left and the pylorus to the right side of the screen (Fig. 3).

5. Rocking of the transducer dorsally (Fig. 4a) and ventrally (Fig. 4b) allows examination of the stomach in long axis.

When examining the stomach, it is a good idea to keep the transducer still for one minute to observe the gastric contractions and evaluate their strength and frequency.

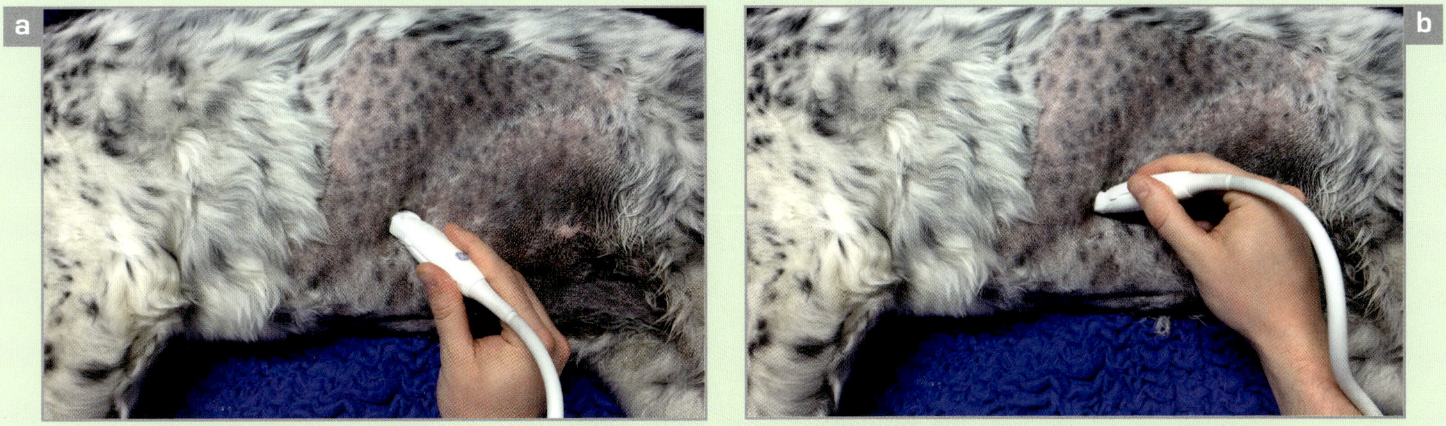

Figure 2. After identifying the stomach on the screen, and with the marker pointing to the head of the animal, the transducer is fanned up (a) and down (b) to evaluate the stomach in short axis.

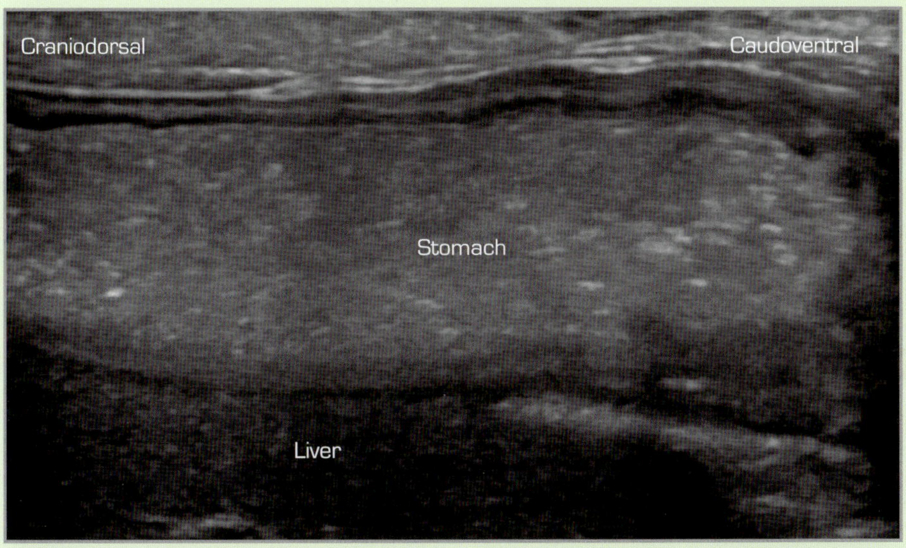

Figure 3. View along the long axis of the stomach. The gastric wall layers are clearly visible.

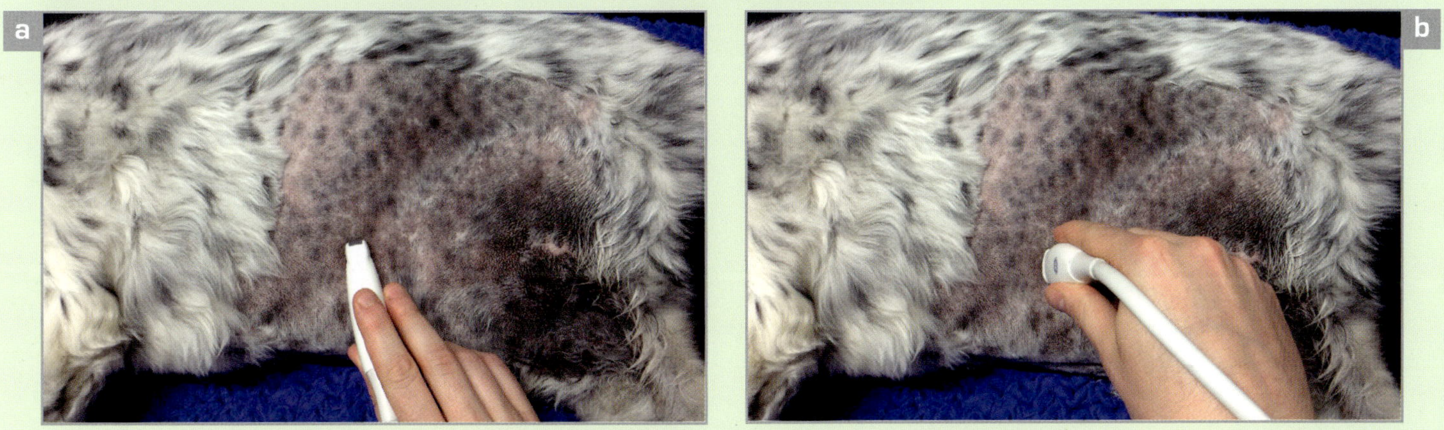

Figure 4. The stomach is evaluated along its long axis by rocking the transducer up (a) and down (b).

Small intestine

1. It is almost impossible to ultrasonographically follow all the small intestine from the duodenum to the ileum, so the objective is to follow a specific pattern and try to examine any loop that is visible.

2. With the marker pointing to the head of the animal, and starting from the stomach, slide the transducer in a caudal direction following a "castle" pattern (Fig. 5), until you see the urinary bladder on the screen.

3. Examine every loop that comes into view on the screen and try to identify the lumen and layers of the intestine (Fig. 6).

4. If a loop appears thickened, measure the intestinal wall thickness from the inner mucosa to the inner serosa.

5. The duodenum can be identified and evaluated. The technique to identify the duodenum will be described in the Pancreas chapter.

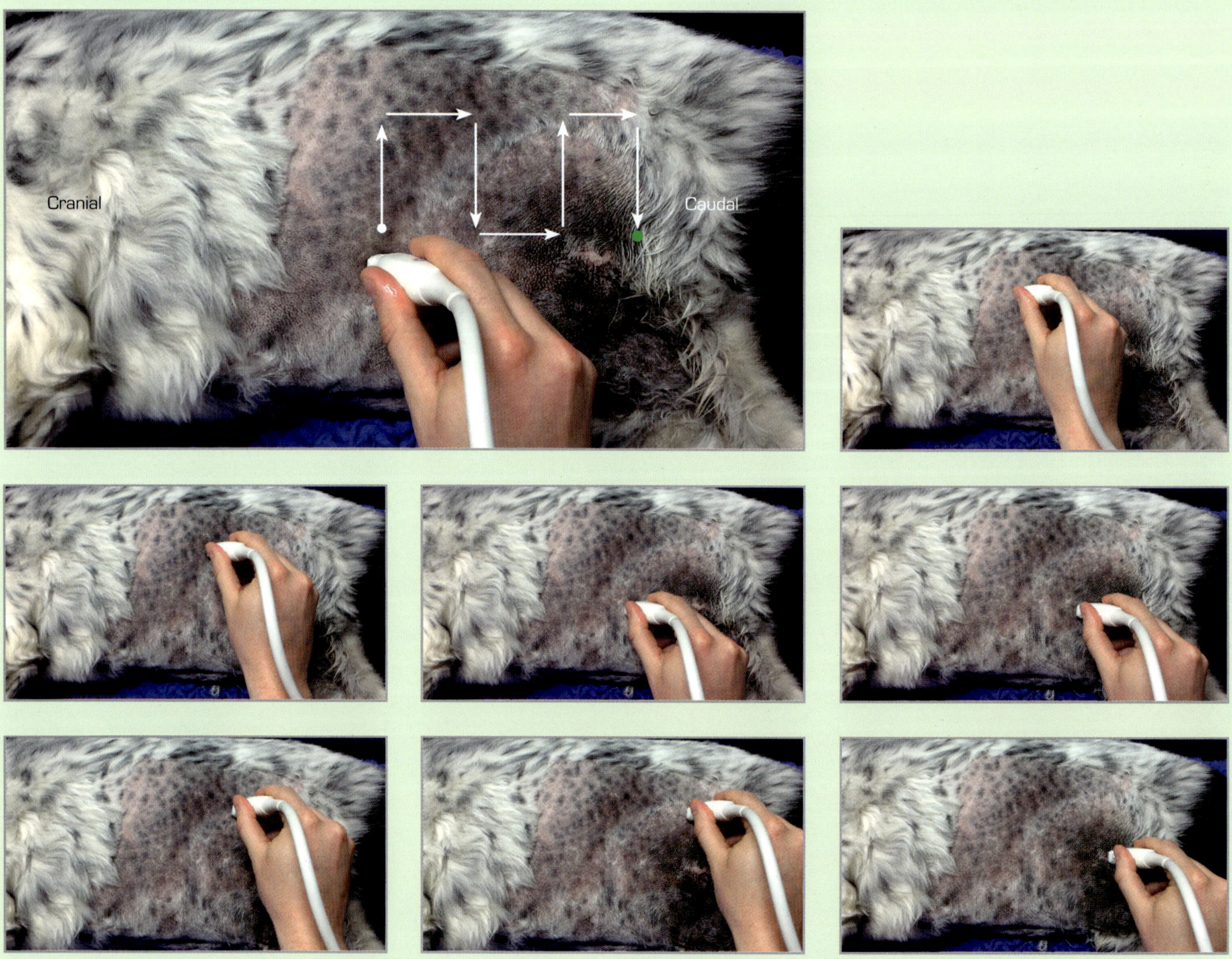

Figure 5. To evaluate the intestine, hold the transducer with the marker pointing to the head of the animal. Then, start at the level of the stomach and slide the transducer dorsally, caudally, ventrally, caudally and then dorsally again. Repeat the movement following a "castle" pattern in a caudal direction, until you reach the level of the urinary bladder. While sliding the transducer, any loop of intestine, lymph node and mesenteric tissue that comes to view is evaluated.

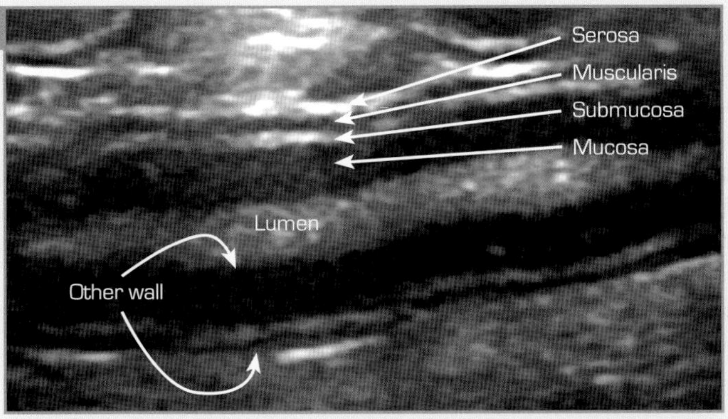

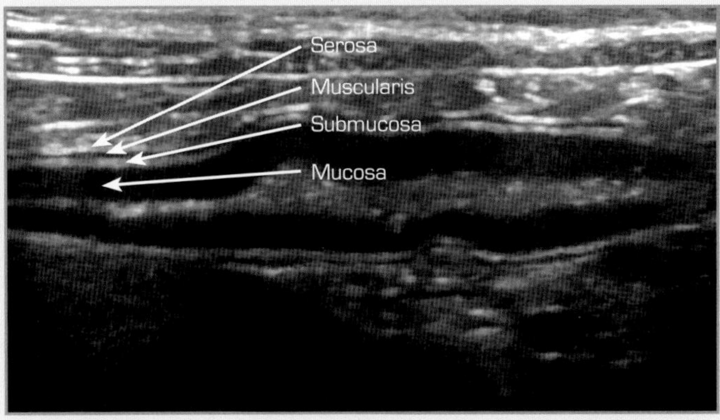

Figure 6. [a] Jejunal loop in a healthy cat. Intestinal layering is clearly visible in this normal intestine (hypoechoic mucosa, hyperechoic submucosa, hypoechoic muscularis and hyperechoic serosa). [b] Duodenum in a healthy dog. The layers of the wall are clearly identifiable.

Large intestine

1. Identify the urinary bladder and slide the transducer (with the marker pointing to the head of the animal) dorsally, towards the spine, and identify the descending colon, which is dorsal to the urinary bladder (Fig. 7). The descending colon can be identified by its location, thin wall and the artefacts caused by the gas and faeces in it.

The lumen of the colon usually contains faeces and gas that produce artefacts.

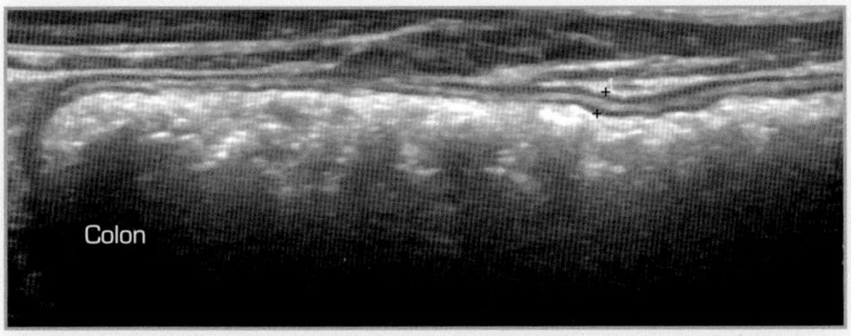

Figure 7. Normal colon in a dog. Its wall (between callipers) is thin (up to 2 mm thick) compared with the small intestine. The layers of the colon (hypoechoic mucosa, hyperechoic submucosa, hypoechoic muscularis and hyperechoic serosa) are clearly visible.

2. Slowly slide the transducer cranially to follow the descending colon and then examine the transverse and ascending colon. At the level of the transverse colon, some rotation of the transducer is required to achieve optimal alignment.

3. When at the level of the transverse to ascending colon, some rotation of the transducer will be required again to achieve optimal alignment.

4. Following the ascending colon caudally, the ileocaecocolic junction (Fig. 8) appears on the screen, where the small intestine (with a more prominent, thicker wall and a thicker mucosa) is visible in contrast to the colonic wall which is thinner.

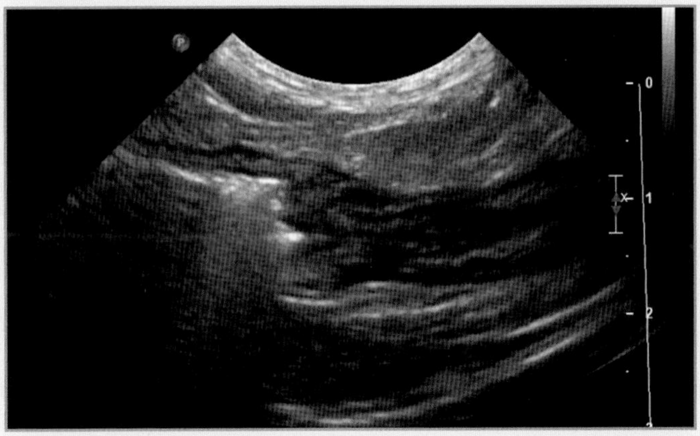

Figure 8. The normal ileocaecocolic junction in a 7-year-old Yorkshire Terrier.

Normal appearance

Wall thickness should be evaluated in order to establish whether the gastrointestinal tract is ultrasonographically normal (Table 1).

Table 1. Maximum normal wall thickness of the gastrointestinal tract in the dog and cat.

Segment of the gastrointestinal tract	Dog	Cat
Stomach	5 mm	2 mm
Small intestine (duodenum)	5 mm	2-3 mm
Small intestine (rest of the segments)	4 mm	4 mm
Large intestine	2 mm	2 mm

Stomach

The stomach varies in size depending on the amount of ingesta it contains. The normal thickness of the gastric wall is up to 5 mm in the dog and up to 2 mm in the cat (see Table 1).

Gastric wall thickness should be measured between the gastric rugal folds.

The layers of the gastric wall can usually be identified. The mucosa is hypoechoic, the submucosa is hyperechoic, the muscularis is hypoechoic and the serosa is hyperechoic (see Figs. 1 and 3). The rugal folds are commonly visible and more clearly identifiable in an empty stomach. The stomach contracts on average once every 12 seconds or approximately 5 times a minute during feeding.

Small and large intestine

The intestinal layers can be easily identified in the normal intestine. The mucosa is hypoechoic, the submucosa is hyperechoic, the muscularis is hypoechoic and the serosa is hyperechoic (see Figs. 6 and 7). The intestinal wall should be measured from the inner mucosal margin to the inner serosal margin (Fig. 9).

The duodenum has the thickest wall and can normally measure up to 5 mm in the dog and up to 3 mm in the cat. The duodenal papilla can also be identified as a small tubular structure in longitudinal view and as a rounded structure in transverse view (Fig. 10). Mucosal indentation corresponding to the Peyer patches can be seen sometimes in the antimesenteric border of the duodenum (Fig. 11). The rest of the small intestine has been reported to be up to 3 mm thick (especially in cats), although the author prefers 4 mm as a cut-off measurement for normal for dogs and cats. The ileum in cats has a distinctive "wagon wheel" appearance in transverse view.

The ileocaecocolic junction can, and should, be evaluated in dogs and cats. It is commonly easy to identify in dogs and cats (Fig. 8) though in dogs sometimes gas in the caecum creates difficulties.

The small intestine normally has one to three peristaltic contractions per minute, while no peristaltic contractions are usually seen in the colon.

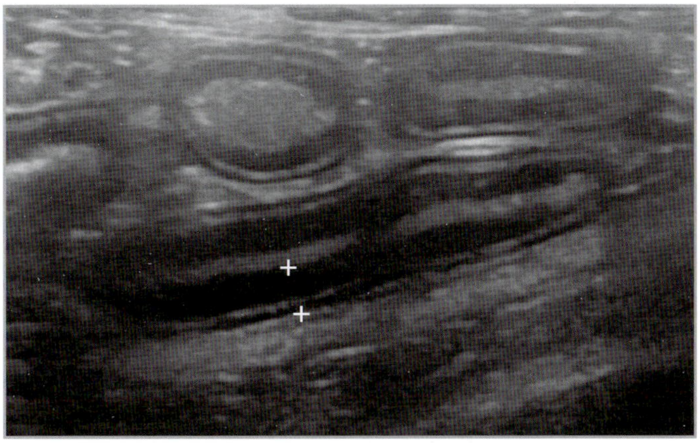

Figure 9. Wall measurement of a normal jejunal loop in a cat. The callipers are placed from the mucosal surface to the inner serosa.

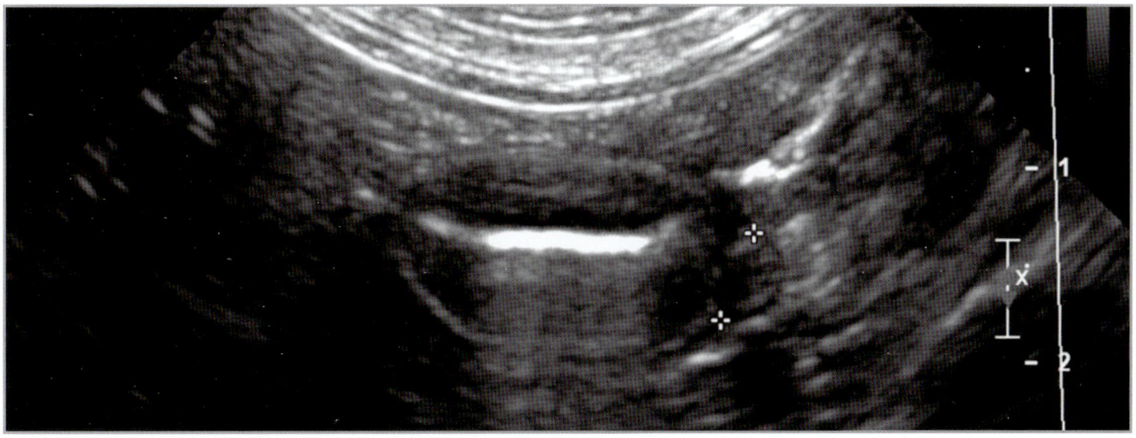

Figure 10. Normal duodenal papilla (between callipers) in a 9.5-year-old, Staffordshire Bull Terrier, transverse view.

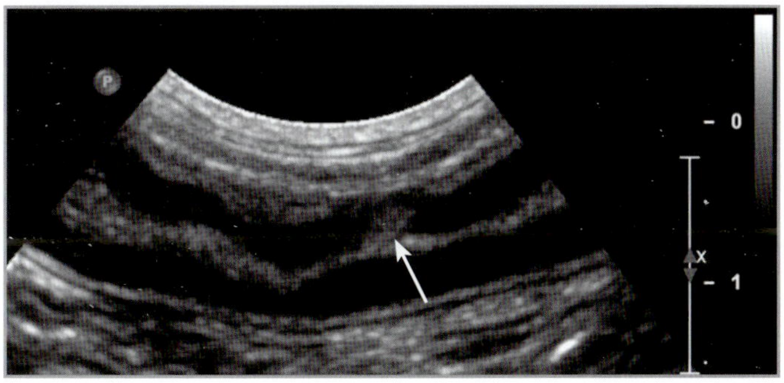

Figure 11. Mucosal indentation at the antimesenteric border of the duodenum from a dog, corresponding to a Peyer patch.

Variations from normal

Stomach

As the stomach can be filled with gas, fluid, ingesta or any combination of these, it can appear more or less distended on ultrasound examination. In a distended stomach it is important to assess the frequency of any contractions and to search for any evidence of obstruction and/or wall thickening. The pylorus should also be evaluated for adequate passing of gastric contents to the duodenum.

Gastric foreign bodies can be diagnosed as an incidental finding or as the cause of the clinical signs exhibited by the patient (vomiting, anorexia, etc.). Foreign bodies commonly have a hyperechoic surface and acoustic shadowing (Fig. 12). Linear foreign bodies may appear as a hyperechoic line that can extend caudally to the duodenum and the rest of the small intestine.

Gastric wall thickening can be associated with malignant and non-malignant diseases. Malignant diseases usually cause focal thickening with disruption or loss of the layers (Fig. 13), while non-malignant diseases commonly cause a more generalised wall thickening with retention of the wall layers (Fig. 14).

Uraemic gastritis appears ultrasonographically as a thickened gastric wall with prominent rugal folds and a hyperechoic line in the inner mucosa (luminal side) consistent with mucosal mineralisation (Fig. 15).

Gastric ulceration can be identified on ultrasound as a hyperechoic defect within the mucosa due to the accumulation of gas microbubbles and blood clots (Fig. 16). If the ulcer is perforated, hyperechoic mesentery around the area may be seen along with free peritoneal gas and fluid.

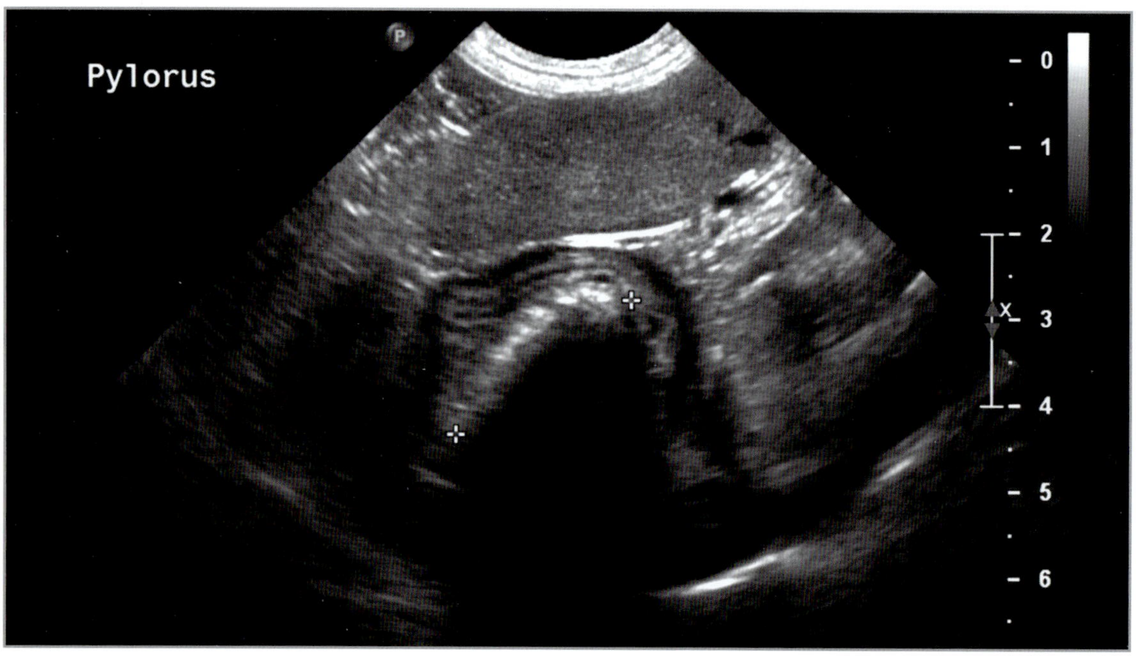

Figure 12. Gastric foreign body (between callipers) in the stomach of a 7-year-old Springer Spaniel. This foreign body with the hyperechoic surface and the strong acoustic shadowing was a corncob in the pylorus of the stomach.

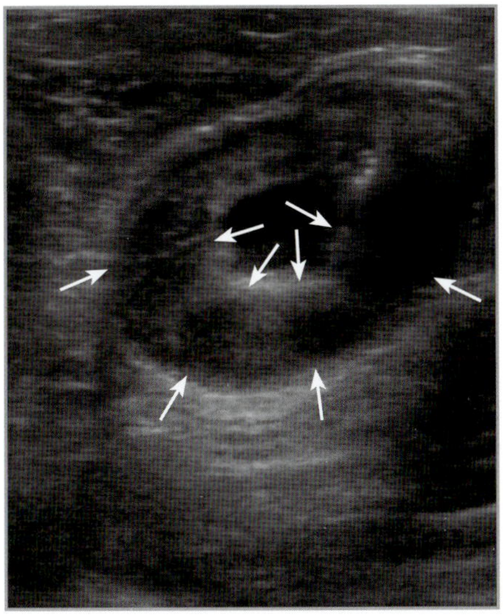

Figure 13. 11-year-old cat diagnosed with gastric lymphoma. There is focal thickening of the gastric wall, which appears hypoechoic with loss of layering (between arrows).

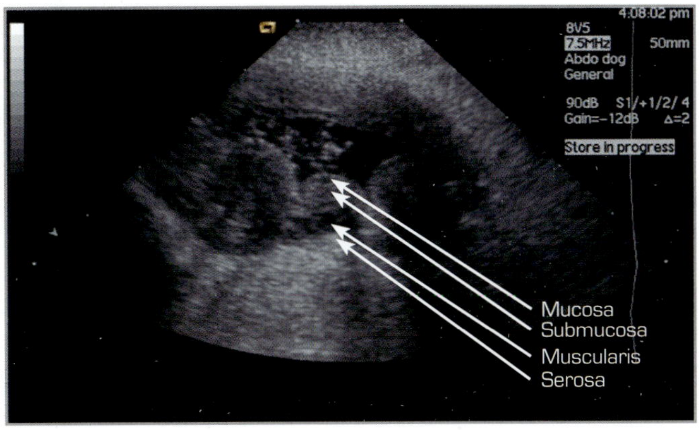

Figure 14. Image along the short axis of the stomach in a dog presented with gastritis. Note the increased thickness of the gastric wall, especially the thickness of the submucosa and the muscularis, with a retained, although abnormal, layered appearance.

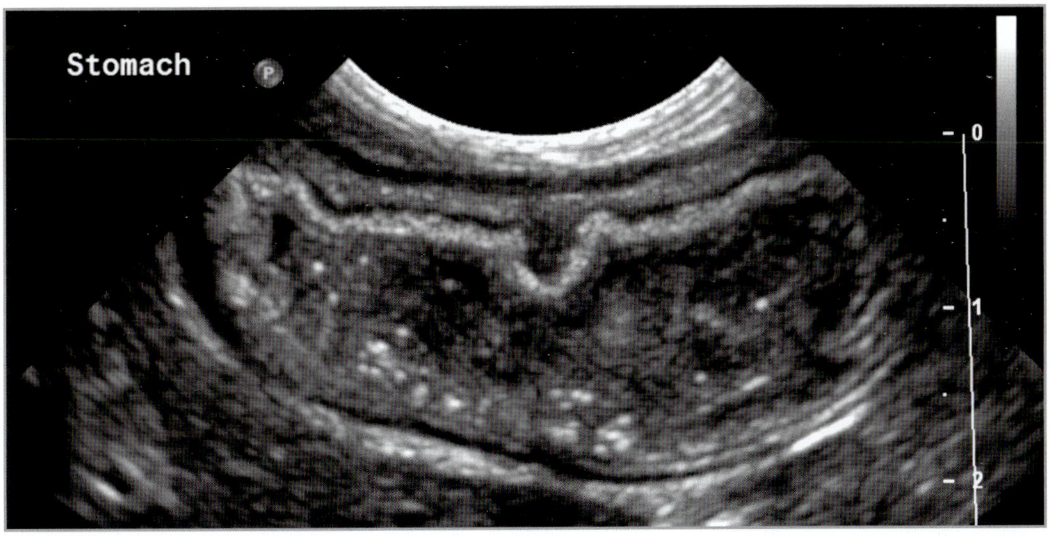

Figure 15. Uraemic gastritis in a 19-month-old dog.

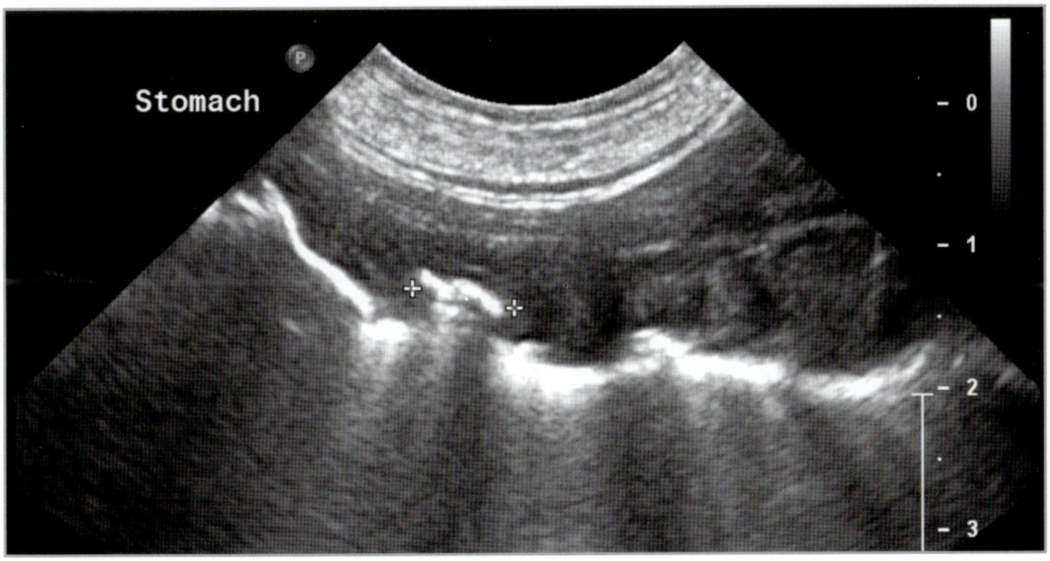

Figure 16. Gastric ulcer in the stomach a 5.5-year-old male German Shepherd dog. Flat hyperechoic depression in the gastric wall is present (between callipers).

Small and large intestine

Ultrasonography is very sensitive in the identification of intussusception. The intussusceptum and intussuscipiens create a multilayered appearance ("multiple rings" sign on transverse views and "too many layers" sign on longitudinal views) (Fig. 17). Occasionally, fat and lymph nodes may also be involved in the intussusception.

Although it may be more challenging to identify, gastroduodenal or duodenogastric intussusception can also be identified on ultrasound examination.

Intestinal dilatation can be associated with functional (Fig. 18) or mechanical ileus (Fig. 19):

- Functional ileus: generalised intestinal dilatation may be seen in cases of severe gastroenteritis, generalised peritonitis, postoperative abdomen, pain, drugs, or electrolyte imbalances. In these cases, a relatively uniform intestinal dilatation can be seen.
- Mechanical ileus: it commonly causes local dilatation of the intestine; however, it can also result in a more generalised dilatation if it is located more caudally. Partial intestinal obstruction causes less marked dilatation of the intestine cranial to the obstruction. Artefacts caused by the material lodged cranial to the obstruction sometimes obscure the identification of the exact cause. Intestinal foreign bodies are a common cause of mechanical ileus and can often be identified ultrasonographically (Fig. 19A). The ultrasonographic appearance is that of a hyperechoic surface with distal acoustic shadowing. The geometric shape or pattern can provide information as to the exact shape and type of foreign body. A linear foreign body commonly appears in the ultrasound image as a linear hyperechoic line in the lumen involving many loops and causing plication of the bowel (Fig. 20). Gastrointestinal parasites can appear as linear foreign bodies; however, acoustic shadowing is usually not observed with adult parasites.

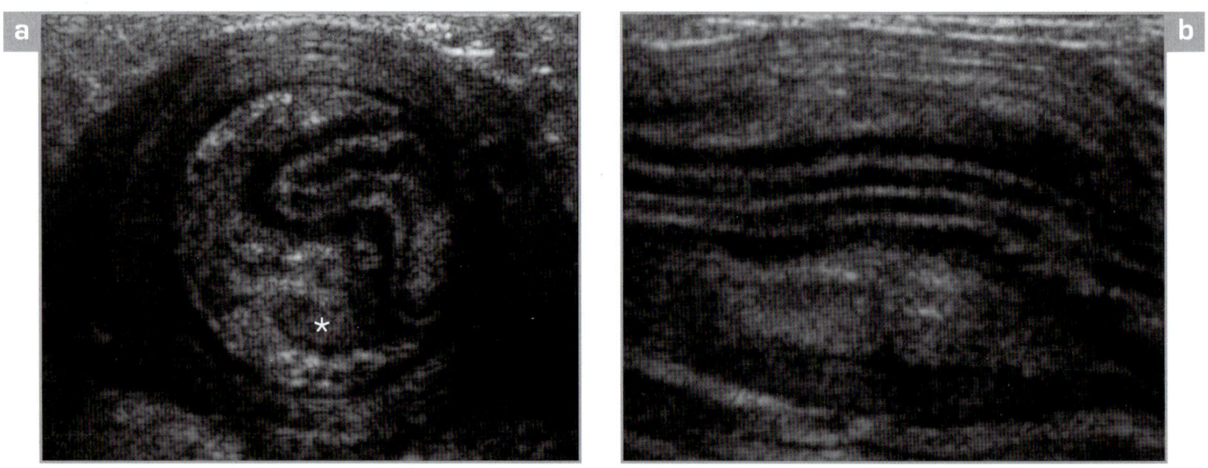

Figure 17. Intussusception in a dog. **(a)** Observe the "multiple rings" sign on the transverse image with a loop of intestine within another. A lymph node (*) and mesenteric tissue are visible within the intussuscipiens. **(b)** Longitudinal view of the same intussusception where the "too many layers" sign is visible.

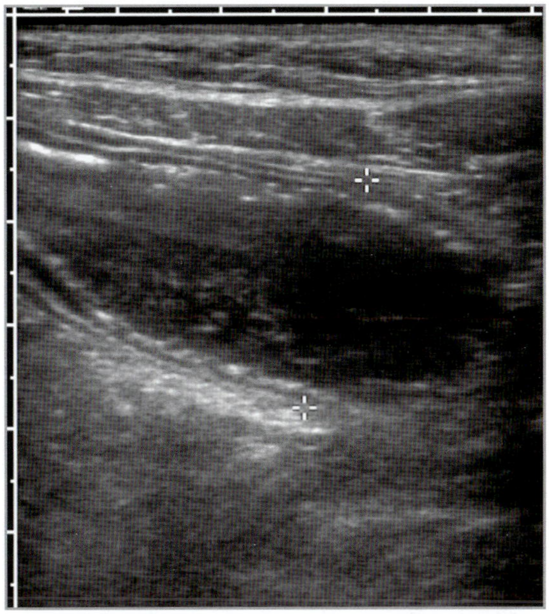

Figure 18. Dilated and fluid-filled loop of jejunum (between callipers) in a dog that had generalised small intestinal dilatation with fluid-filled bowel, compatible with functional ileus.

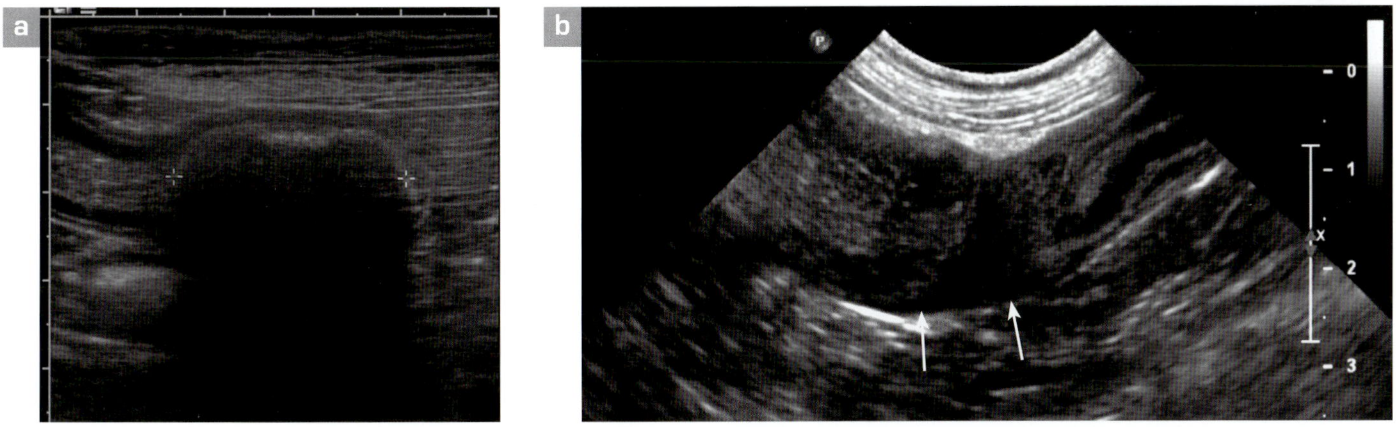

Figure 19. (a) Small intestinal foreign body (fruit stone, between callipers) in a dog causing partial small intestinal obstruction. Note the hyperechoic surface and distal acoustic shadowing. **(b)** Annular jejunal mass (arrows) associated with mechanical ileus in a 10-year old Labrador Retriever. The mass was confirmed on histopathology as adenocarcinoma.

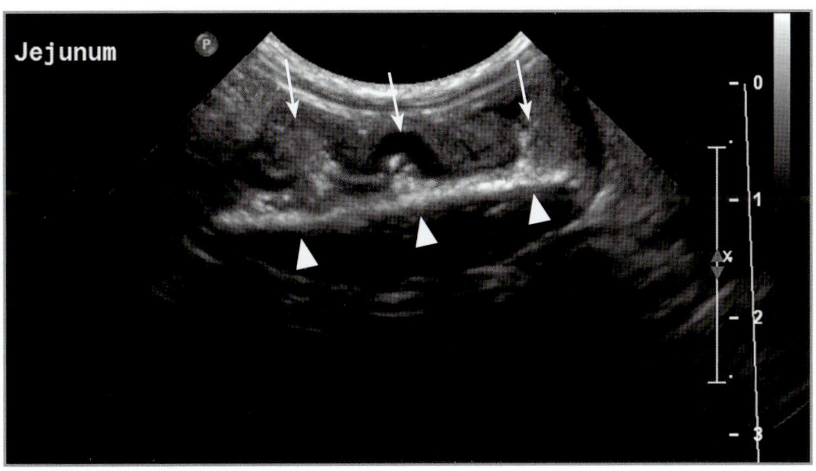

Figure 20. Jack Russel Terrier 7-year-old with a linear foreign body (rope). The foreign body is visible in the jejunum as a linear hyperechoic structure in the lumen (arrowheads), causing plication (long thin arrows).

Corrugated intestinal wall can be seen in cases of enteritis, peritonitis, pancreatitis (Fig. 21), neoplasia, intestinal wall ischaemia and intestinal lymphagiectasia.

Intestinal wall thickening can be seen with malignant and non-malignant diseases. Malignant lesions are usually focal and cause loss or disruption of the intestinal wall layers (Fig. 22), while non-malignant lesions tend to cause a more diffuse thickening with preservation of the intestinal wall layering. However, lymphosarcoma can be either diffusely infiltrative or cause focal lesions. In cases of rupture of the intestinal wall, focal peritoneal changes may be detected ultrasonographically.

Finally, another pattern worth mentioning is the linear mucosal hyperechoic lines perpendicular to the long axis of the intestine. This appearance has been associated with lacteal dilatation (Fig. 23), mucosal inflammation and protein-losing enteropathy, lymphagiectasia and, occasionally, with diffusely infiltrative tumours.

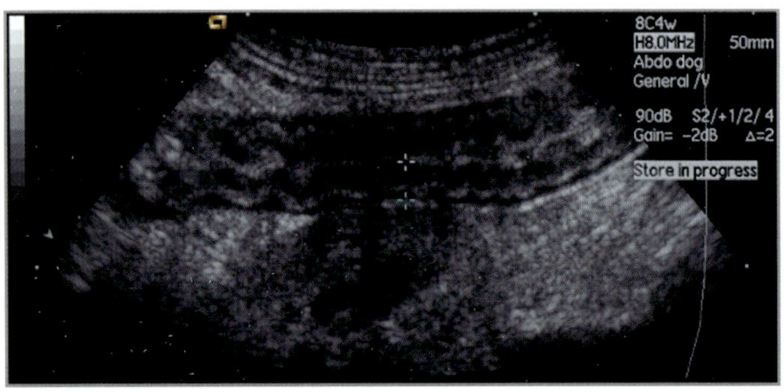

Figure 21. Corrugated duodenal wall in a dog diagnosed with pancreatitis.

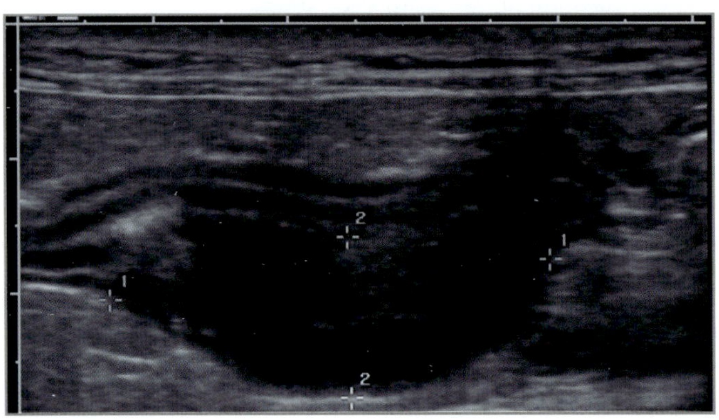

Figure 22. Intestinal lymphoma in a cat. Note the focally thickened, hypoechoic small intestine wall (between callipers) with loss of the normal layered appearance that is still preserved in other parts of the wall of this loop.

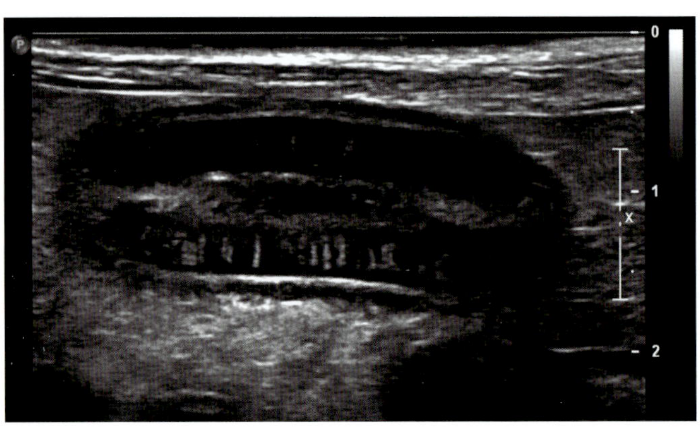

Figure 23. Linear mucosal hyperechoic lines perpendicular to the long axis of the intestine in a dog. These likely represent dilated lacteals.

7

CHAPTER

PANCREAS

Scanning technique

The animal is placed in lateral recumbency with the head towards the ultrasound machine. The pancreas can also be evaluated with the animal in dorsal recumbency that may be more convenient for left-handed ultrasonographer. The technique in dorsal recumbency is similar.

Usually, a transducer greater than 5 MHz is required for the evaluation of the canine and feline pancreas depending on the animal's size. An 8–12 MHz linear, microconvex or convex transducer is commonly preferred for small dogs and cats, while a 5–8 MHz microconvex or curvilinear transducer is preferred for medium and large size dogs.

The pancreas is a V-shaped structure forming a body and two lobes, right and left (Fig. 1).

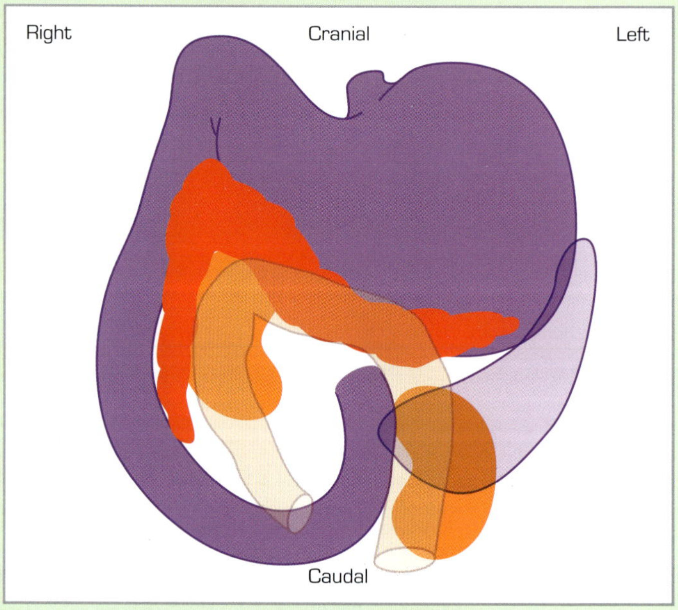

Figure 1. Diagram of the location of the pancreas in the abdomen: the pancreas is shown in red, the stomach in purple and descending duodenum, the spleen in light purple, the kidneys in orange and the colon in light brown.

- The right kidney, descending duodenum and pancreaticoduodenal vein can be used as landmarks for the identification of the right lobe of the pancreas.
- The pyloric antrum, portal vein and right pancreatic lobe can be used as landmarks for the identification of the body of the pancreas.
- The splenic vein and portal vein mainly (and the stomach, spleen and transverse colon) can be used for the identification of the left lobe of the pancreas.

For the body and left lobe of the pancreas, the technique is similar in small and large-sized breeds of dogs, and in cats. However, the technique for scanning the right lobe of the pancreas in lateral recumbency is different depending on the size of the dog.

Right pancreatic lobe

Small dogs and cats

1. Position the animal in right lateral recumbency with the head towards the ultrasound machine and the limbs towards the examiner.
2. Ask the assistant to lift the animal approximately 45°.
3. Place the transducer parallel to the tabletop with the marker pointing to the head of the animal at the level of the umbilicus near the middle of the right flank (Fig. 2).

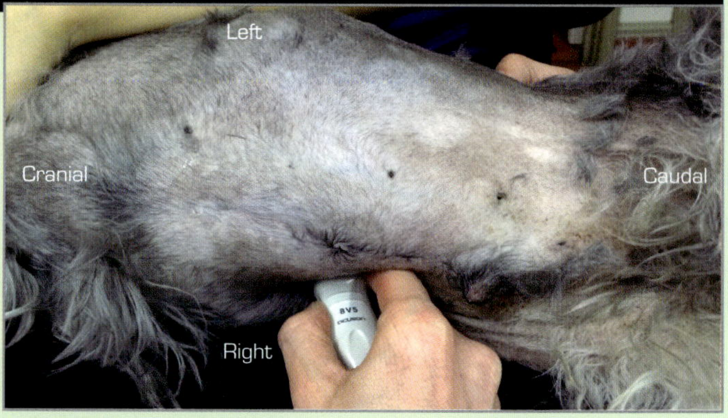

Figure 2. Transducer positioning to identify the right lobe of the pancreas in small dogs and cats.

4. Ask the assistant to position the dog in right lateral recumbency while you maintain the transducer parallel to the tabletop, pointing towards the last right rib.

5. Ask the assistant to place a hand at the back of the animal so that position can be maintained when you press. Then, apply some pressure to identify the right kidney, keeping the transducer with the same orientation (Fig. 3).

> If you think the transducer is oriented correctly but cannot see the right kidney on the screen, fan the transducer towards the tabletop (you may need to press harder or increase the visible depth). You should identify the right kidney during the fanning movement. If not, check the orientation of your transducer and try again.

6. Once you have identified the right kidney, release the pressure slowly and the descending duodenum will appear along the top of your screen (Fig. 4).

> If unsure or if you see too many intestinal loops (this would mean you have fanned the transducer upwards while releasing the pressure), fan your transducer all the way towards the tabletop, to the point where you cannot see any intestinal loops, and then fan very slowly upwards (towards the left of the animal). The first small intestinal loop to come into your view should be the descending duodenum.

7. Fan your transducer up or down slightly to identify the right lobe of the pancreas on the screen just below the duodenum or in the area of the duodenum (depending on the orientation of your transducer). The visualisation of the pancreaticoduodenal vein confirms it is the right lobe of the pancreas (Fig. 5).

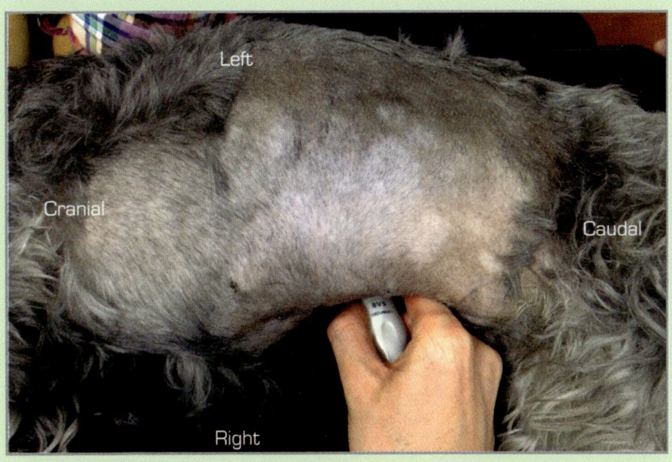

Figure 3. After positioning the transducer, its orientation is maintained, and pressure is applied until the right kidney is identified.

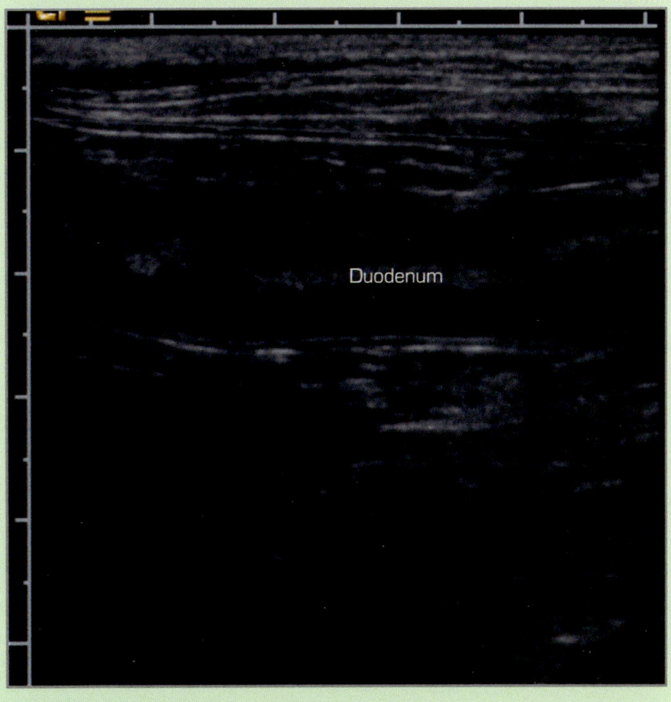

Figure 4. Image of the descending duodenum in a dog, after the right kidney has been identified and the pressure on the transducer has been released slowly.

8. In cats, the technique is the same (Fig. 6); however, much less pressure should be applied (the same applies in very small-sized dogs).

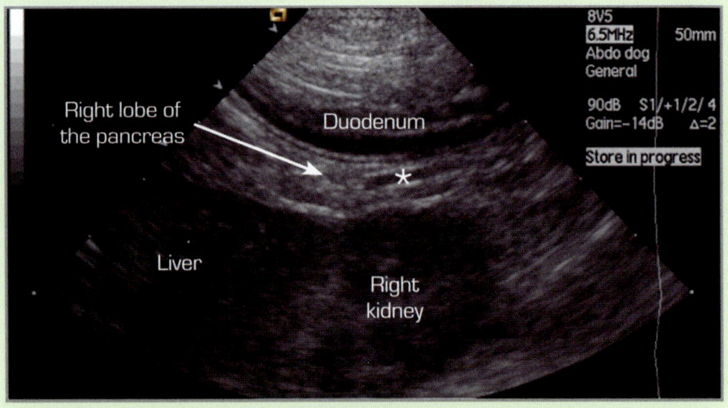

Figure 5. The right lobe of the pancreas in a small dog. After identifying the descending duodenum, the transducer is fanned slightly and slowly, and the right lobe is identified just below the duodenum and confirmed by the presence of the pancreaticoduodenal vein (*). The right caudal liver and right kidney are also visible in this image.

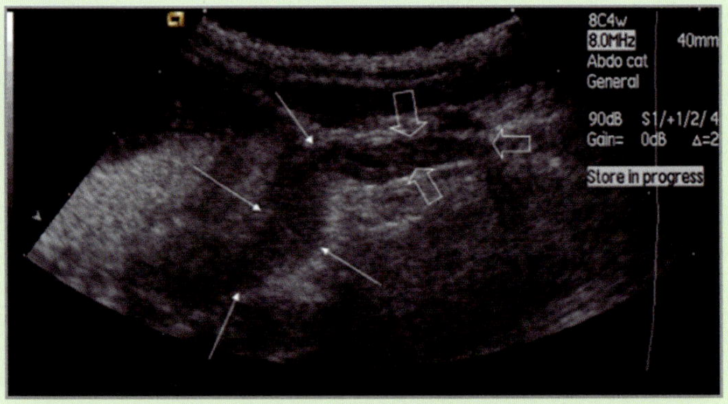

Figure 6. Pancreas in a healthy cat. The right lobe (thin arrows), the body and the left lobe (thick arrows) are visible. In cats, the margin of the pancreas is more obvious than in dogs.

Large dogs

1. Position the animal in left lateral recumbency with the head towards the ultrasound machine and the limbs away from the examiner.

2. Wide clipping of the area of the last two intercostal spaces from the spine to, at least, midway down the right lateral wall, is necessary.

3. Place the transducer with the marker pointing to the head of the animal in a dorsal orientation, aligned with the spine, at the level of the right kidney.

> For beginners, it may be advantageous to place the transducer perpendicular to the skin within the intercostal space (last or one before the last intercostal space) and not caudal to the last rib (Fig. 7).

4. After you have identified the right kidney, slide the transducer ventrally following the rib (Fig. 8).

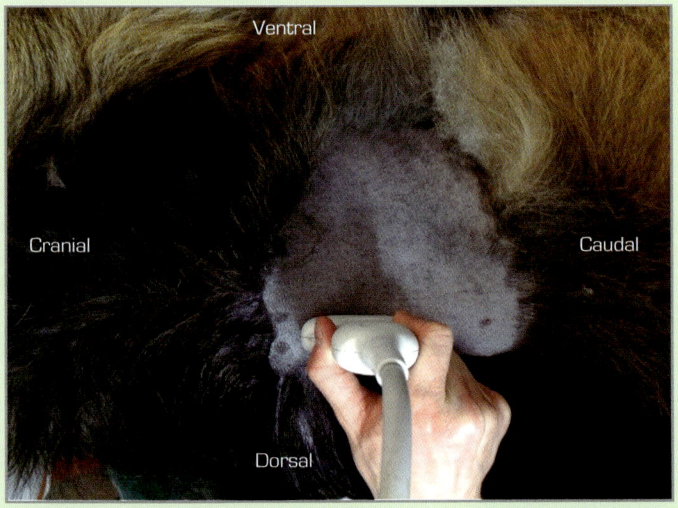

Figure 7. Transducer positioning for the identification of the right kidney in a large-sized breed of dog. The view is from the position of the ultrasonographer.

5. The first small intestinal loop identified at the top of the screen is the descending duodenum. Although this is commonly the first loop imaged at the top of the screen, in some animals, the colon can be seen first, and then the descending duodenum as you continue sliding ventrally. The colon can be easily distinguished by its thin wall compared with the small intestine.

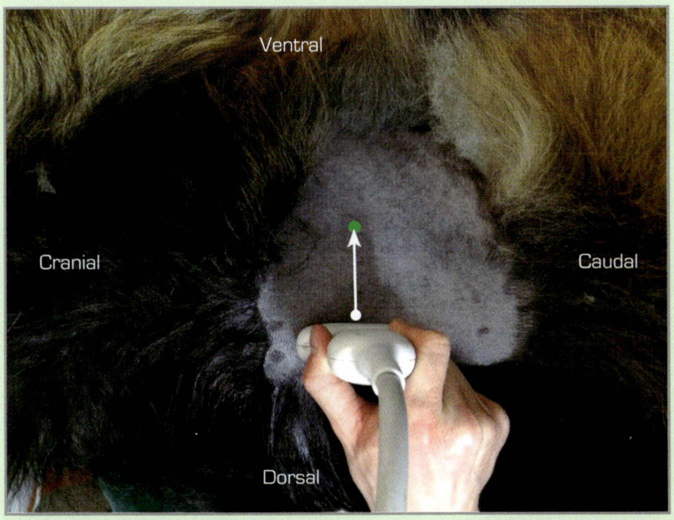

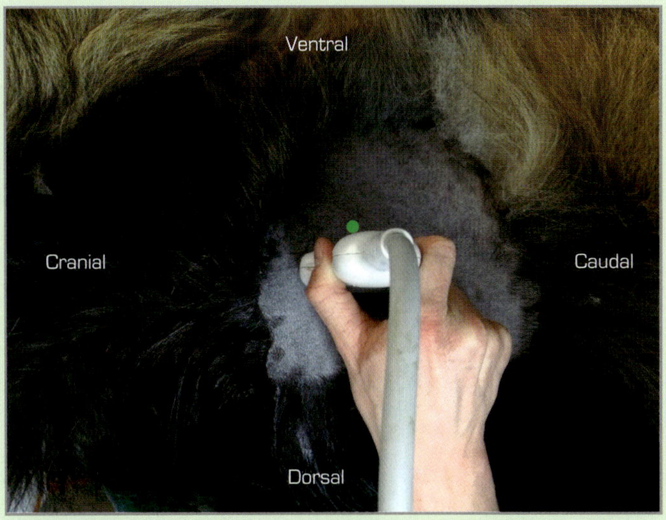

Figure 8. The transducer is slid ventrally from the level of right kidney until visualising the duodenum. The duodenum is the first loop of small intestine seen at the top of the screen.

6. Fan your transducer up or down slightly to identify the right lobe of the pancreas just below the duodenum. The visualisation of the pancreaticoduodenal vein confirms it is the right lobe of the pancreas.

7. If excessive gas in the descending duodenum may be interfering with the examination, the transducer can be rotated counterclockwise (transducer marker points to the spine), to create a transverse image of the duodenum and pancreas. The pancreas is then visible next to the descending duodenum at 7 o'clock position (Fig. 9). Sliding the transducer cranially and caudally allows to examine the right pancreatic lobe.

> This technique can also be used in small dogs.

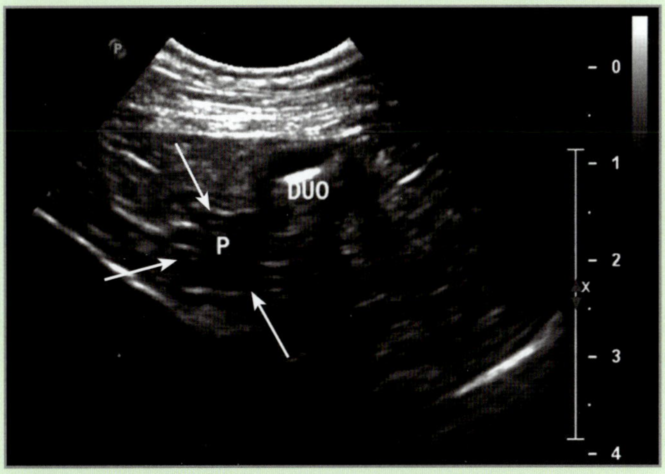

Figure 9. Transverse image of the right pancreas from the right dorsal approach in the large breeds of dogs. By rotating the transducer counterclockwise, so the marker points to the spine, the right lobe of the pancreas can be identified (P, between arrows) bellow and to the left of the descending duodenum (DUO) at approximately 7 o' clock position on the screen. Sliding the transducer cranial and caudal allows the examination of the pancreas. This orientation can be used if there are artefacts interfering from material and gas in the duodenal lumen.

Body of the pancreas

1. Position the animal in right lateral recumbency with the head pointing towards the ultrasound machine and the limbs towards the examiner.

2. Place the transducer on the ventral midline and identify the stomach caudal to the liver (Fig. 10).

3. Apply a steady and marked pressure (Fig. 11) and fan your transducer ventrally towards the pylorus.

4. Looking carefully at the screen, you will be able to identify the portal vein (most ventral large vessel in the abdomen) below the pylorus. Look at the area between the pylorus and the portal vein to find the body of the pancreas (Fig. 12). Using the analogy of a 12-hour clock, for the visible stomach, the body of the pancreas is commonly seen at 4 o'clock (3–6 o'clock). The body of the pancreas is slightly hypoechoic to the surrounding structures.

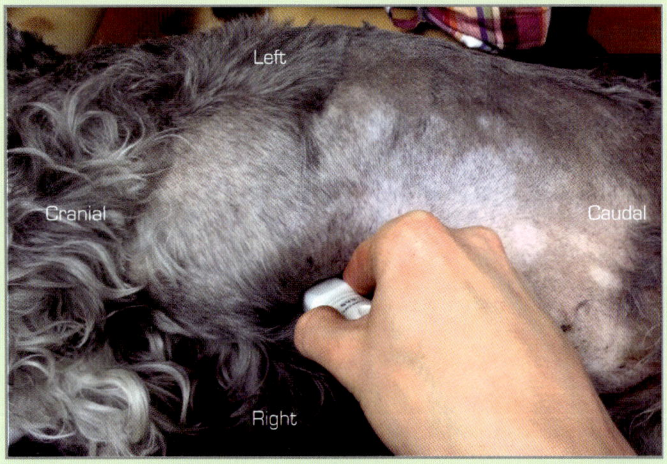

Figure 10. Transducer positioning for the identification of the body of the pancreas.

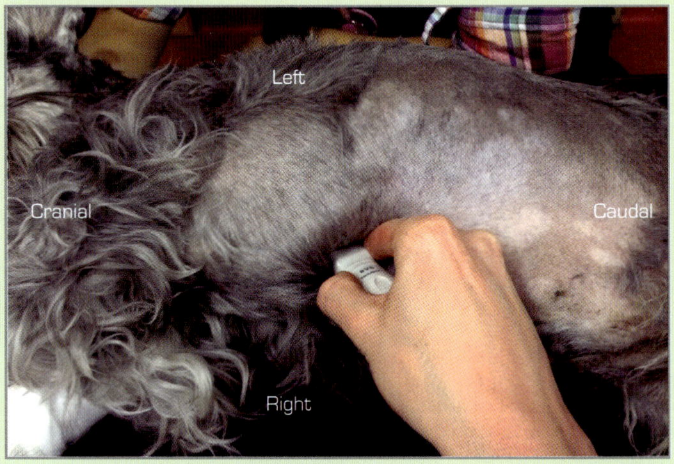

Figure 11. Pressure is applied to the transducer, which is fanned ventrally on this image to identify the pylorus and portal vein. The body of the pancreas is identified between these two structures.

The body of the pancreas is commonly identified between the stomach and the portal vein.

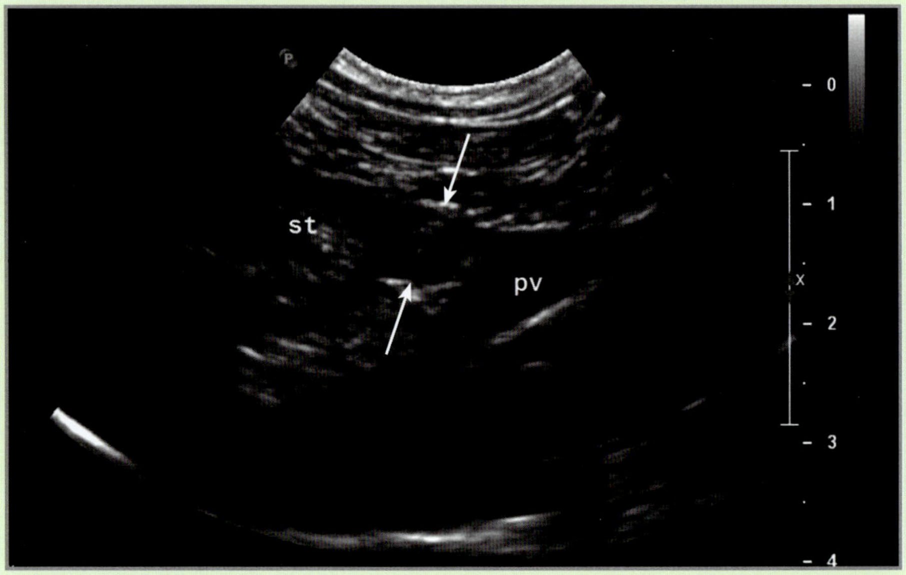

Figure 12. The body of the pancreas (between arrows) in a dog, located between the stomach (st) and the portal vein (pv), at 3 o'clock (considering the pylorus as a clock).

Left pancreatic lobe

1. Position the animal in right lateral recumbency with the head pointing towards the ultrasound machine and the limbs towards the examiner.

2. Identify the spleen by following the last rib dorsally from the liver as described in the Spleen chapter (Fig. 13).

> The left pancreatic lobe is more difficult to identify than the other two parts of the pancreas.

3. The splenic vein is identified below the spleen as a small, rounded anechoic area.

4. Maintain the same orientation of the transducer and slide it dorsally towards the spine, keeping the splenic vein in the middle of the screen (Fig. 14).

5. Stop the sliding movement as soon as you see the portal vein (most ventral large vessel in the abdomen).

6. Look between the splenic vein and the portal vein to identify the left pancreatic lobe (Fig. 15).

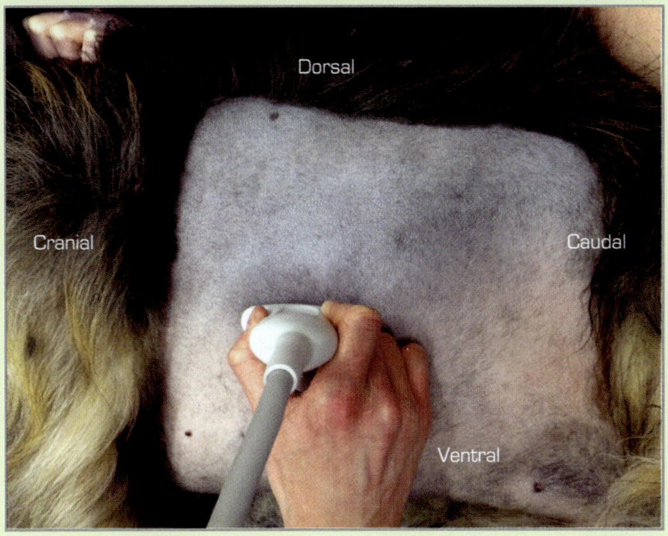

Figure 13. Transducer positioning for the identification of the spleen and splenic vein, after sliding the transducer dorsally and to the left along the last rib.

7. The left pancreatic lobe is adjacent to the greater curvature of the stomach, medial to the spleen, cranial to the transverse colon and can extend to the cranial pole of the left kidney.

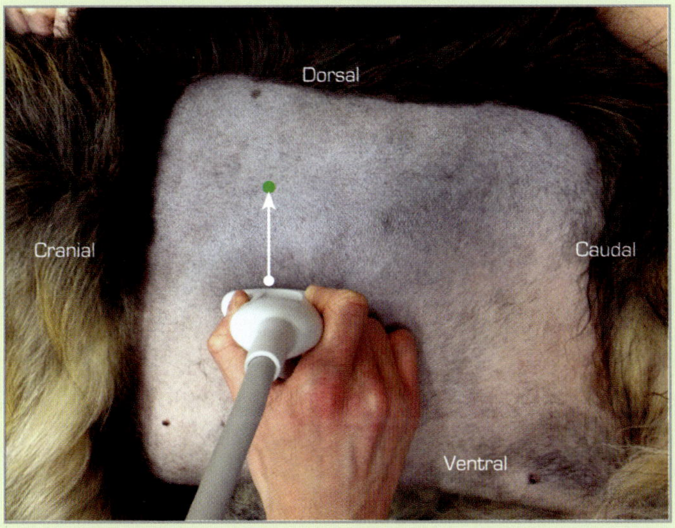

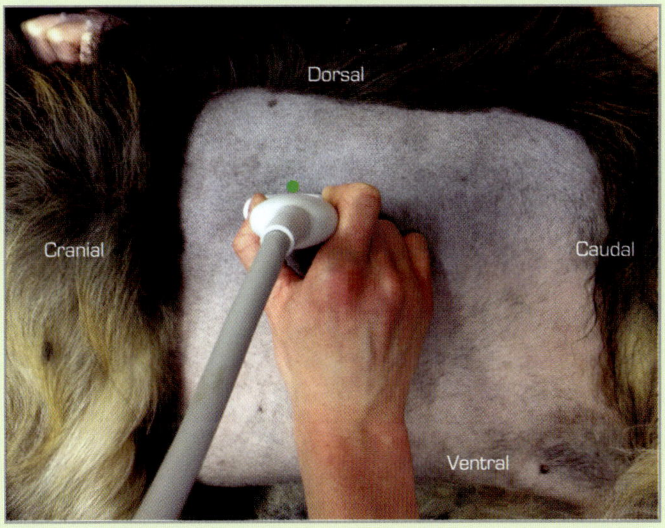

Figure 14. Dorsal sliding of the transducer to visualise the portal vein. The left lobe of the pancreas is visible in the area between the splenic vein and the portal vein.

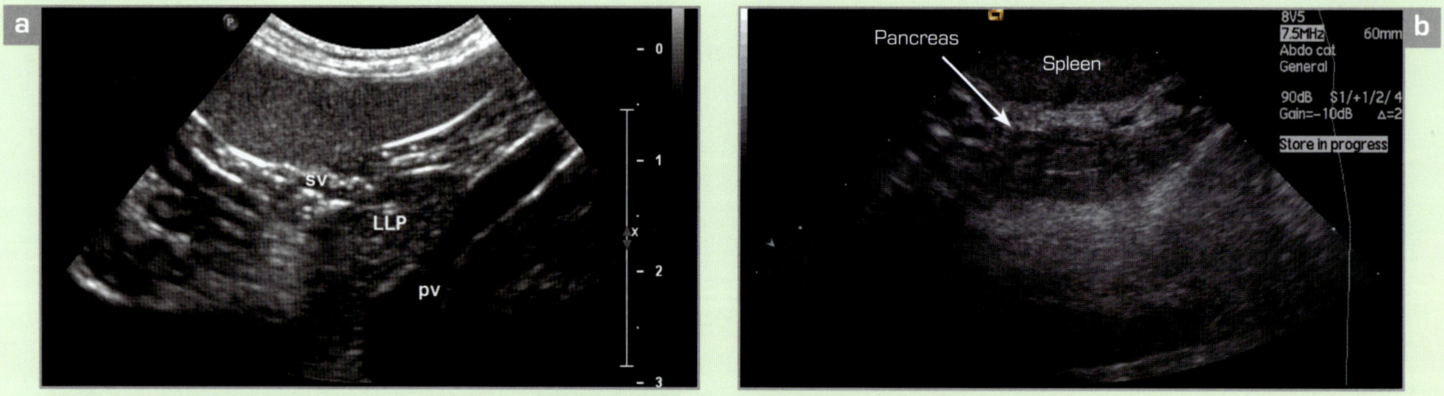

Figure 15. Normal left lobe of the pancreas (LLP) in a dog (a) and in a cat (b). sv: splenic vein, pv: portal vein.

Normal appearance

The normal pancreas is a thin, poorly marginated organ with homogeneous echogenicity and echotexture (see Figs. 5 and 6). It is usually isoechoic to slightly hyperechoic to the caudate liver lobe. The pancreas may rarely appear uniformly hypoechoic. To the authors experience, the normal pancreas is uniform in echogenicity, mildly hypoechoic to the surrounding tissues, and it does not stand out as an organ with very distinct margins.

The pancreaticoduodenal vein is visible in the right lobe of the pancreas and can confirm that you are examining the right lobe of the pancreas (see Fig. 5). The pancreatic body is seen between the pyloric antrum and portal vein and is usually hypoechoic to the surrounding mesenteric fat (see Fig. 12). The left pancreatic lobe is hypoechoic to the spleen and to the surrounding mesenteric fat (Fig. 15). The anechoic tubular structure visible in the left pancreatic lobe corresponds to the pancreatic duct (more consistently visible in cats). The lack of Doppler flow signal differentiates it from a vessel.

In dogs, the normal pancreatic thickness can reach 10 mm and the pancreatic duct measures up to 1 mm. In cats, the thickness of the pancreas has been reported to be up to 9 mm for the body and left lobe and up to 6 mm for the right lobe, while the pancreatic duct in the left lobe of the pancreas can measure up to 2.5 mm in diameter. The mean pancreatic duct diameter increases with age in cats.

Variations from normal

Pancreatitis can have a variety of appearances including variable echogenicity (hypoechoic, hyperechoic or mixed echogenicity) and possibly containing cyst-like lesions (Fig. 16). The appearance most commonly expected in cases of acute pancreatitis is a thicker and hypoechoic pancreas (Fig. 16a). Cyst-like lesions may be identified with acute pancreatitis. An abnormal appearing pancreas of normal or smaller size and without evident clinical signs or pain in the pancreatic region may indicate subclinical disease. In chronic pancreatitis, some areas of scarring and calcification may be seen. The typical appearance of chronic pancreatitis is that of a mildly thickened pancreas with increased echogenicity and with less obvious or no changes in the surrounding mesentery. Localised free peritoneal fluid, hyperechoic adjacent mesenteric fat (Fig. 16a and 16c), gastric

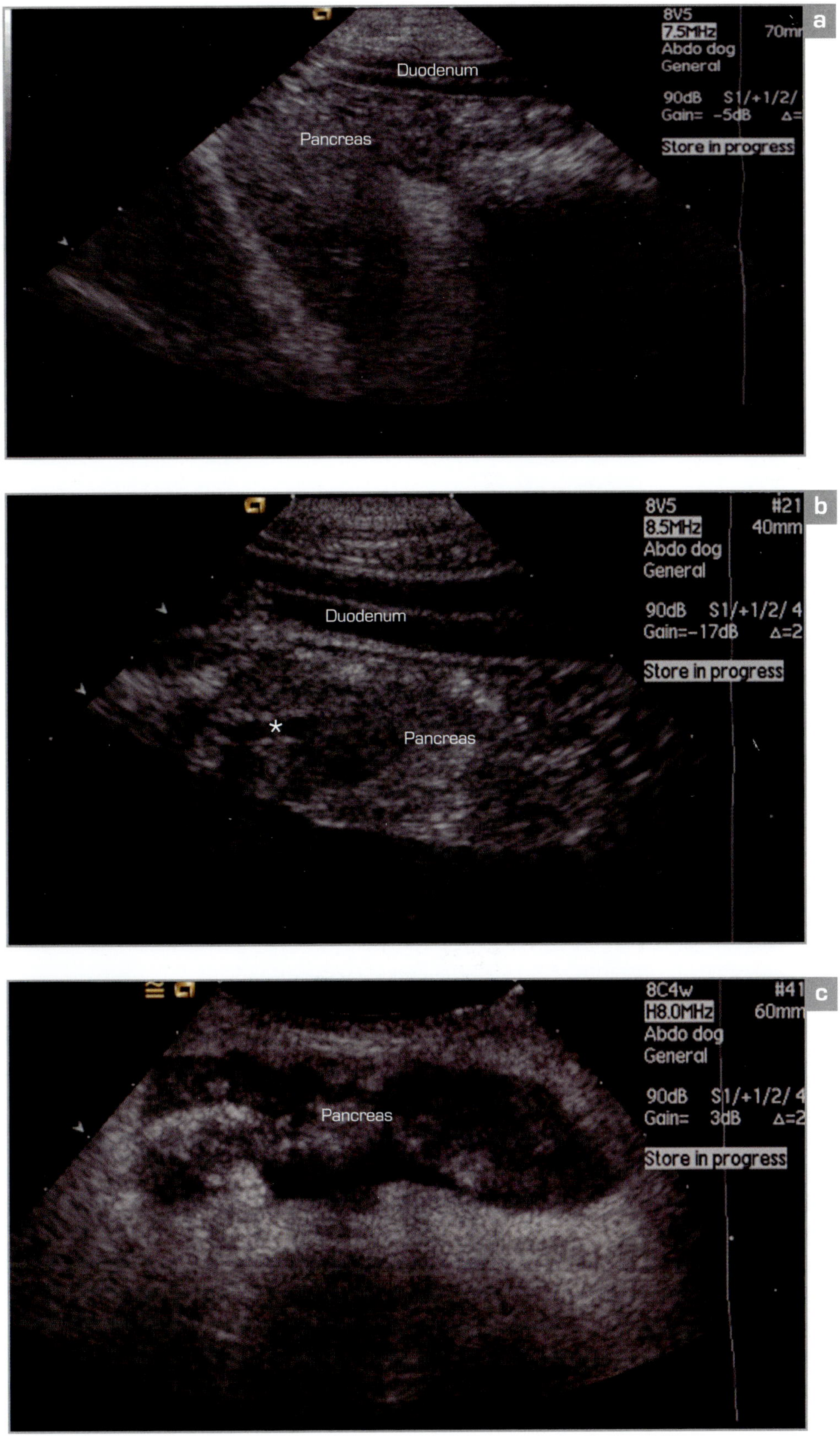

Figure 16. Pancreatitis in three different dogs. **[a]** The whole pancreas is thick and uniformly hypoechoic while the surrounding mesentery is hyperechoic. **[b]** The right lobe of the pancreas has mixed echogenicity. The pancreaticoduodenal vein (*) is visible. **[c]** The right lobe of the pancreas has mixed echogenicity and the surrounding mesentery is markedly hyperechoic. Minimal peripancreatic free fluid is also visible. The hyperechoic surrounding mesentery indicates peri-pancreatic inflammation (peritonitis).

and duodenal wall thickening may be present in acute and subacute phases. Other signs seen with pancreatitis may include corrugated appearance of the duodenum (see Fig. 21 in Chapter 6), focal lymphadenopathy and common bile duct dilatation (see Fig. 19 in Chapter 4) and gallbladder enlargement. In the dogs the right pancreatic lobe is more commonly affected.

In cats the findings are usually less obvious than in dogs with the body and the left lobe showing the most severe changes. Feline pancreatitis has been associated with hepatic lipidosis, inflammatory bowel disease and cholangiohepatitis. Regional ascites and thickening of the duodenal and/ or gastric wall may also be observed in feline pancreatitis.

In haemorrhagic, necrotising pancreatitis, the pancreatic margins are ill defined and irregular hypoechoic to anechoic areas can be seen, while the adjacent mesentery is hyperechoic and hyperattenuating.

Differentiating acute from chronic pancreatitis can be as challenging as it is difficult to evaluate the clinical relevance of unexpected pancreatic lesions seen on ultrasound in dogs and cats.

Pancreatic cystic lesions (Figs. 17 and 18) can include true cysts, pseudocysts, retention cysts, abscesses and cystic dilatation of the pancreatic duct. They cannot be differentiated only by ultrasound.

- A true pancreatic cyst was described in a cat as septate with a thick wall and pedunculated. Multiple recurrent cysts associated with pancreatitis, atrophy and endocrine dysfunction, have also been described in a cat. Blockage of the pancreatic duct causes retention cysts which cannot be ultrasonographically differentiated from pseudocysts or congenital cysts. Retention cysts are commonly incidental findings and tend to have a larger quantity of anechoic fluid compared with inflammatory pseudocysts.

- Pseudocysts (Fig. 17) can be seen in both dogs and cats. They are fluid-filled lesions associated with pancreatitis. Pseudocysts are anechoic or poorly echogenic cystic lesions often displaying acoustic enhancement. They can spontaneously disappear or persist and require surgical drainage. Large pseudocysts may cause extrahepatic biliary obstruction. Pseudocysts contain viscous fluid with high trypsin-like immunoreactivity, which confirms their pancreatic origin.

- Pancreatic abscesses (Fig. 18) are usually a complication of pancreatitis, and they are more common in dogs than cats. They contain pus and may appear as cystic lesions with echogenic to almost anechoic fluid. They may even appear as masses if the fluid they contain is very echogenic. Abscesses contain exudate composed mainly of degenerative neutrophils.

> Definitive diagnosis of the type of cystic lesions and differentiation between cysts and neoplasms requires a fine-needle aspirate.

Pancreatic oedema has a characteristic ultrasonographic appearance as the pancreas contains hypoechoic or anechoic fissures that highlight the lobulation throughout the enlarged pancreas (Fig. 19). Pancreatic oedema may be associated with pancreatitis, but it can also be caused by portal hypertension or hypoalbuminemia.

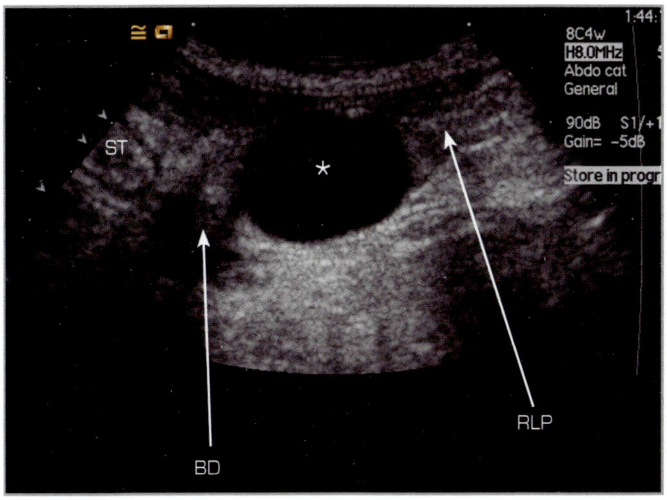

Figure 17. Pancreatic cystic lesion in a cat (*). The appearance is not specific to a particular type of fluid and aspiration is usually required to distinguish the type of cystic lesion. In this case, the results from the aspiration suggested a pseudocyst. ST: stomach; BD: body of the pancreas; RLP: right lobe of the pancreas.

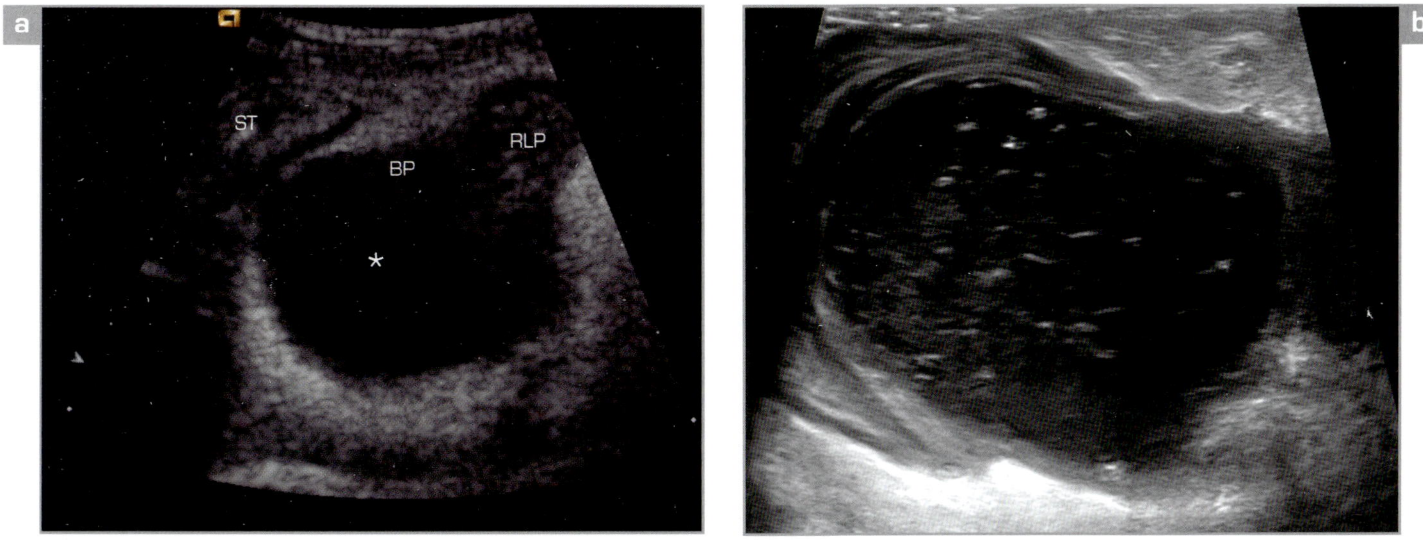

Figure 18. **(a)** Pancreatic abscess (*) in a dog visible in the area of the body of the pancreas (BP). The beginning of the right lobe of the pancreas (RLP) and part of the stomach (ST) are also visible. **(b)** A 5 cm pancreatic abscess in a dog. The wall is thick, and the fluid appears echogenic.

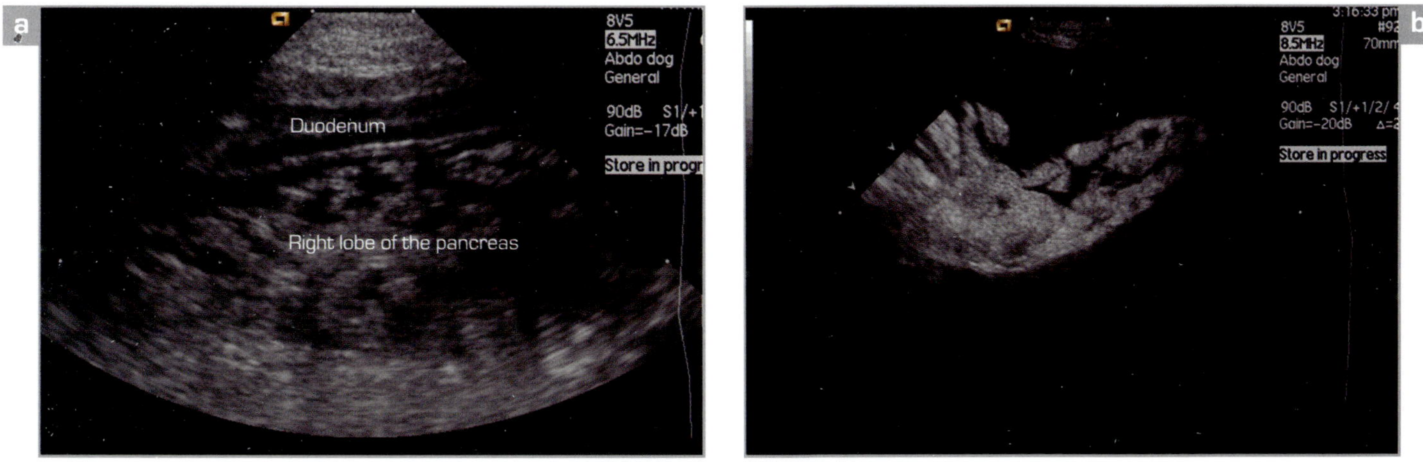

Figure 19. Pancreatic oedema. **(a)** Right lobe of the pancreas with pancreatic oedema in a dog. Mild ascites is also visible. **(b)** Pancreatic oedema is visible in the left lobe of the pancreas of another dog. Marked ascites is also visible.

Pancreatic nodular hyperplasia (Fig. 20) is commonly found in older dogs and cats. It appears as, relatively well defined hypoechoic or isoechoic nodules of variable size in the pancreas. Nodular hyperplasia cannot be distinguished from neoplasia based solely on ultrasound findings. Neoplasia should be included in the differential diagnosis when pancreatic nodules are identified. Aspiration and/ or biopsy for cytology and/ or histopathology are required to distinguish pancreatic nodular hyperplasia from neoplasia.

Exocrine pancreatic tumours, such as adenocarcinomas (Fig. 21), are rare but they are the most common type of pancreatic neoplasia in small animals. They usually affect older dogs and cats. The Airedale Terrier is considered to be predisposed to pancreatic adenocarcinoma. Adenocarcinomas usually metastasise before the appearance of clinical signs. They may compress the common bile duct, invade the adjacent gastric or duodenal wall and metastasize to the liver. Other tumours that may be seen in the pancreas of the dogs and cats include cystadenomas, adenomas, lymphomas and metastatic carcinomas.

Pancreatic endocrine tumours, such as insulinomas, gastrinomas and glucagonomas, are uncommon. Insulinomas are difficult to identify and, when seen, as single or multiple hypoechoic nodules that can be ill-defined and most are less than 2.5 cm in size (Fig. 22). A normal appearance of the pancreas on ultrasound does not exclude the presence of insulinomas. Most endocrine tumours are malignant and spread to liver and regional lymph nodes. Insulinomas are extremely rare in cats.

Pancreatic bladder refers to the cystic dilatation of the pancreatic duct and it has been reported in cats. A cat with pancreatitis and pancreatolithiasis along with a pseudobladder (this termed was used instead of pancreatic bladder) has also been described.

Pancreatolithiasis is the presence of calculi in the pancreatic ducts. They appear as hyperechoic structures associated with acoustic shadowing.

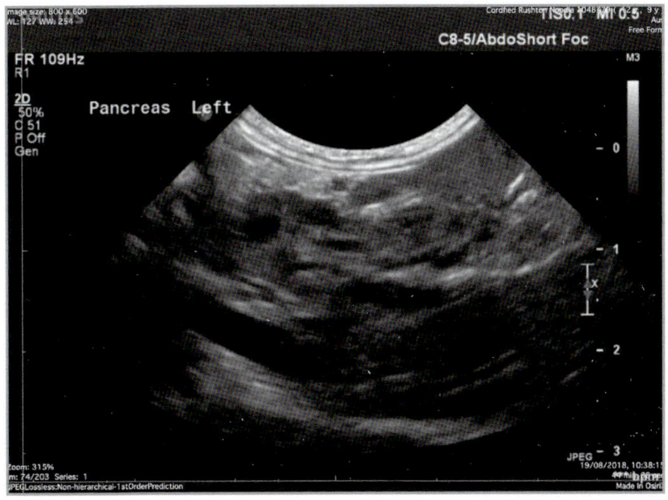

Figure 20. Hypoechoic nodules in the left lobe of the pancreas (between arrows) in a 9-year-old Siamese cat with nodular hyperplasia.

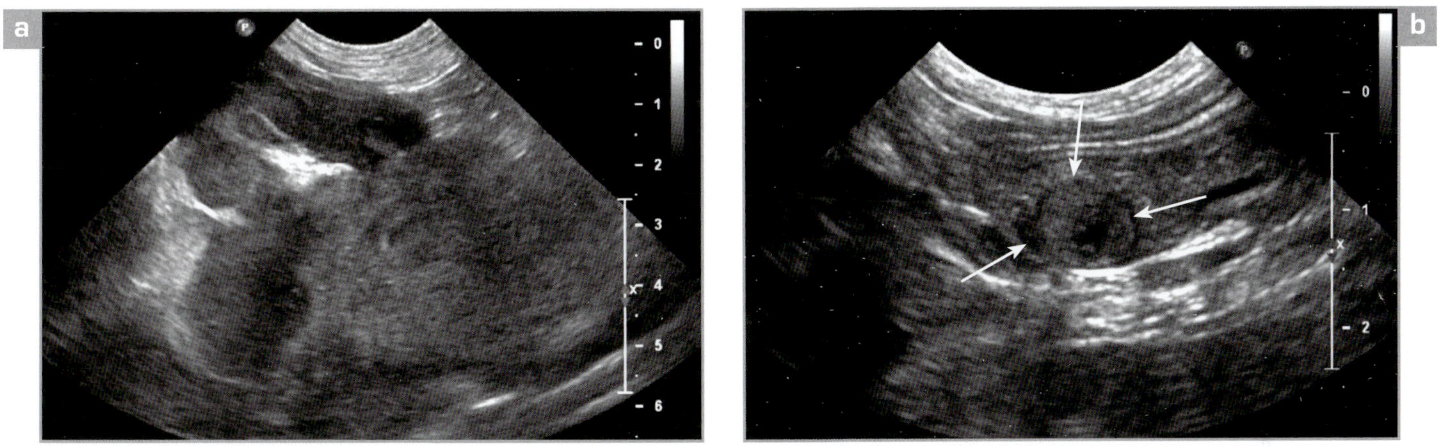

Figure 21. (a) Pancreatic adenocarcinoma in a 17-year-old, male neutered Labrador retriever. A large mixed echogenicity mass is visible. **(b)** Pancreatic adenocarcinoma (between arrows) in the right lobe of the pancreas of a 10-year-old, male neutered Persian cat.

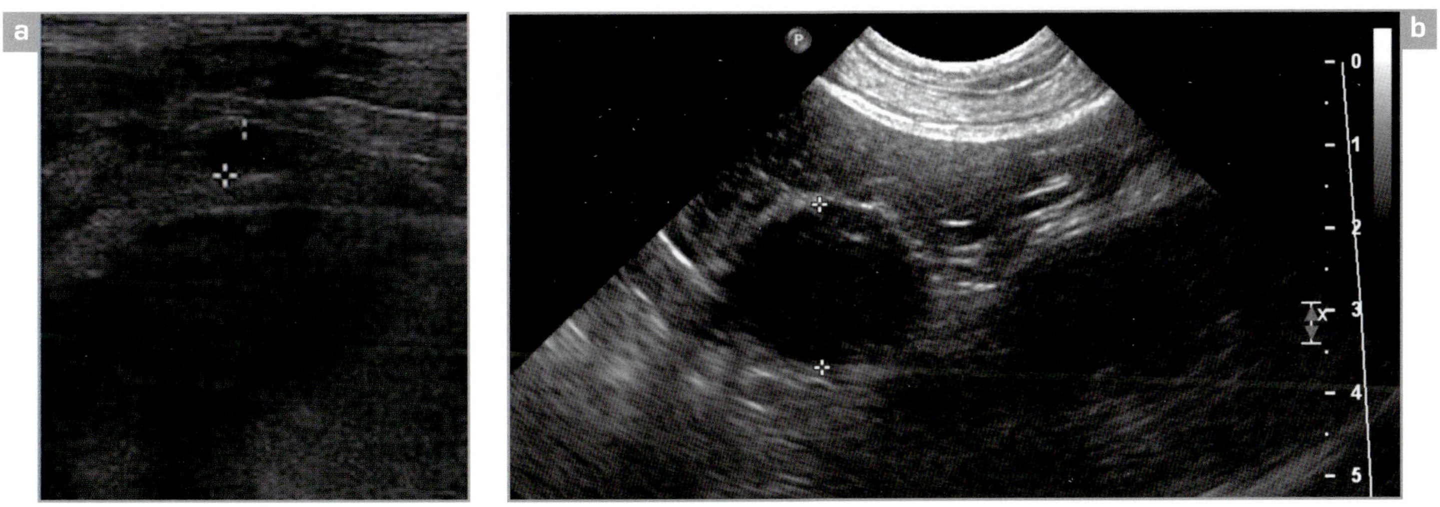

Figure 22. (a) Hypoechoic nodular area (between callipers) is visible in the right lobe of the pancreas of a dog with insulinoma. **(b)** Larger hypoechoic mass (between callipers) in a dog with a large insulinoma near the body of the pancreas.

8

CHAPTER

KIDNEYS AND URETERS

Scanning technique

A high-frequency transducer is required to evaluate the kidneys. In dogs, a 5–10 MHz transducer is usually adequate, while for cats a transducer higher than 8 MHz (commonly 10 MHz or more) should be employed.

In cats, high-frequency linear transducers are ideal for imaging the kidneys due to the relatively more caudal position of these organs in comparison with those in dogs. High frequencies linear transducers can also be ideal for imaging the kidneys in small dogs.

Left kidney

Place the animal in right lateral recumbency with the head towards the machine and the limbs towards the examiner.

1. To locate the left kidney, place the transducer with the marker pointing to the head of the animal, caudal to the last rib in the dorsal abdomen (Fig. 1). Cranial rocking and/or sliding of the transducer is sometimes required if the kidney is more cranial than expected. The kidneys are easy to identify because they have a characteristic appearance (Fig. 2). Alternatively, slide the transducer dorsally from the caudal edge of the spleen towards the spine until you see the left kidney.

2. Rotate the transducer slightly clockwise or anticlockwise to image the kidney in its long axis. When the kidney is almost in its longest view, the peripelvic hyperechoic stranding appears on the screen as parallel lines closer or further away from each other depending on the angle of the ultrasound beam (Fig. 2).

3. After achieving a view of the kidney in its longest axis, fan the transducer dorsally and ventrally until you cannot see renal tissue on each side of the movement (Fig. 3).

4. Rotate the transducer 90° clockwise and fan the transducer all the way cranially and all the way caudally until you cannot see renal tissue on each side of the movement (Fig. 4) to evaluate the kidney in transverse orientation.

5. While performing these movements, evaluate the kidney and compare its echogenicity to that of the liver and spleen.

6. Measure the maximum length of the kidney in three different images and accept the longest measurement as correct. (Fig. 5).

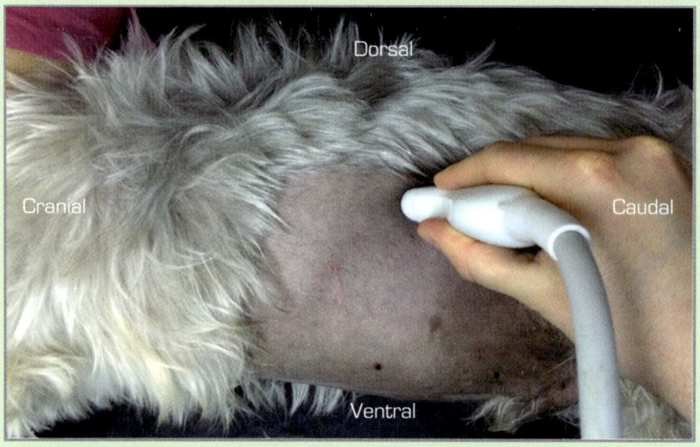

Figure 1. Initial position of the transducer for evaluation of the left kidney: caudal to the last rib or in the last intercostal space, parallel to the spine, with the marker pointing to the head of the animal. The transducer plane is commonly between dorsal and sagittal.

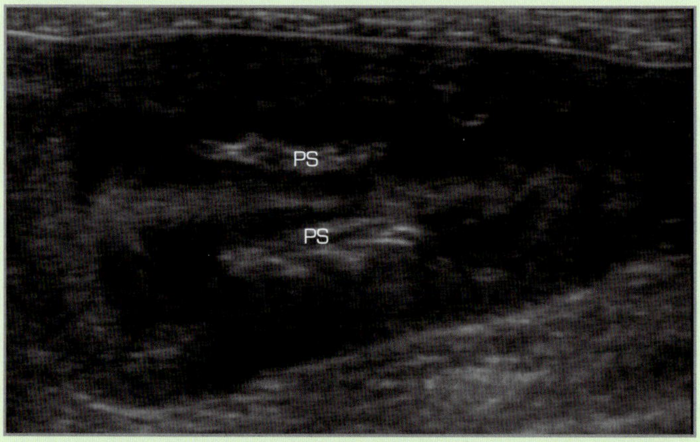

Figure 2. Image of a normal canine left kidney in a sagittal plane. The more echogenic cortex and the less echogenic medulla are visible. The peripelvic hyperechoic stranding (PS) is visible.

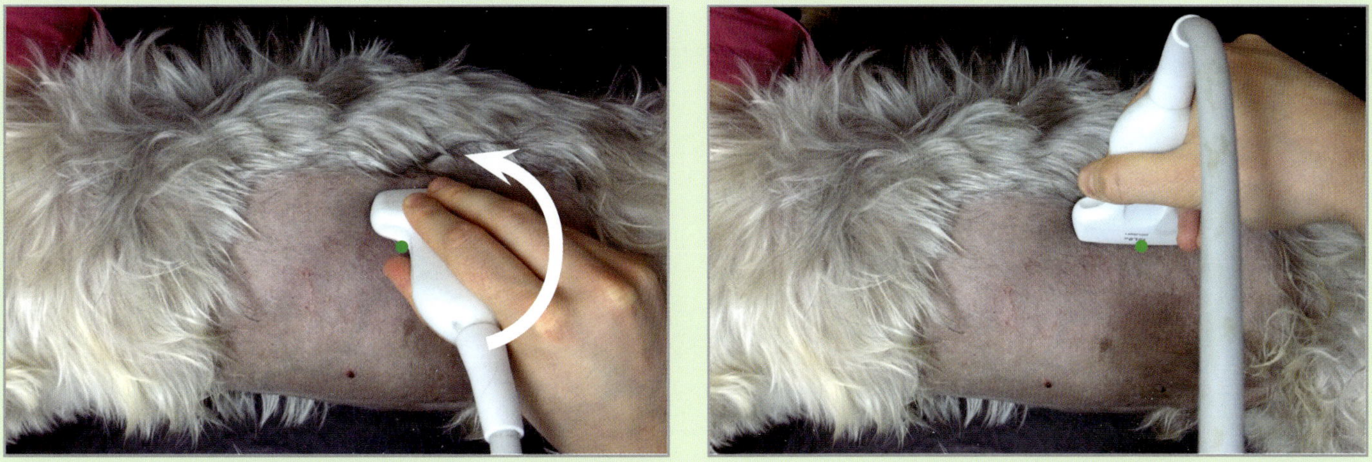

Figure 3. After the transducer is rotated to visualise the kidney in its longest axis, it should be fanned dorsally and ventrally to examine the entire kidney.

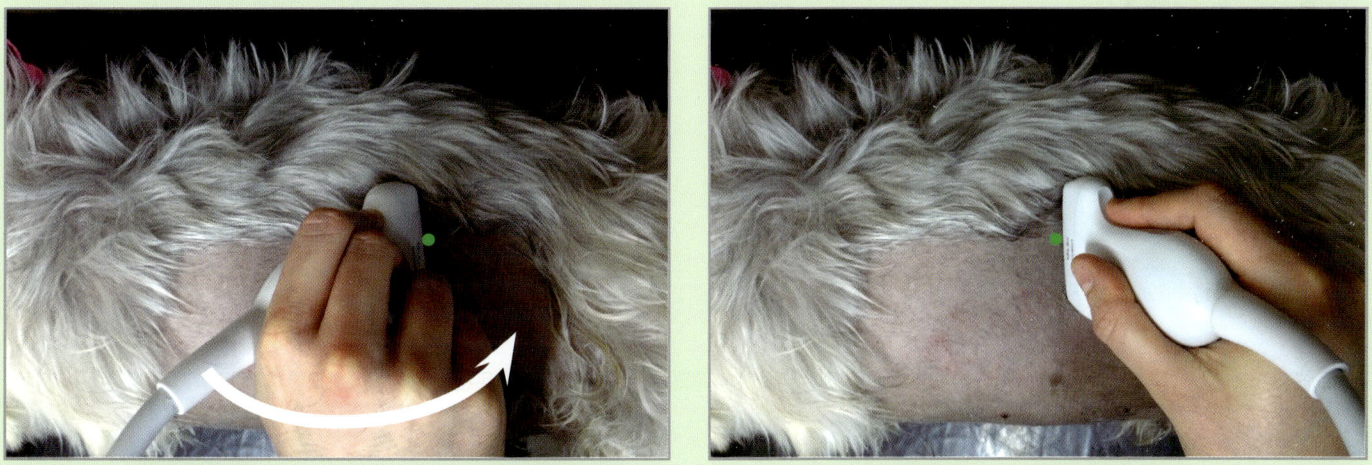

Figure 4. Following examination of the kidney along its length, the transducer is rotated 90° clockwise and fanned cranial to caudal to assess the kidney a second time in the transverse plane.

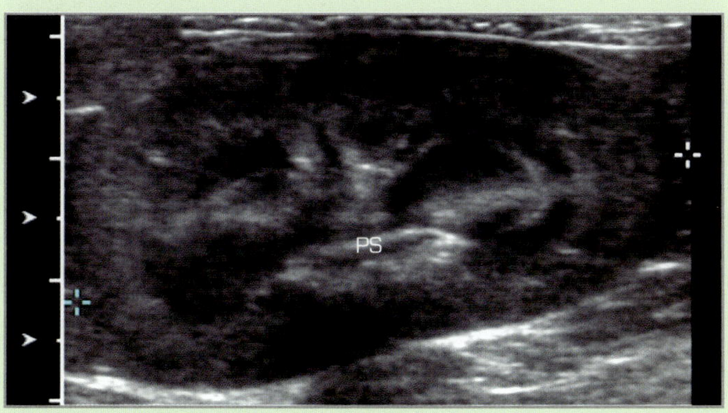

Figure 5. Image of a canine kidney in its near-longest axis. Three measurements in three different images of the kidney are required: the longest of the three measurements is considered as the correct one. PS: peripelvic hyperechoic stranding.

Right kidney

Position the animal in left lateral recumbency with the head towards the ultrasound machine and the limbs away from the examiner (Fig. 6a).

1. To locate the right kidney, place the transducer with the marker pointing to the head of the animal at the level of the last two intercostal spaces or caudal to the last rib, in the dorsal abdomen and near the spine (Fig. 6a). If you start caudal to the last rib or at the level of the last intercostal space and you do not see the right kidney, slide the transducer cranially. Make sure that you are near the spine and that the depth is set up adequately to see the right kidney, especially in large dogs.

2. In cats and small dogs, the right kidney can be imaged and evaluated from the right side with the animal in right lateral recumbency (the transducer is placed under the animal). The technique is similar to that used to identify the right lobe of the pancreas (see in Chapter 7 for more information on how to locate the right kidney).

3. Once you have identified the right kidney and placed it in the middle of the screen, rotate the transducer slightly clockwise or anticlockwise to image the right kidney in its long axis (same technique as for the left kidney).

4. After visualising the kidney in its longest axis, fan the transducer all the way dorsally and all the way ventrally until you cannot see kidney on each side of the movement (same technique as for the left kidney).

5. Rotate the transducer 90° clockwise and fan the transducer cranially and caudally until you cannot see kidney on each side of the movement (same technique as for the left kidney).

6. While performing these movements, evaluate the kidney and compare its echogenicity to the liver.

7. Measure the maximum length of the kidney in three different images and accept the longest one as correct.

8. If the acoustic shadowing from the ribs is interfering with the evaluation of the right kidney (Fig. 6b), slide caudally and rock your transducer cranially, or slide cranially and rock your transducer caudally to avoid the interference.

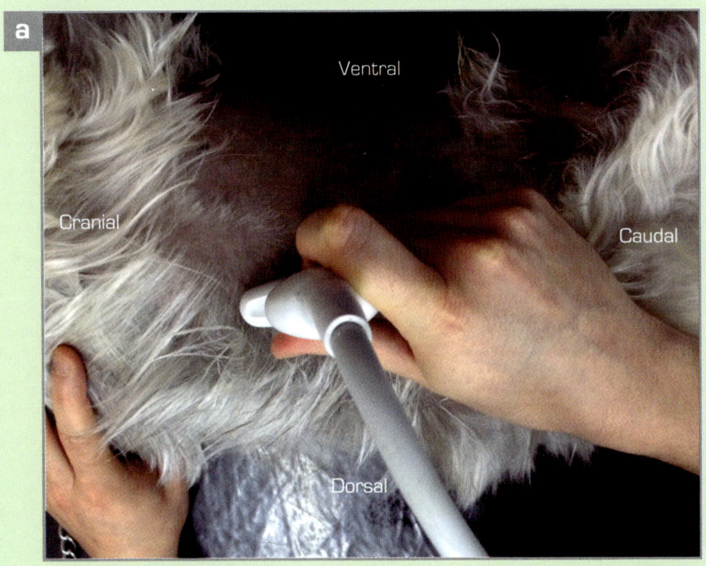

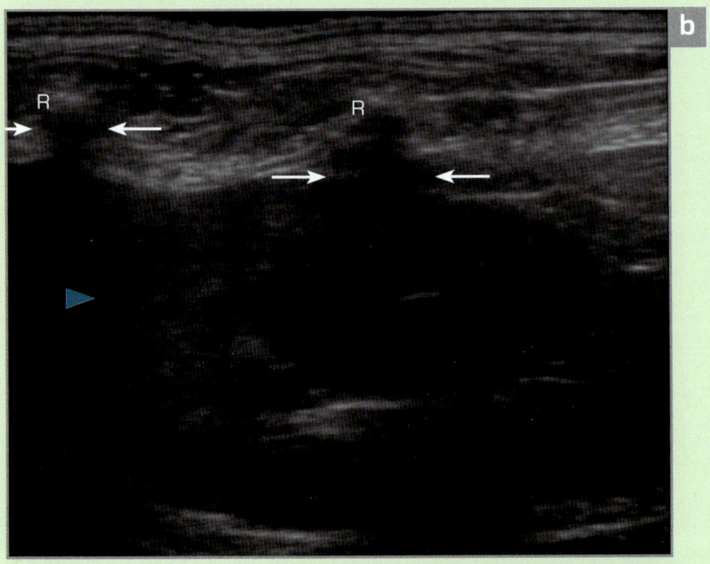

Figure 6. (a) Initial position of the transducer for evaluation of the right kidney: caudal to the last rib or in the last two intercostal spaces, parallel to the spine, with the marker pointing to the head of the animal. (b) Image of the right kidney (between blue arrowheads) in a dog with the transducer in dorsal orientation. The ribs (R) are visible causing acoustic shadowing (white arrows) that leads to poor visualization of the right kidney.

Normal appearance

The kidney has a characteristic ultrasonographic appearance that most novices can immediately identify. It has the renal sinus, a cortex and a medulla. The cortex is moderately echogenic and hyperechoic to the medulla (see Fig. 2), with some age-related variations:

- In young dogs and cats, the medulla is almost anechoic.
- In older dogs and cats, the medulla becomes more hyperechoic; however, it is always possible to distinguish the margin between cortex and medulla (Fig. 7).

Linear echogenicities can be seen in the medullary area (Fig. 7 and 8) reflecting the diverticula with the interlobar arteries and veins. The arcuate and interlobular arteries may be seen in the corticomedullary junction.

If the corticomedullary junction is unclear, focally or generally, then the kidney does not have a normal ultrasonographic appearance. The renal cortical echogenicity in a healthy patient is equal to, or slightly less or

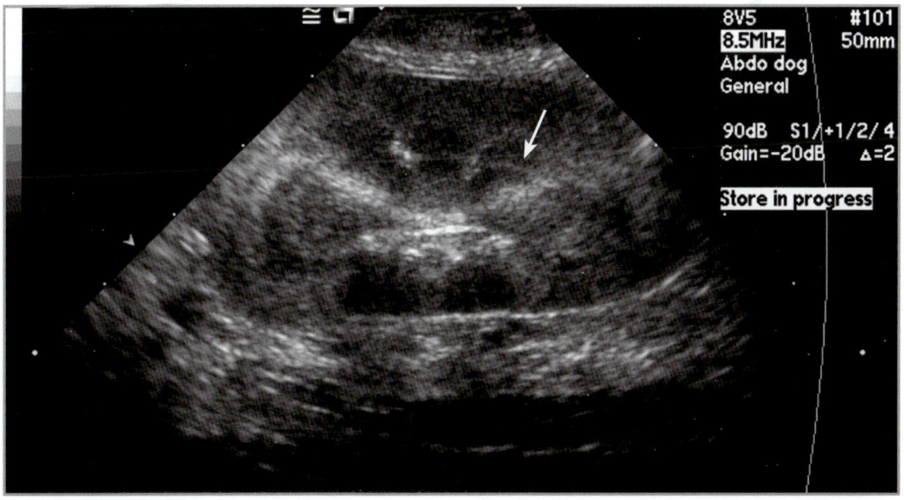

Figure 7. Sagittal view of the kidney in an eight-year-old dog. The renal medulla is mildly hyperechoic; however, there is clear differentiation between the cortex and the medulla. This appearance is normal in older dogs and cats. A medullary rim sign, an incidental finding in this case, is also visible (arrow).

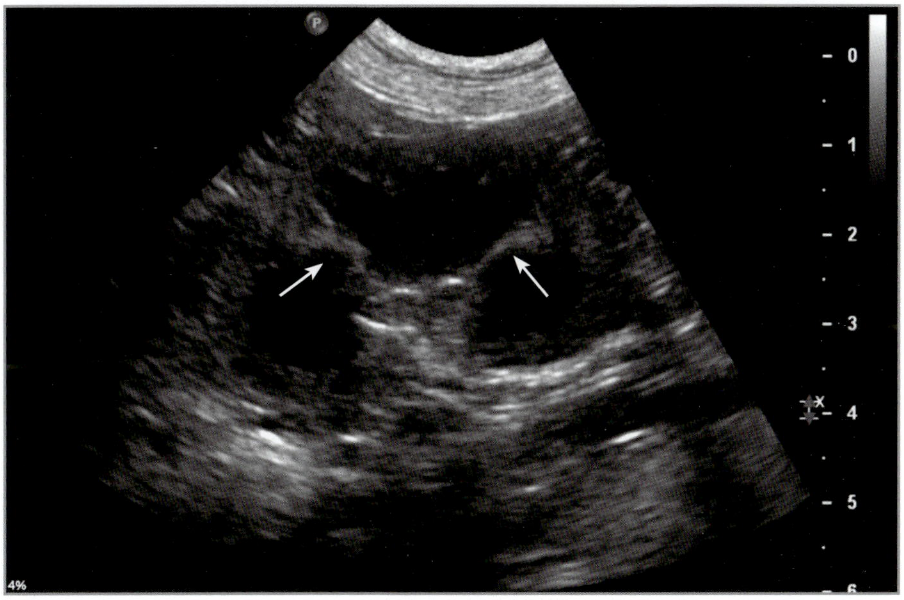

Figure 8. Image from the left kidney of a 3-year-old Boston terrier in an orientation between dorsal and sagittal. Linear echogenic areas (arrows) correspond to the diverticula and interlobar vessels are visible.

slightly more than the hepatic echogenicity, and significantly less than the splenic echogenicity (Fig. 9). A thin or thick echogenic rim, called the renal medullary rim sign, can sometimes be seen just inside the medulla, parallel to the corticomedullary junction (Figs. 7 and 10).

The renal medullary rim sign is a non-specific ultrasonographic sign in dogs and cats which can be seen in clinically normal animals.

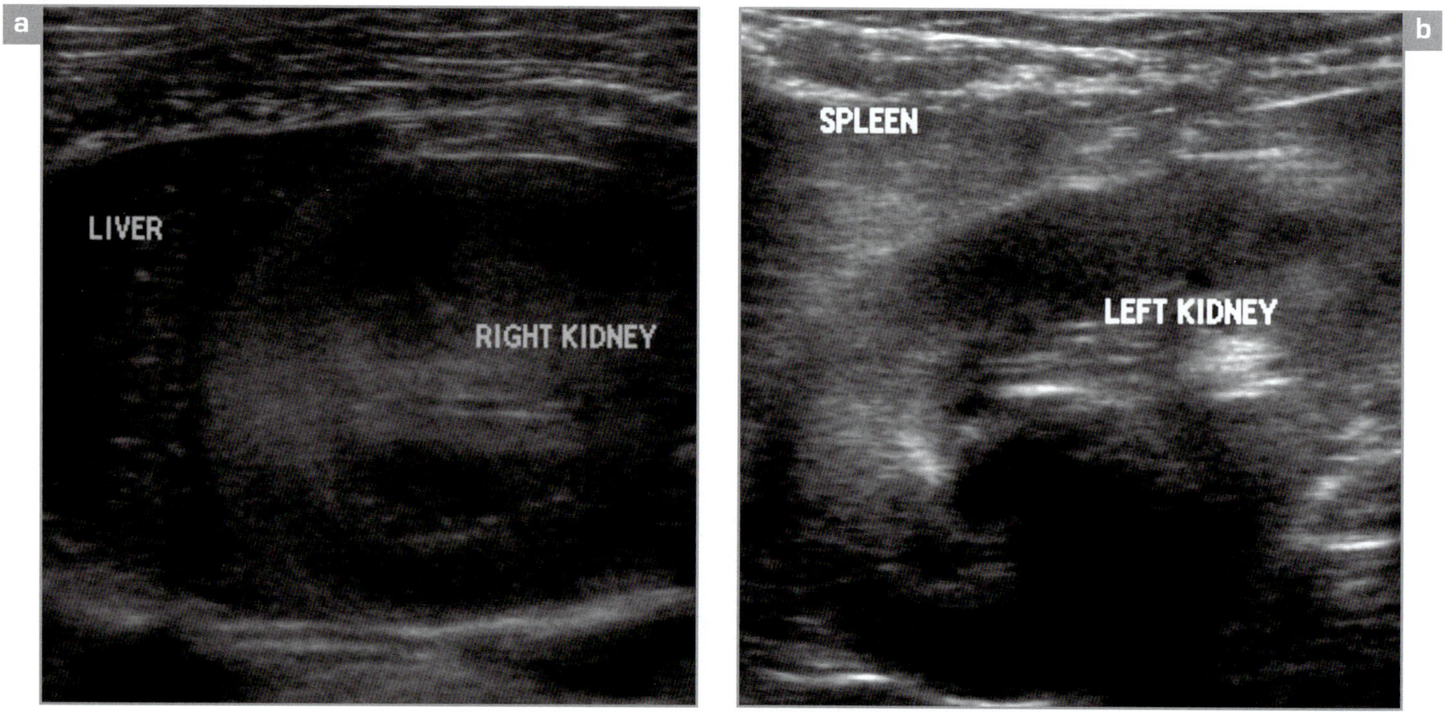

Figure 9. (a) The renal cortex is mildly hyperechoic to the liver in this healthy dog. It can also be isoechoic or hypoechoic to the hepatic parenchyma. (b) The renal cortex is normally hypoechoic to the spleen.

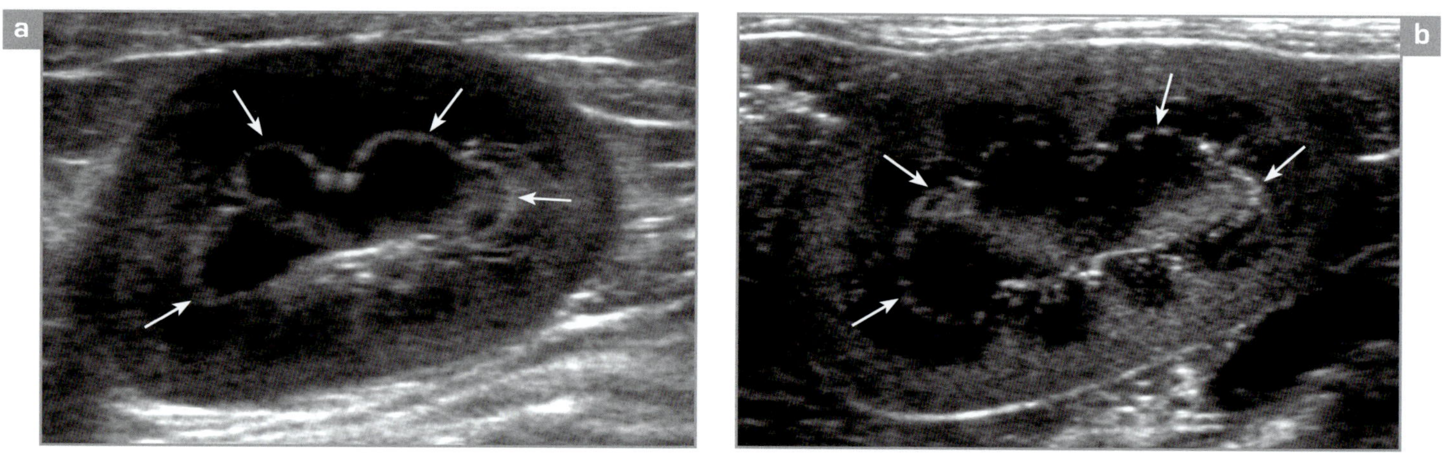

Figure 10. (a, b) Feline kidneys. The medullary rim sign is visible (arrows). These cats had no evidence of renal disease.

There is no method for accurate determination of the normal renal ultrasonographic size in the dog. However, the ratio between aortic diameter and renal length has been investigated, concluding that a normal ratio is between 5.5 and 9.1. Tables have been published that correlate the normal renal length with the weight of the dog. They may be useful until the novice ultrasonographer becomes experienced with renal size differences in different breeds and sizes of dogs. A method to evaluate renal size variations in different breeds and sizes of dogs is to measure the renal length on ventrodorsal radiographs of the abdomen, where normal renal length should be 2.5–3.5 times the length of the L2 vertebra. This can be used until the examiner gains experience with the size of the kidneys in different sizes and breeds of dogs.

In cats, the renal length has been reported to range from 3.8 cm to 4.4 cm (Fig. 11). Very few large-sized cats may have a renal length up to 5 cm. According to the author's experience, Persian, Angora, Abyssinian and Chinchilla cats tend to have smaller kidneys than other breeds and their length can be as low as 3.5 cm. In these breeds, if the kidneys appear otherwise ultrasonographically normal and there are no clinical or biochemical indications of renal disease, a smaller size, as low as 3.5 cm in length, could be considered normal.

The renal pelvis cannot normally be imaged (Fig. 12), so if fluid is seen in the renal pelvis, it means that it is dilated. When the animal is polyuric or receives (or has recently received) intravenous fluids, the renal pelvises commonly appear slightly dilated and triangular in shape (Figs. 13).

Finally, the ureters are very small (less than 2 mm in diameter) and difficult to see and follow when not dilated.

Variations from normal

A normal ultrasonographic appearance of the kidneys does not exclude the possibility of renal disease. Furthermore, the ultrasonographic appearance of renal abnormalities is not specific to a particular disease or aetiology, even though other findings can help reduce the possible differential list for the renal abnormalities observed.

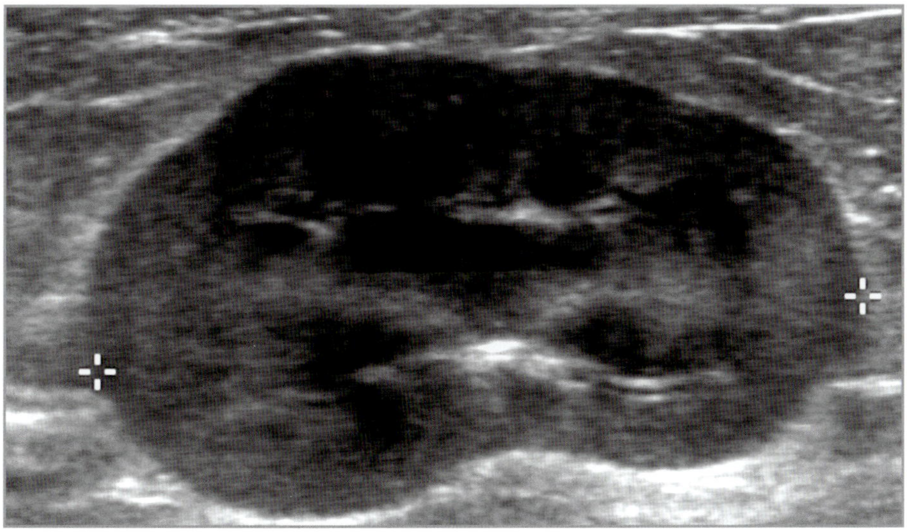

Figure 11. Measurement of the right renal length in a cat. The size of this kidney was 4.1 cm, which is considered within the normal range. Note that the callipers are placed at maximum length and parallel to the peripelvic hyperechoic stranding.

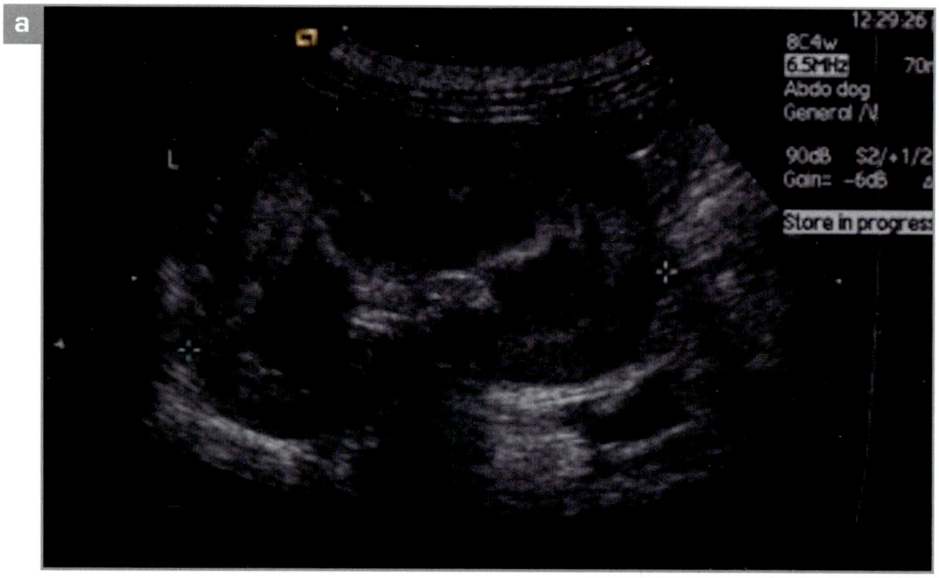

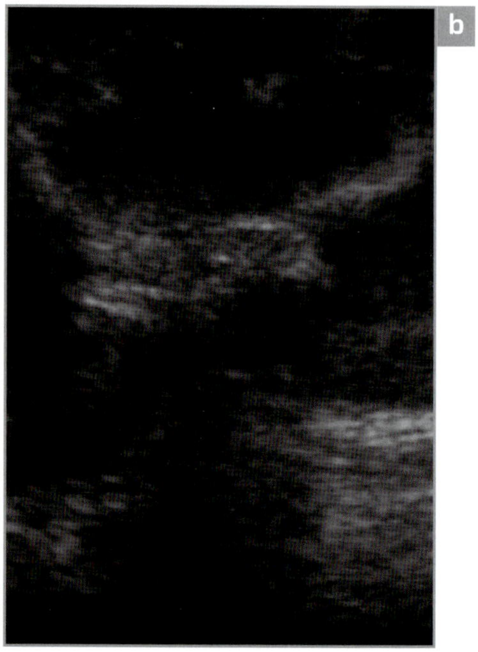

Figure 12. (a) Right kidney in a healthy dog. The normal renal pelvis is not visible. (b) Close-up view of the area of the pelvis.

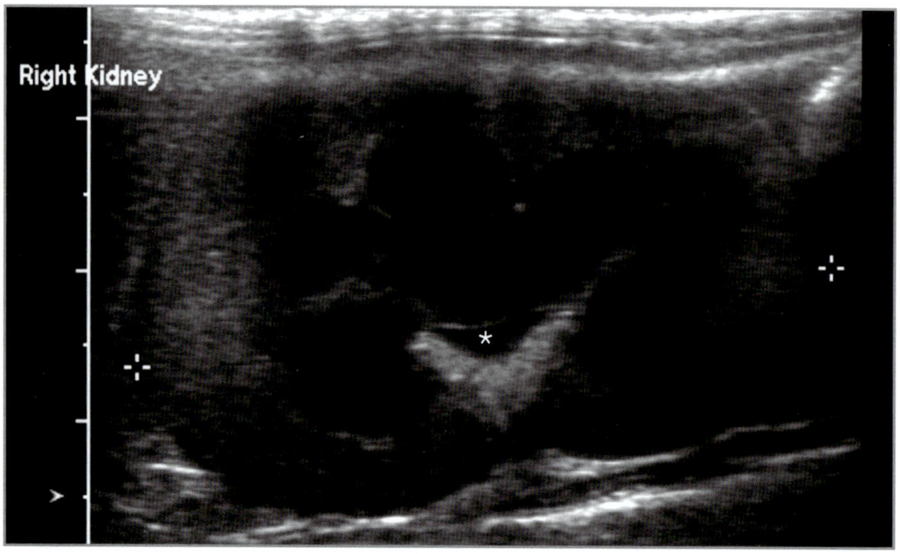

Figure 13. Sagittal view of the right kidney in a dog receiving intravenous fluids with no evidence of renal disease. The renal pelvis (*) is mildly dilated and almost triangular in shape. A similar appearance can also be observed in polyuric animals or in animals with renal disease (e.g. pyelonephritis).

Absent kidney

In renal agenesis or if a kidney has been removed by previous nephrectomy, the missing kidney cannot be found on ultrasound. However, ultrasonography is not sensitive enough to confirm renal agenesis, or absent kidney (e.g. previously removed), as a very small and/or a very abnormal kidney may not be identified ultrasonographically. Intravenous urography (excretory urography) is required to confirm the absence of a kidney. The remaining kidney may be enlarged, but normal in echogenicity and echotexture, due to compensatory hypertrophy.

Ectopic kidneys

Kidneys may be located in an abnormal position. In the animals that the kidneys are not readily identifiable in the expected normal position, a thorough search of the abdomen and other locations (e.g. pelvic inlet) may be required to locate them. Intravenous urography or computed tomography may help in identifying the location of ectopic kidneys.

Focal and multifocal lesions

Focal lesions and masses in the kidneys may be easily identified on ultrasound as they commonly cause distortion of the renal margin and/or have different echogenicity to the renal parenchyma. However, the ultrasonographic appearance of a mass is not specific to a disease and a fine-needle aspirate or a biopsy is required for the final diagnosis.

- Renal cysts may be solitary or multiple (Fig. 14a), congenital or acquired. They are thin-walled and have a circular shape. Their contents are usually anechoic with distal acoustic enhancement. Polycystic renal disease is commonly seen in Persian cats, but it also affects other breeds of cats (Fig. 14a) and has also been reported in dogs. Abscesses (Fig. 14b), haematomas and tumours may look similar to cysts; however, they commonly have thick walls and may contain septa.

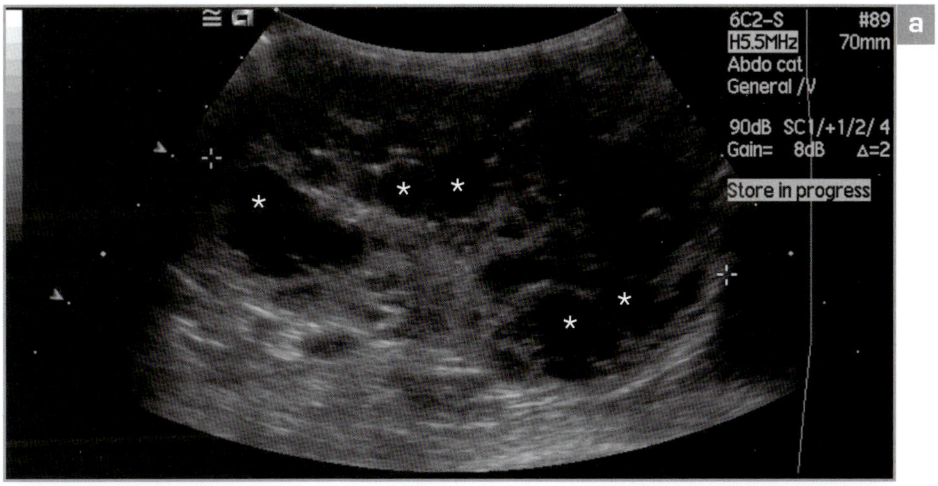

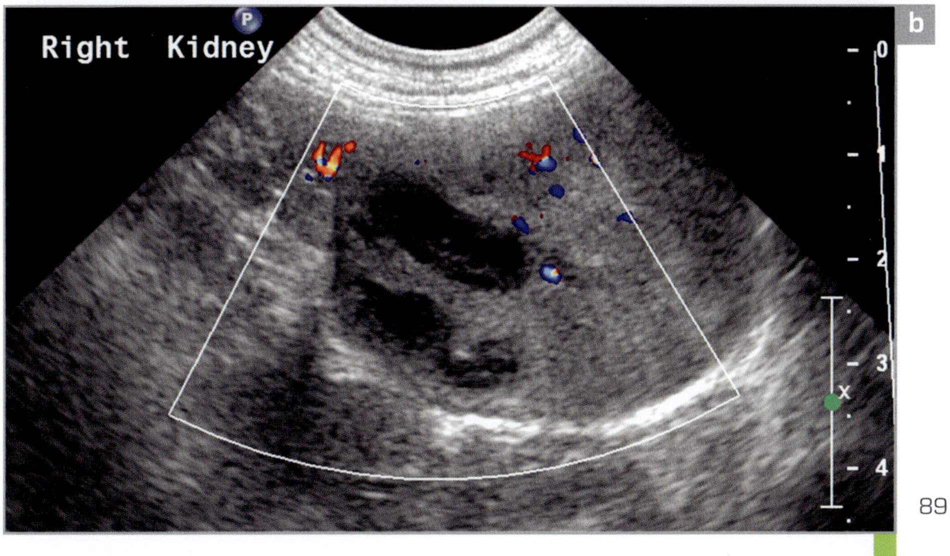

Figure 14. (a) Sagittal view of the left kidney of a British blue cat with polycystic renal disease. Multiple large (*) and smaller cysts are visible. (b) Renal abscessation in a 5-year-old Golden Retriever. Colour-flow Doppler shows lack of blood flow in the cavitary lesion.

- Renal masses may be either solid or cystic. Their echogenicity varies from hypo- to hyper- to iso-echoic to the renal parenchyma. They can also have a mixed echogenicity. Isoechoic masses can be seen only if they distort the renal margin or renal architecture or if their echotexture is different to that of the kidney. Renal carcinomas and renal haemangiomas are the most common malignant and benign neoplasms affecting canine kidneys, respectively. In cats, renal lymphoma is the neoplasm most commonly identified in the kidneys (Fig. 15), although other tumours may also be observed (Fig. 16). The ultrasonographic appearance is not specific to a tumor type. Uniformly hypoechoic masses though have been associated with lymphoma. Non-neoplastic renal masses, such as granulomas, may also be seen. Haematomas or abscesses appear as cavitary lesions.

> The ultrasound appearance of a renal mass varies, and it is not specific to a tumour type.

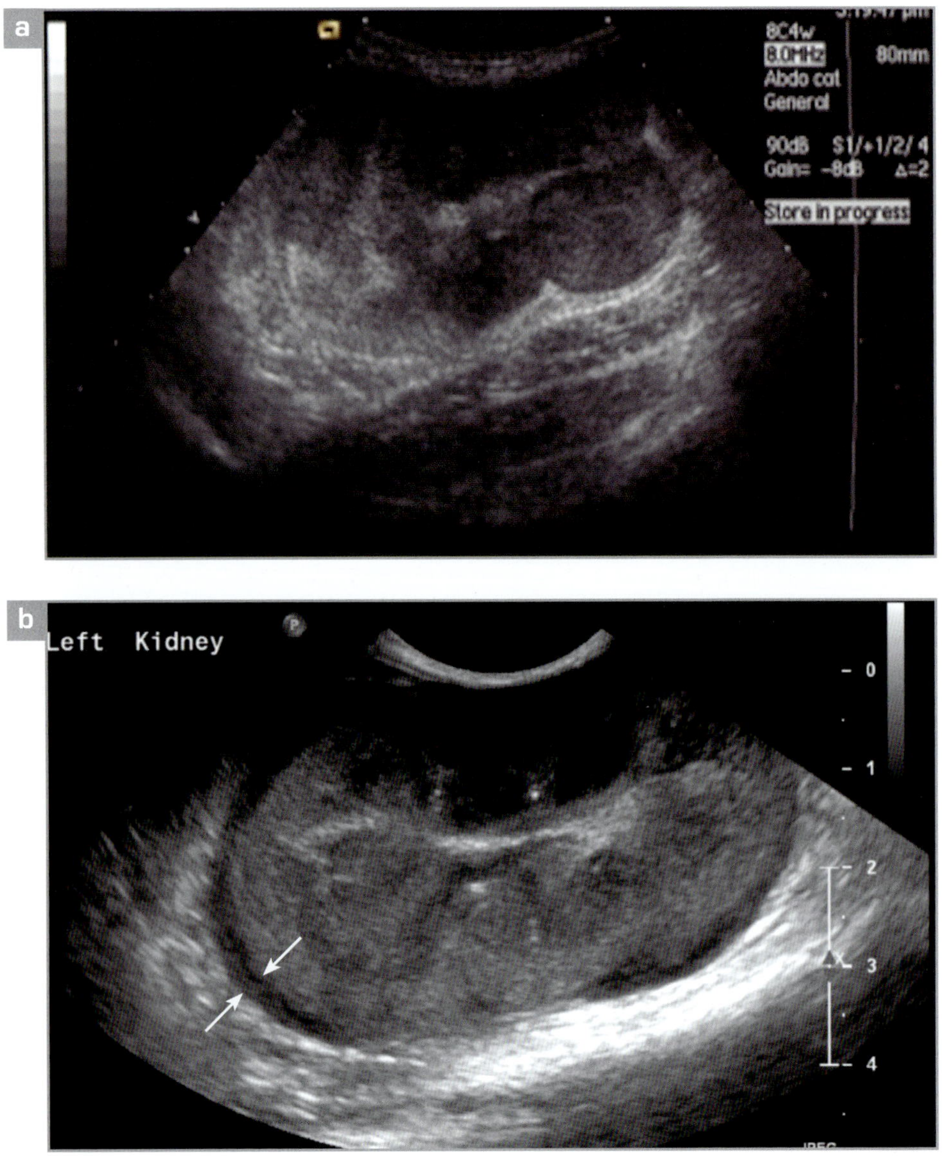

Figure 15. (a) Domestic shorthair cat diagnosed with lymphoma. The kidney is enlarged with a hyperechoic medulla, reduced corticomedullary differentiation and a nodule in the caudal pole isoechoic to the renal cortex, giving the kidney an irregular outline. **(b)** Another domestic shorthair cat diagnosed with lymphoma. There is nephromegaly with increased cortical and medullary echogenicity. A thin hypoechoic rim is visible around the kidney (arrows). This last feature is sometimes seen with renal lymphoma.

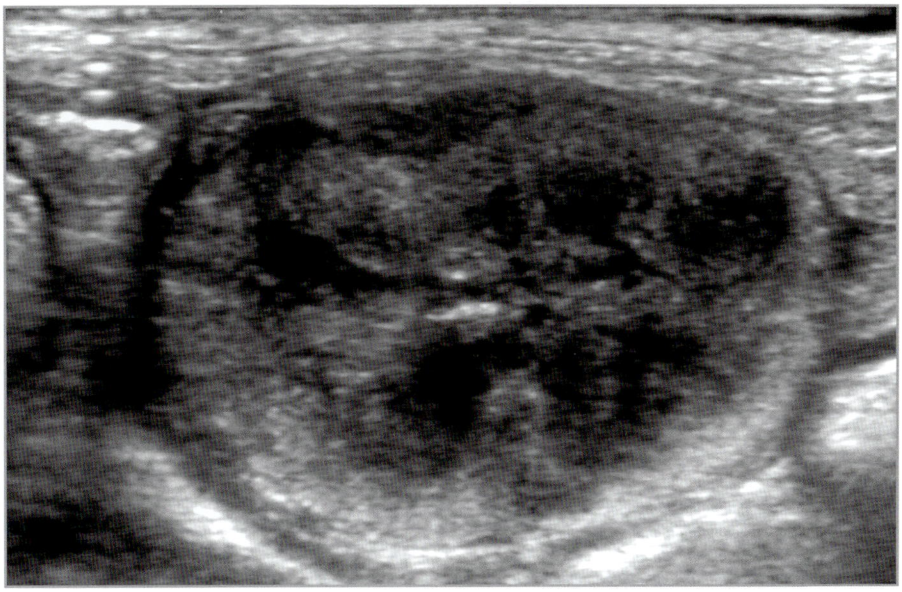

Figure 16. Domestic shorthair cat diag- nosed with renal carcinoma. The kidney is enlarged and has an irregular shape and outline, an increased medullary echogenicity and a hypoechoic peripheral rim surrounding the kidney.

- Focal mineralised areas with distal acoustic shadowing may be imaged associated with nephrolithiasis (Fig. 17) and nephrocalcinosis, but also with calcification within an abscess, cyst or haematoma. Fibrosis or calcification in the renal parenchyma and/or collecting system appear as hyperechoic areas in the kidney. Causes of hyperechoic lesions in the renal cortex include old renal infarcts, calcification, presence of gas, fibrosis and infection.

- Renal infarcts tend to be hypoechoic or isoechoic initially and hyperechoic later. They are triangular in shape with the apex of the triangle towards the corticomedullary junction and the base at the cortical surface (Fig. 18). In chronic cases, there is peripheral depression of the renal cortex in that area, with focally- reduced renal cortical thickness.

- A hyperechoic band within the medulla close and parallel to the corticomedullary junction is a non-specific sign that could also be seen also in dogs and cats with no evidence of renal disease. This band is called the medullary rim sign (see Figs. 7 and 10). A similar band can also be seen in dogs with hypercalcaemic nephropathy and has been reported with acute tubular necrosis, leptospirosis, chronic interstitial nephritis, and pyogranulomatous vasculitis due to feline infectious peritonitis. Thus, the clinical significance of the medullary rim sign seen on ultrasound must be interpreted in relation to the clinical and biochemical findings.

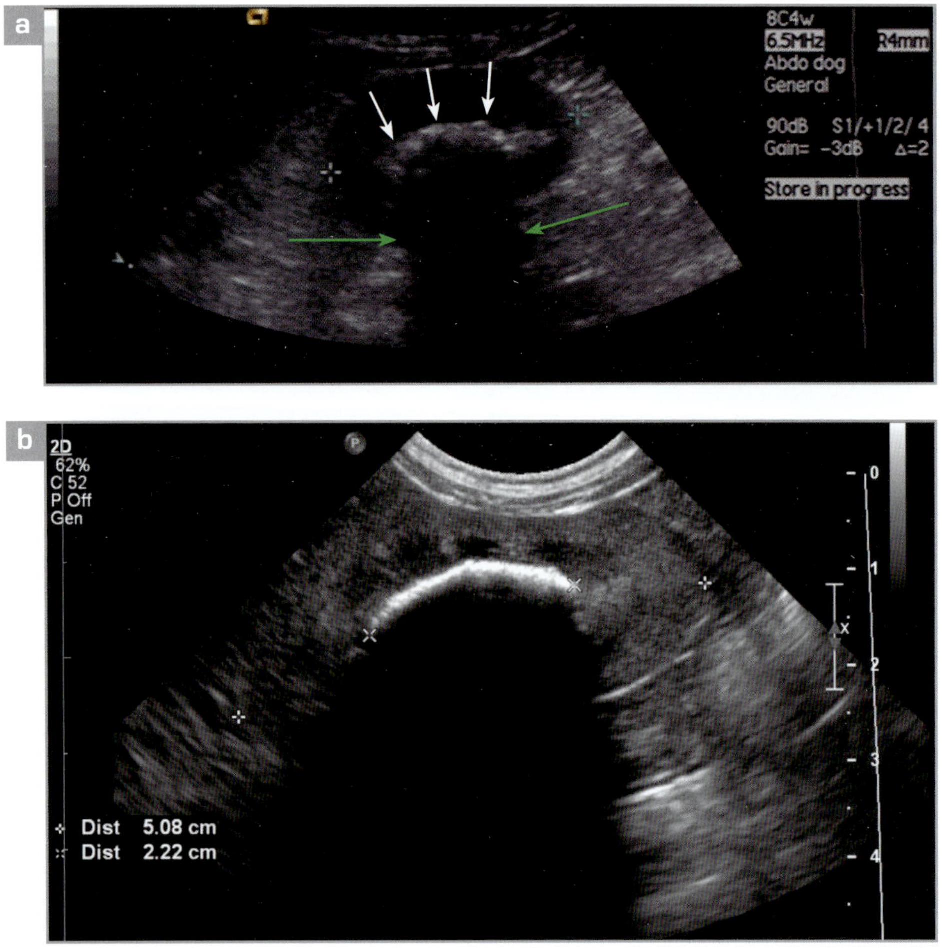

Figure 17. (a) Nephroliths (white arrows) in the renal pelvis of the left kidney in a dog. Note the distal acoustic shadowing (green arrows). (b) Large nephrolith (between callipers) in a 10-year-old crossbred.

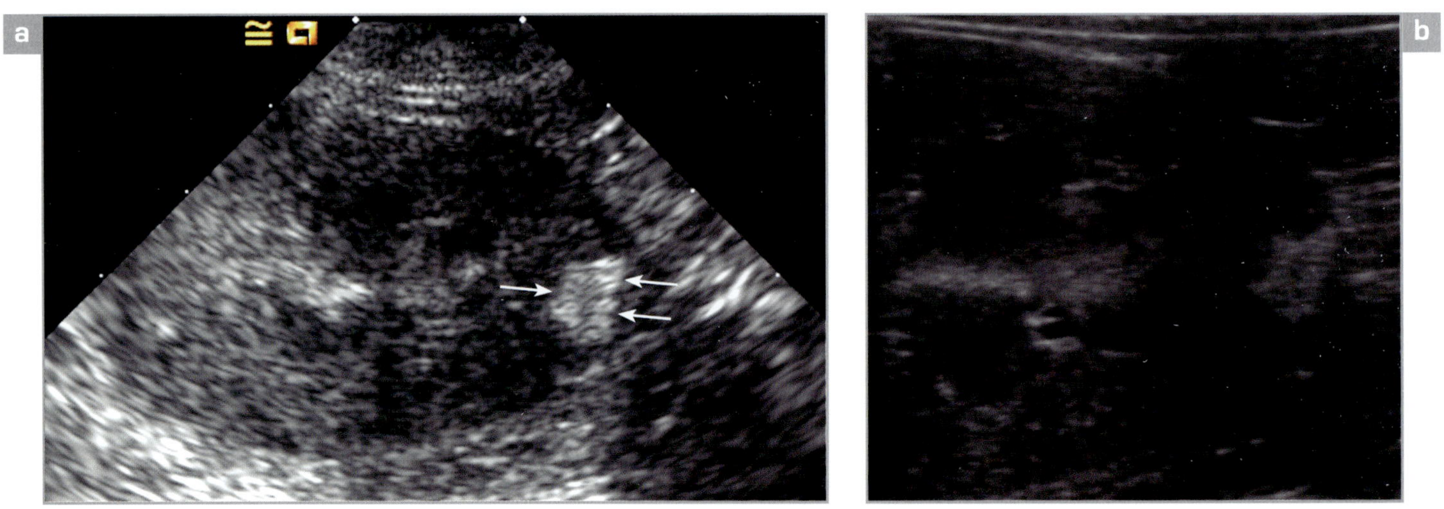

Figure 18. (a) Oblique view of the left kidney in a dog. The hyperechoic cortical lesion in the caudal pole (arrows), with the base towards the periphery represents an infarct. (b) Close-up image of a renal cortical infarct from another dog.

Diffuse changes

- In renal dysplasia (Fig. 19), the kidneys appear small, irregular and hyperechoic on ultrasound. In chronic inflammatory disease or end-stage renal disease, the kidneys may be similar to those observed in renal dysplasia, depending on how advanced the disease is. The confirmation comes only from histological analysis.

- In end-stage renal disease, kidneys are typically small, irregular and diffusely echogenic with poor visualisation of the corticomedullary junction and internal renal architecture (Fig. 20).

- Increased cortical and/or medullary echogenicity (Fig. 21) are non-specific signs that may be seen in different nephropathies including interstitial nephritis, glomerulonephritis and ethylene glycol toxicity (Fig. 21a).

Renal dysplasia should be suspected in young dogs with clinical renal insufficiency and abnormally shaped kidneys.

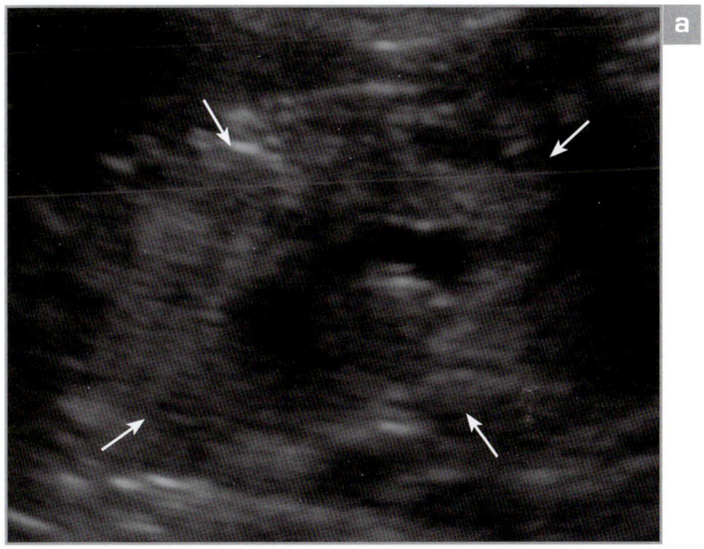

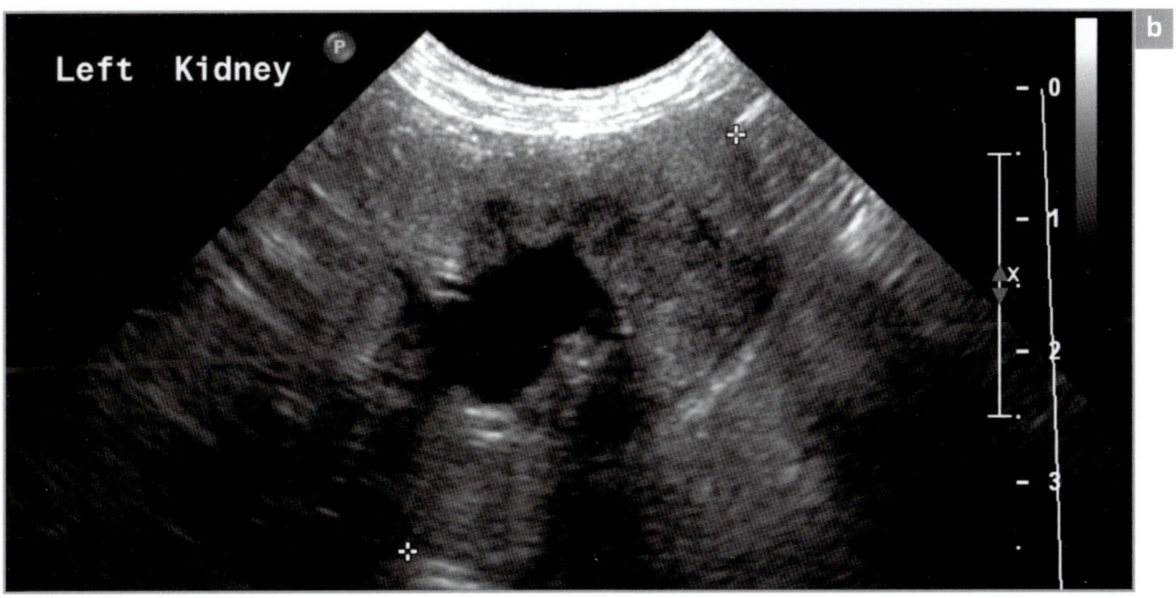

Figure 19. (a) Renal dysplasia in a young Labrador Retriever. The kidney (arrows) is difficult to identify as it is small, hyperechoic and irregular in outline. **(b)** Renal dysplasia in a young Cavalier King Charles Spaniel. The kidney (between callipers) is small in size, irregular in outline with hyperechoic cortex and medulla and with moderate pyelectasia.

- It is difficult to differentiate acute from chronic renal disease by ultrasound. Furthermore, normal- appearing kidneys on ultrasound can be seen in dogs with clinically evident renal disease. Renal neoplasia can also appear on ultrasound as diffuse renal changes (Figs. 15b and 16), instead of focal or multifocal changes. Renal lymphosarcoma may appear ultrasonographically as reduced cortical echogenicity in the dog. In cats, lymphosarcoma most commonly appears as diffuse increased cortical echogenicity, but it can also appear as reduced cortical echogenicity.

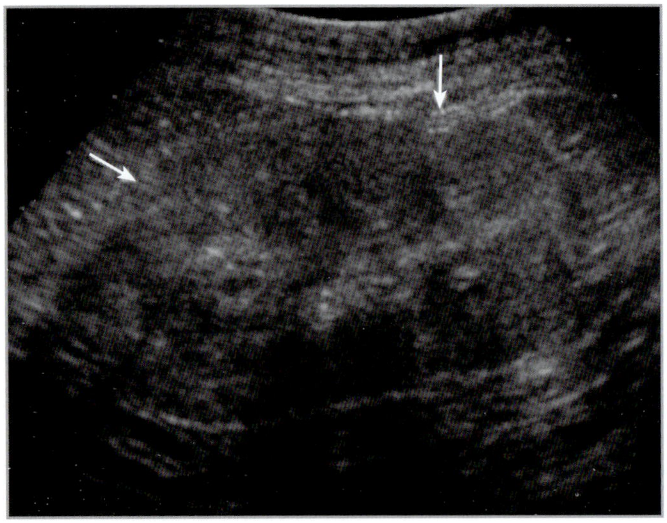

Figure 20. End-stage renal disease in a dog. The kidney is small, diffusely increased in echogenicity and with an irregular outline (arrows).

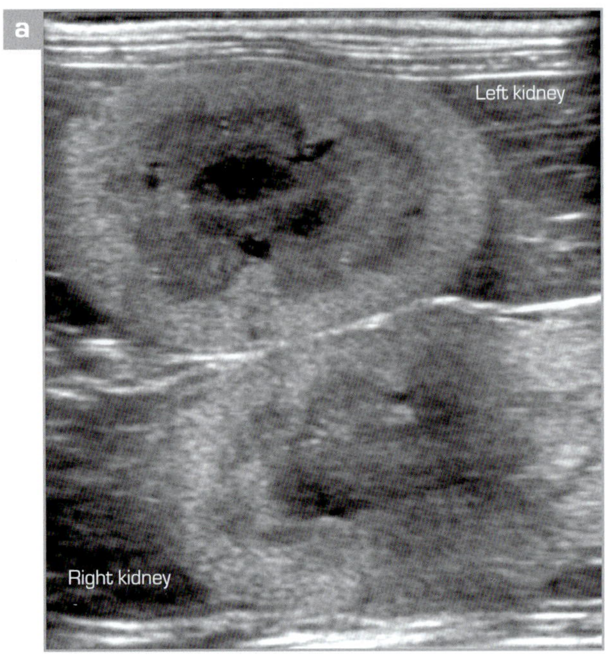

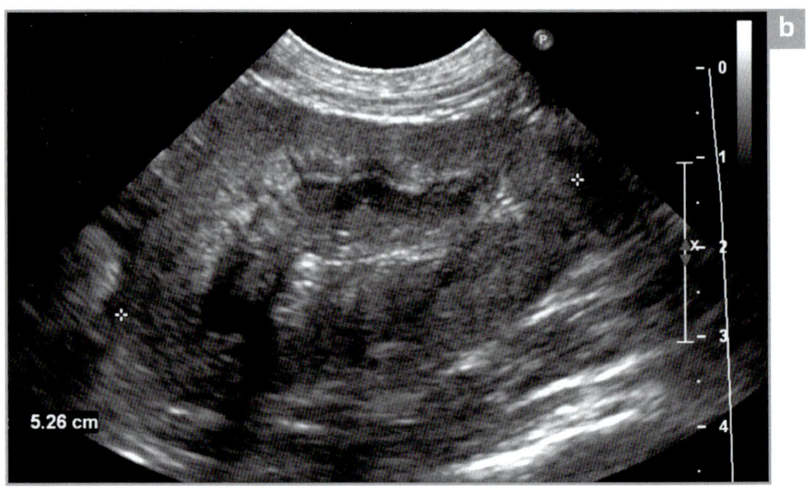

Figure 21. (a) Ethylene glycol toxicity in a cat. Both kidneys are diffusely hyperechoic. (b) Renal amyloidosis in a 5-year-old, male Shar-Pei dog. There is increased echogenicity of the cortex and medulla with reduced corticomedullary differentiation.

Disorders of the renal pelvis and ureters

- Pyelectasia (Fig. 22) is the dilatation of the renal pelvis. If the renal pelvis is slightly dilated, it is visible, and its shape becomes triangular on ultrasound. This is commonly seen in animals with polyuria and/or in animals receiving intravenous fluid therapy.

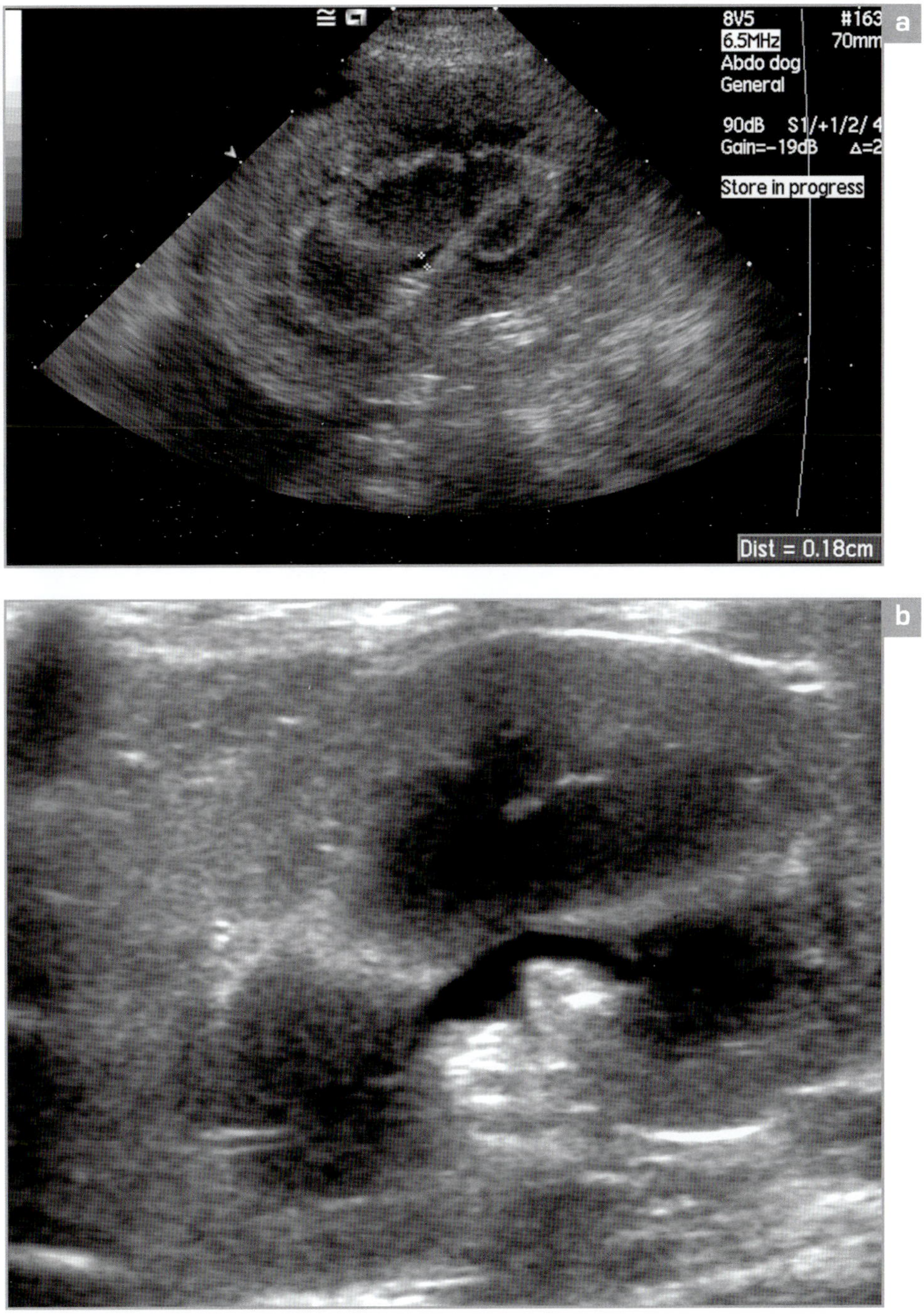

Figure 22. (a) Mild pyelectasia (between callipers) in a polyuric dog. **(b)** Mild pyelectasia in another dog.

- Hydronephrosis (Fig. 23) is the dilatation of the renal pelvis secondary to the obstruction of the renal collecting system. This can progress to severe dilatation with the kidney appearing as a cystic, thin-walled structure (Fig. 23d). The attachments of the renal capsule, along with the location, may give an indication that you are looking at a hydronephrotic kidney. Once hydronephrosis has been identified, the ureters should be followed up to the urinary bladder to identify the area of obstruction.

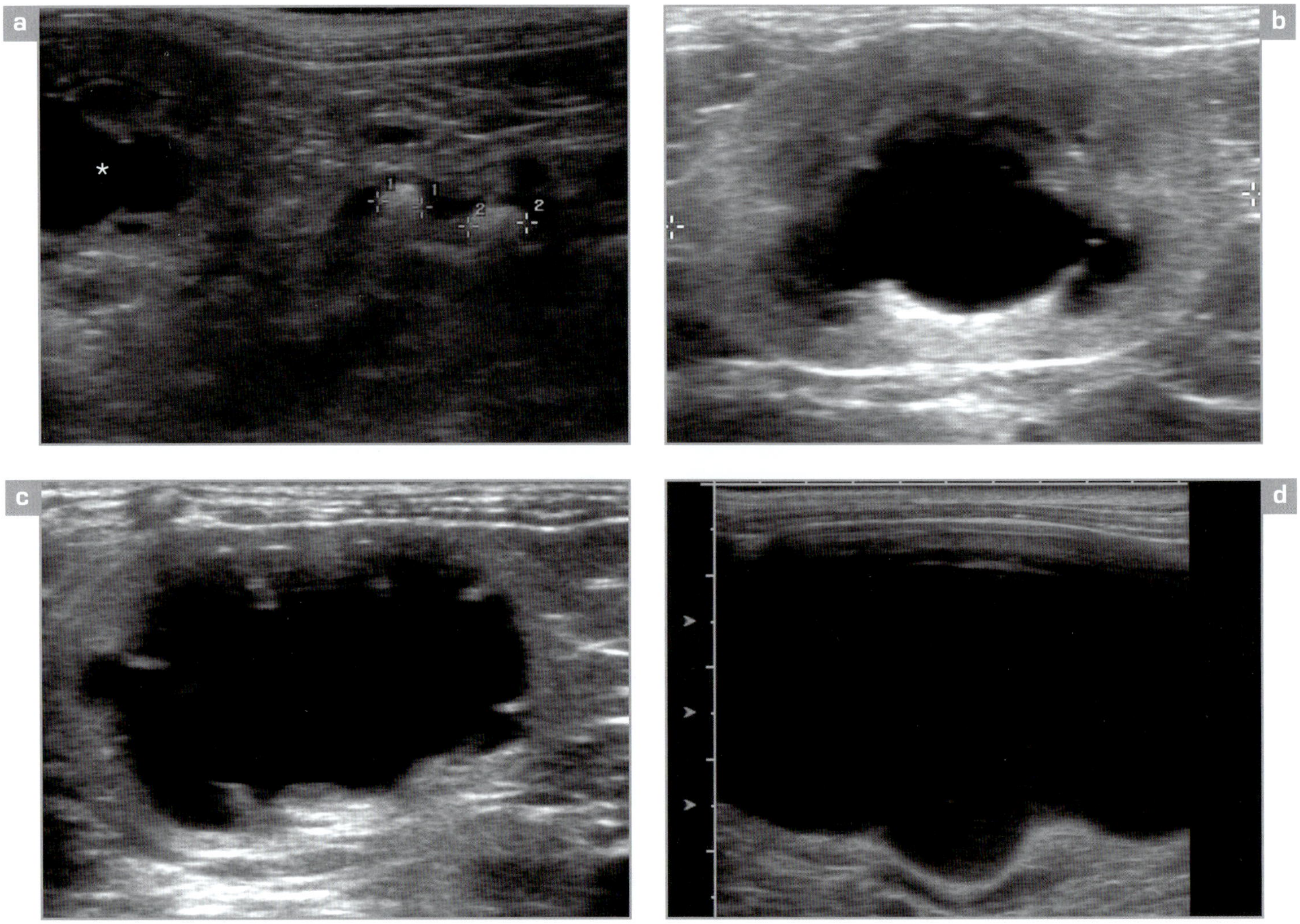

Figure 23. **(a)** Hydronephrosis secondary to ureteric obstruction. Two calculi are visible in the mildly dilated ureter (between callipers). **(b)** Moderate hydronephrosis secondary to a blocked ureter from a transitional cell carcinoma. **(c)** Moderate to severe hydronephrosis secondary to ureteric obstruction from a calculus. **(d)** Severe hydronephrosis secondary to a ligated ureter post-ovariohysterectomy.

- Ectopic ureters (Fig. 24) can be unilateral or bilateral. It is common to see dilated ureters on ultrasound secondary to infection and these can thus be followed to the level of their termination or caudal to the urinary bladder. In case of ectopic ureter, the renal pelvis may also be dilated. It is difficult to diagnose ectopic ureters with double opening on ultrasound since they can be followed to the urinary bladder, so if there is a second opening is in the segment continuing caudally, they may not be identified.

- When a ureter is dilated it is termed a hydroureter. This may be secondary to ureteral obstruction or inflammation. Normograde pyelography (contrast injection in the dilated renal pelvis after removal of equal amount of urine) under ultrasound guidance may be useful in highlighting the ureter and confirming the obstruction.

- A ureterocoele (Fig. 25) is a congenital dilatation of the distal part of the ureter. Ureterocoeles appear as cystic structures projecting to the urinary bladder lumen. They can occasionally accompany ectopic ureters or ureteral obstruction.

- Ureteroliths (Fig. 23a) appear as hyperechoic structures with distal acoustic shadowing. Ureteroliths may cause complete or partial obstruction or may be small enough not to cause obstruction of the ureter.

- Gas bubbles may be seen in the ureter, or even the renal pelvis, and it is usually secondary to double contrast cystography or pneumocystography. It may also be secondary to infection with gas forming bacteria, though this is less common. Gas bubbles appear as hyperechoic foci with "dirty" shadowing.

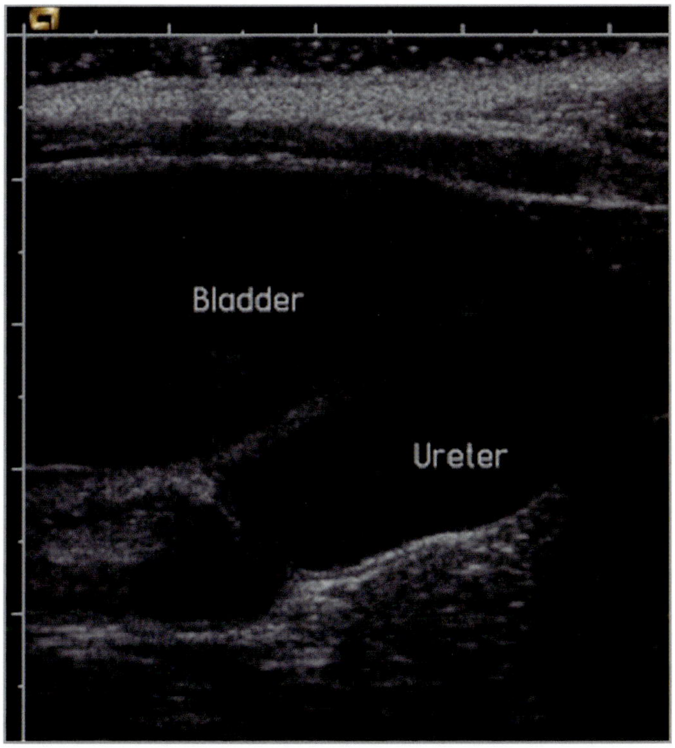

Figure 24. Parasagittal view at the level of the urinary bladder. The ectopic ureter is markedly dilated and visible bypassing the bladder and terminating at the beginning of the urethra. The cranial aspect of the animal is to the left of the image.

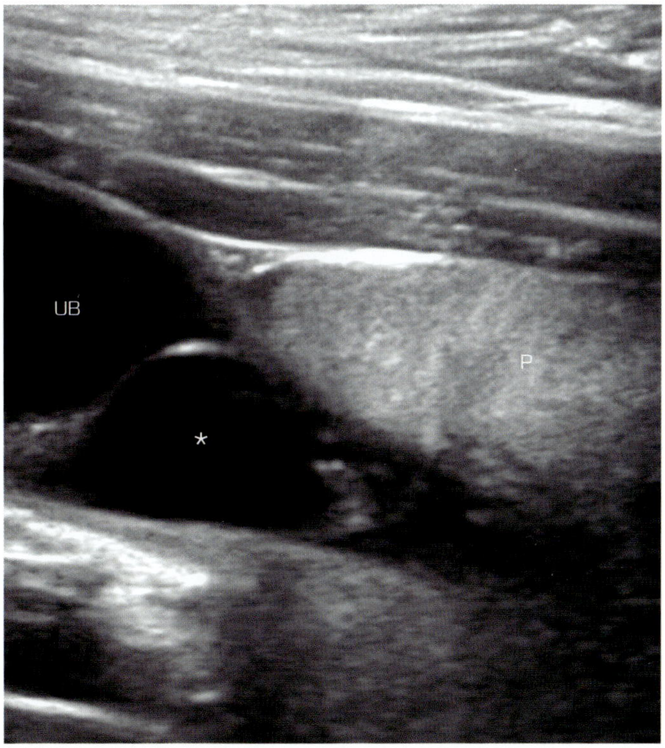

Figure 25. A ureterocoele (*) in a 17-month-old male Labrador. UB: urinary bladder, P: prostate.

Subcapsular or perirenal fluid

- Subcapsular or perirenal fluid can be urine, haemorrhage, transudate or exudate. It is difficult to determine ultrasonographically if the fluid is around the kidney (perirenal with separate wall) or under the renal capsule (subcapsular). Once fluid around the kidney has been seen on ultrasound, the differential diagnosis should include perinephric pseudocyst (Fig. 26), subcapsular haematoma, subcapsular urinoma or abscess.

- Retroperitoneal fluid can be seen in various conditions, including ruptured ureter or kidney, or trauma. As for subcapsular and perirenal fluid, the ultrasonographic appearance of the fluid is not characteristic and ultrasound-guided fine-needle aspirate is needed to identify the nature of the fluid.

Doppler evaluation

The arteries near the renal hilum and at the corticomedullary junction can be evaluated by Doppler (Fig. 27). The resistive index determines renal vascular resistance and is calculated by subtracting the end diastolic velocity from the peak systolic velocity and divide the result by the peak systolic velocity. A resistive index of less than 0.7 is considered normal in dogs, while less than 0.6 is suggested as normal in cats. Further information can be found in the papers and chapters detailed in the recommended further reading list at the end of this book.

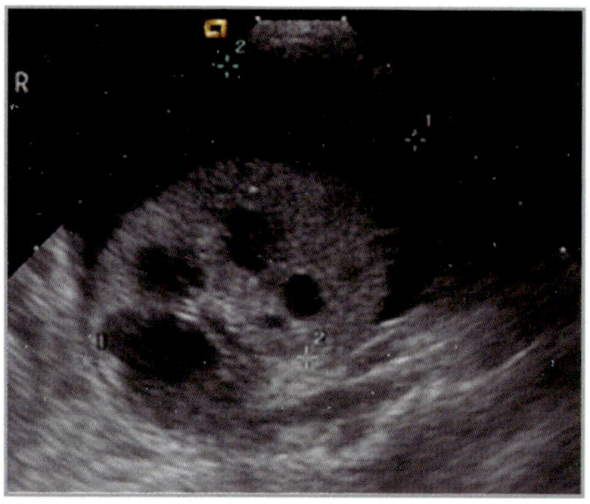

Figure 26. Perinephric pseudocyst confirmed by fluid aspirate in a cat. Fluid around the kidney is visible on this ultrasound scan. Polycystic renal disease is also visible.

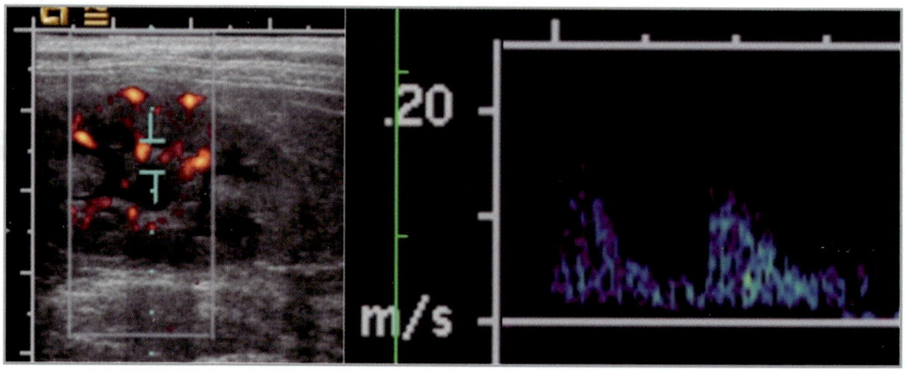

Figure 27. Pulsed-wave Doppler evaluation of the left kidney in a cat.

9

CHAPTER

ADRENAL GLANDS

Scanning technique

The animal is placed in right lateral recumbency with the head towards the ultrasound machine.

Left adrenal

1. Hold the transducer with the marker pointing to the head of the animal (Fig. 1a).

2. Keep the transducer parallel to the spine.

3. Identify the left kidney (Fig. 1b).

4. Fan the transducer towards the spine keeping it with a parallel orientation to the spine and maintaining the transducer at the level of the left kidney (Fig. 2).

5. Without exerting pressure on the probe, slowly fan the transducer ventrally in order to identify the aorta (Fig. 3a). Make sure the aorta is visible across the screen (if not, rotate the transducer to see the aorta across the screen before you continue).

6. With minimal fanning motions of the transducer up and down, identify the renal artery as it originates from the aorta (Fig. 3b).

7. Observe cranial to the corner between the renal artery and the aorta and continue to slowly fan the transducer ventrally while maintaining moderate pressure.

a

b

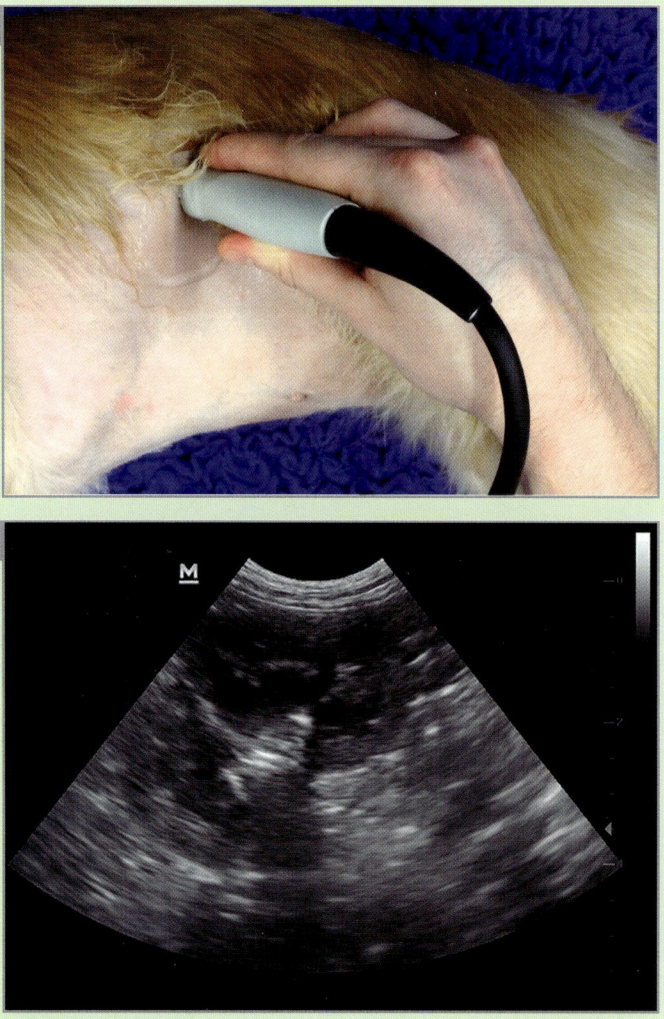

Figure 1. (a) The transducer is positioned parallel to the spine with the marker facing the head of the animal. (b) An image of the left kidney as it is firstly identified when starting the search for the left adrenal.

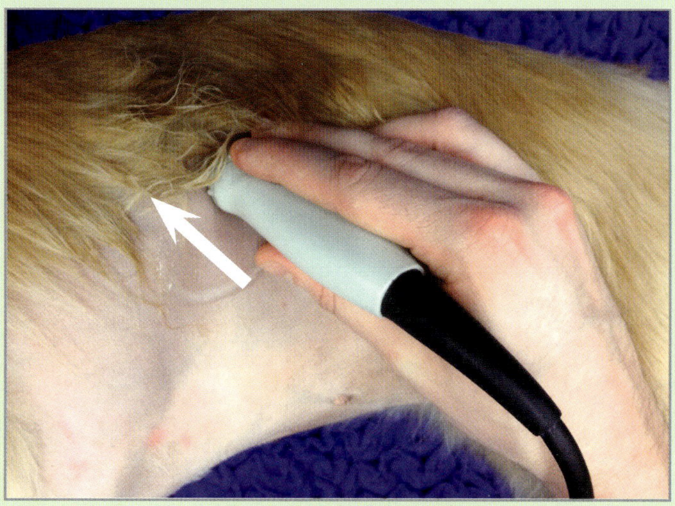

Figure 2. The transducer is angled towards the spine keeping the tip in the same location (fanned up) while the parallel orientation to the spine is maintained.

8. Identify the left adrenal: the normal adrenal appears as a "monkey nut" in the dog (Fig. 4a). In the cat the left adrenal can have a "monkey nut" shape (Fig. 4b), but more often it has a more oval shape. (Fig. 4c).

9. When the left adrenal is identified, the transducer is rotated clockwise or counterclockwise to evaluate the adrenal in full length.

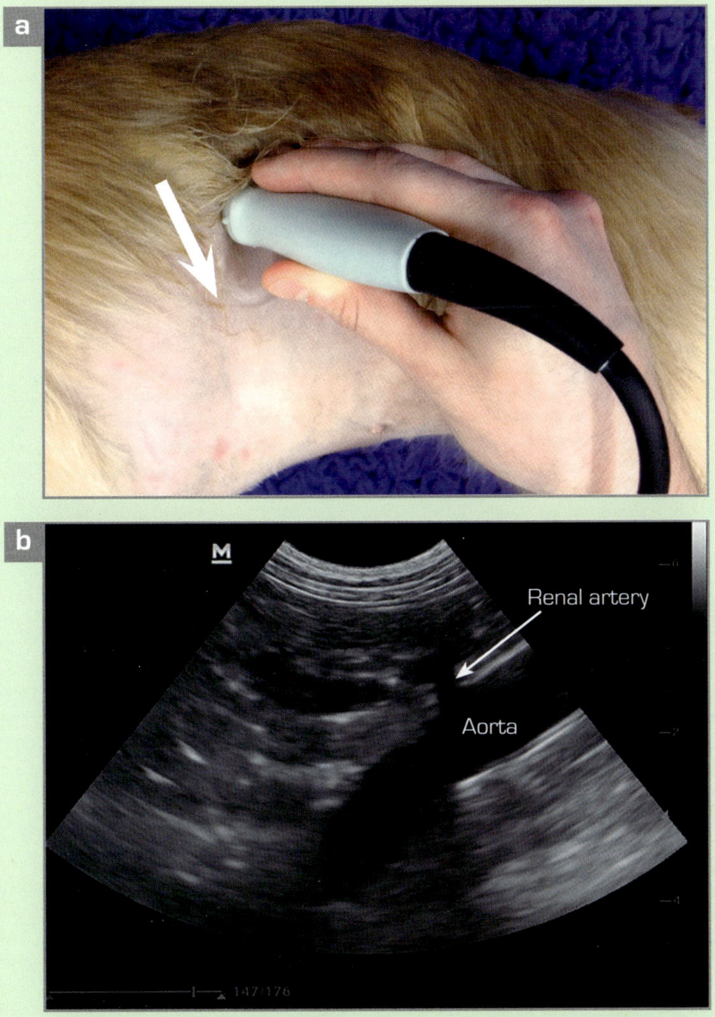

Figure 3. (a) The transducer is angled towards the left kidney (down) keeping the tip in the same location (fanned down) while the parallel orientation to the spine is maintained. (b) The aorta and left renal artery are identified. From this point the transducer is slowly fanned more ventrally looking for the adrenal, cranial to the corner between the renal artery and the aorta.

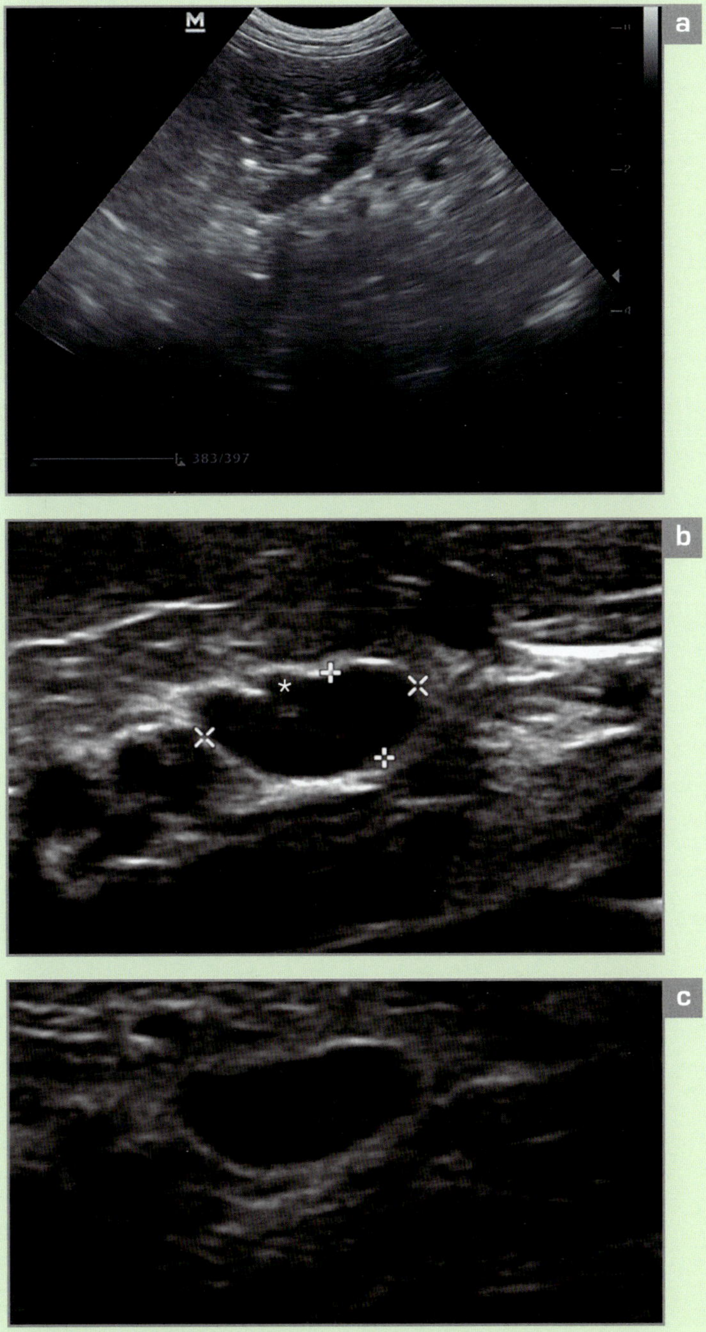

Figure 4. (a) Typical appearance of the left adrenal in the dog, having the characteristic "monkey-nut" shape.
(b) Normal left adrenal (between callipers) in a cat having a "monkey-nut" appearance. The phrenicoabdominal vein (*) is visible.
(c) Normal left adrenal in another cat that has a more oval shape with no distinct waist.

Right adrenal

Small and medium-sized dogs and cats

1. With the patient in dorsal recumbency, ask the assistants to "tilt" the animal at a 45° angle.

2. Keep the transducer with the marker pointing to the head, in a sagittal orientation, parallel to the table and up to a finger above the table (Fig. 5a).

3. Keeping the orientation of the transducer, place it just caudal to the rib cage, two thirds up from the ventral margin of the abdomen.

4. Ask the assistants to position the dog in the proper right lateral recumbency.

5. Ask an assistant to place a hand behind the spine to support the animal while you press.

6. Press with your transducer towards the right kidney (towards the last rib) (Fig. 5b).

7. Identify the right kidney and, while keeping the orientation of the transducer, place the cranial pole of the right kidney in the middle of the screen (Fig. 6).

8. Keeping the orientation of the transducer, fan the transducer upwards until you identify the caudal vena cava (the first large vessel at the top of the screen). A second large vessel may be seen on the screen below the caudal vena cava; it is the aorta (Fig. 7). Make sure the cauda vena cava is visible across the screen (if not, rotate the transducer to see the cauda vena cava across the screen before you continue).

9. As soon as you identify the caudal vena cava, stop fanning dorsally, press midly more and start slowly fanning ventrally (towards the right kidney).

10. The right adrenal can be identified due to its "arrow shape" (or "wedge shape" or "comma shape") near the caudal vena cava and, in many cases, slightly overlapping it (Fig. 8). The cauda vena cava or the right kidney are not necessarily in the view when we see the right adrenal. In cats, also the right adrenal is commonly more oval without distinct waist.

11. When the right adrenal is identified, the transducer is rotated clockwise or counterclockwise to evaluate the adrenal in full length.

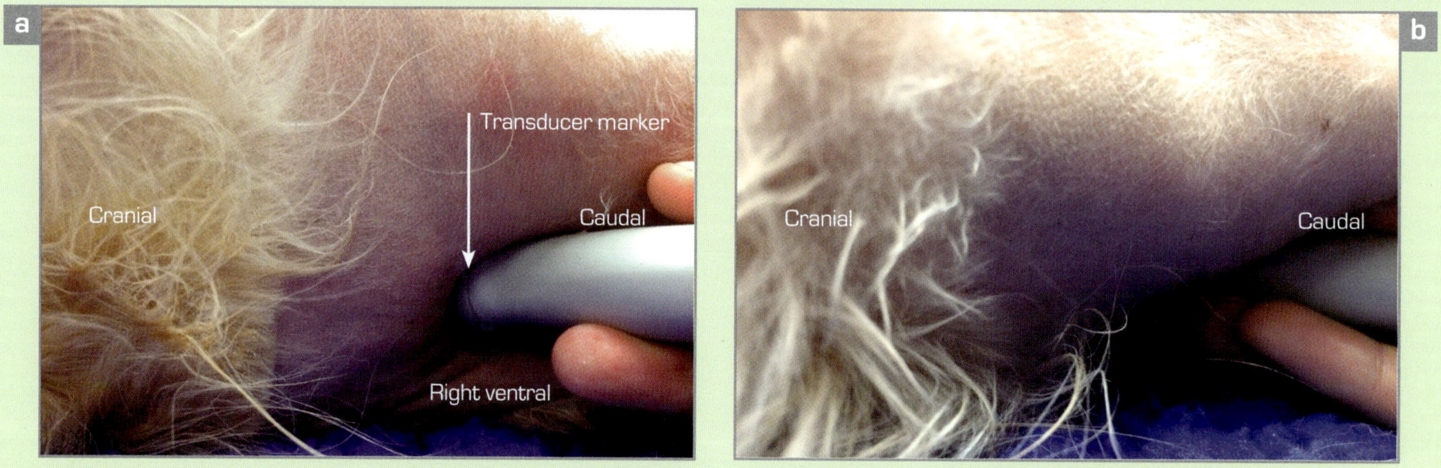

Figure 5. (a) Position and orientation of the transducer for identification of the right adrenal. (b) Pressure is applied to the transducer, while the transducer's orientation and positioning is maintained, under the animal, in order to identify the right kidney.

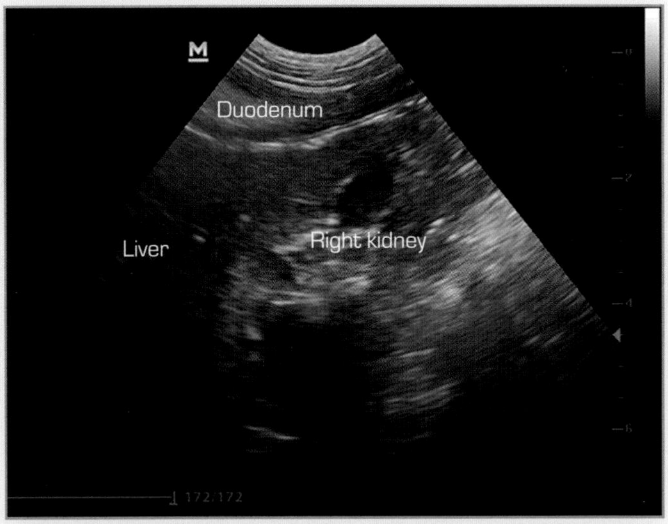

Figure 6. The right kidney is identified by applying pressure to the transducer.
In some cases, the duodenum and liver may also be seen.

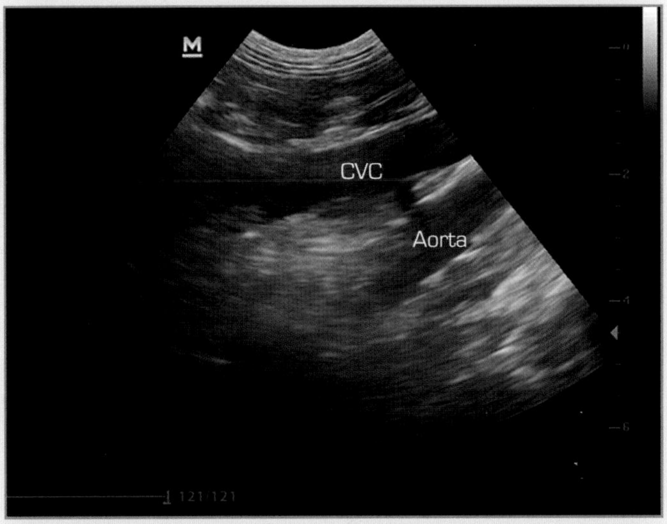

Figure 7. Fanning your transducer upwards, after the right kidney has been identified and the cranial pole has been placed in the middle of the screen, allows identification of the caudal vena cava (CVC). A second large vessel is visible on the screen below the CVC; it is the aorta.

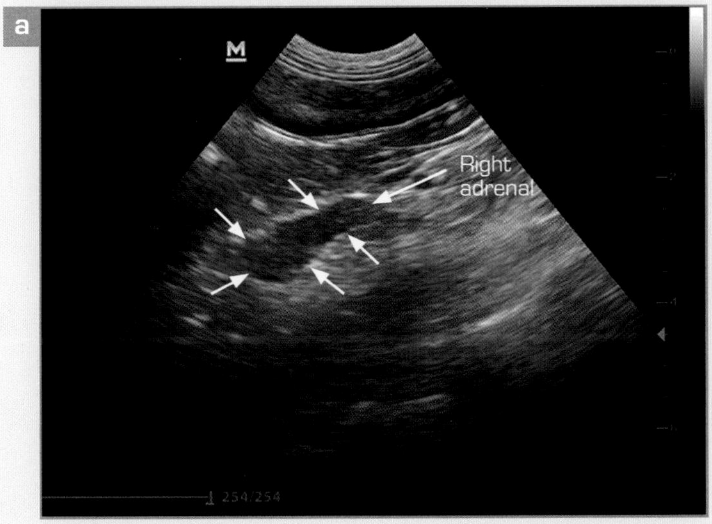

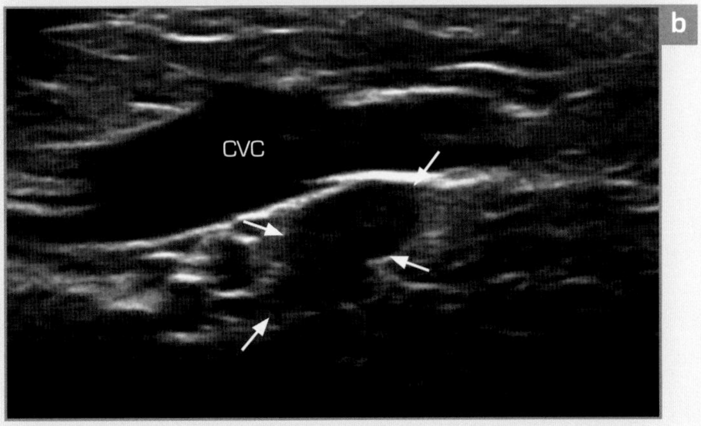

Figure 8. (a) The "arrow-shaped" canine right adrenal is visible (between arrows). (b) Normal feline right adrenal (between arrows). CVC: cauda vena cava.

Large and giant-breed dogs

The animal is positioned in left lateral recumbency with the head towards the ultrasound machine. The hair is clipped at the level of the right kidney (last two intercostal spaces and slightly behind the last rib, just ventral to the spine); the clipped area is extended ventrally to the mid abdomen.

1. With the transducer in a dorsal orientation, parallel to the spine, and the transducer marker pointing to the head, the right kidney is identified (Fig. 9).

2. Slide the transducer ventrally until the caudal vena cava is identified (Fig. 10). Do not press too hard since that may collapse the caudal vena cava and make it difficult to see. Make sure the cauda vena cava is visible across the screen (if not, rotate the transducer to see the cauda vena cava across the screen before you continue to the next step).

3. Slightly fan the transducer dorsally towards the right kidney.

4. As soon as the caudal vena cava almost disappears from the screen, the right adrenal will appear, it looks like a "monkey nut" between the right kidney and the caudal vena cava (Fig. 11). If the transducer is placed behind the last rib pointing dorsally the right adrenal will appear more arrow-shaped.

5. When the right adrenal is identified, the transducer is rotated to evaluate the adrenal in full length.

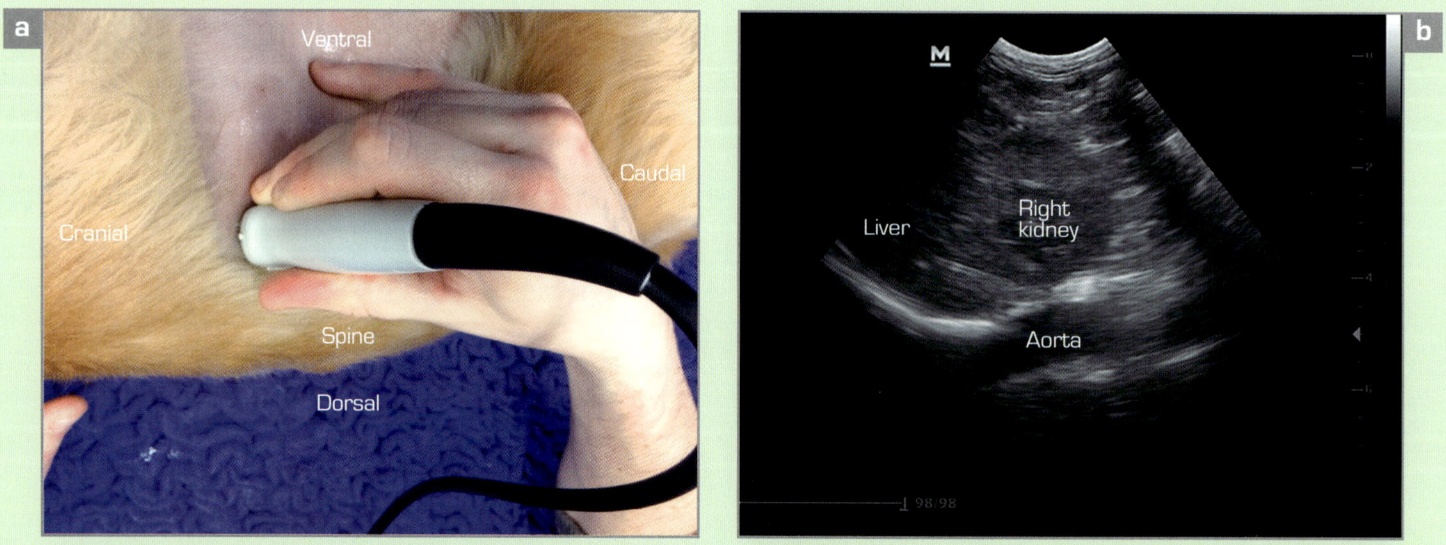

Figure 9. (a) The transducer is positioned in dorsal orientation, parallel to the spine, with the transducer marker pointing to the head. (b) The right kidney and the aorta below are visible after the transducer is positioned as in (a). Some dorsal fanning may be required to identify the aorta in some dogs.

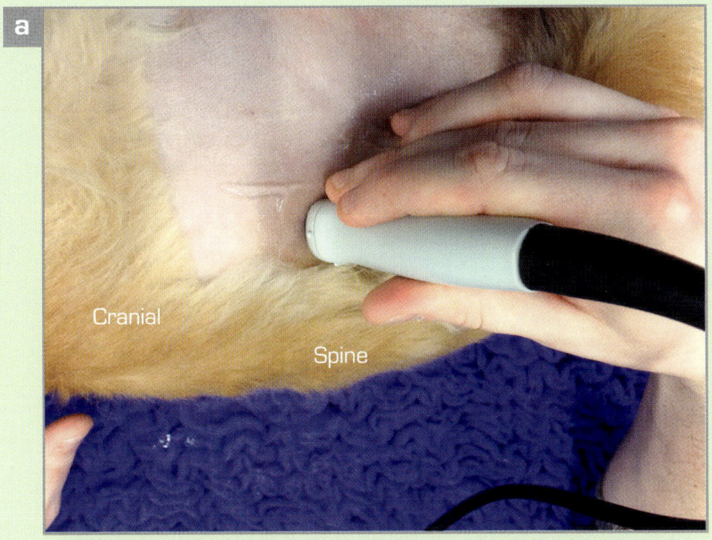

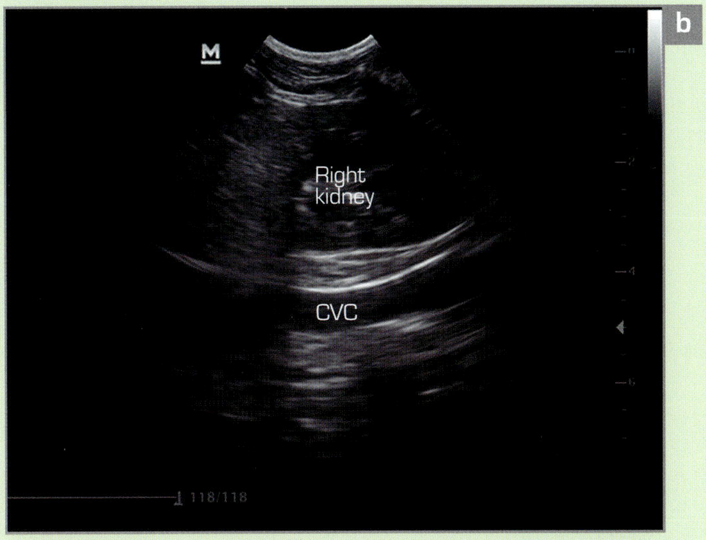

Figure 10. **(a)** The transducer is fanned ventrally while maintaining the same orientation. **(b)** The caudal vena cava (CVC) is identified below the kidney on the screen.

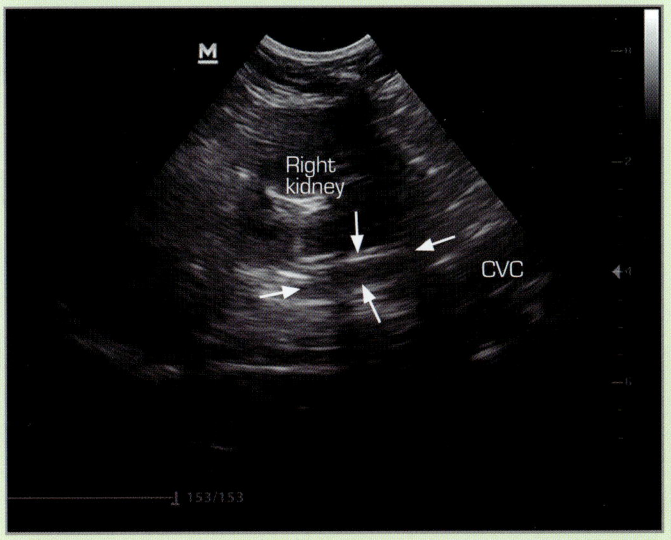

Figure 11. The right adrenal, oblong in shape, is visible between the right kidney and the caudal vena cava (CVC).

Normal appearance

The normal adrenals appear hypoechoic to the surrounding fat (see Figs. 4, 8 and 11). With a high frequency transducer, the junction between the cortex and the medulla can be identified as a thin hyperechoic line. In some situations, the cortex can be clearly distinguished from the medulla, the cortex being hypoechoic to the medulla.

The left adrenal and the right adrenal (when viewed with the technique described for large and giant dogs) appear elongated and bilobed in shape, resembling a monkey nut. The technique for small and medium-sized dogs is used for the right adrenal, which appears arrow-shaped (some describe it as wedge-shaped or comma-shaped). The phrenicoabdominal artery and vein run dorsally and ventrally to the mid body of the each adrenal gland, respectively.

Reference values have been reported for the normal size of the canine adrenals. The maximum diameter of the left adrenal has been reported to range from 3 to 16 mm, while the maximum diameter for the right adrenal has been reported to measure between 3 and 14 mm.

The maximum diameter of the caudal pole of the adrenal gland appears to be the most reliable measurement in size.

The size of 7.4 mm as the maximum normal measurement has been reported to offer a reasonable combination of sensitivity and specificity. The measurements for the adrenals considered normal by the author are as follows:

- **Small dogs**: maximum diameter of the caudal pole of the adrenal up to 8 mm.
- **Medium-sized dogs**: maximum diameter of the caudal pole of the adrenal up to 10 mm.
- **Large and giant breeds of dogs**: maximum diameter of the caudal pole of the adrenal up to 12 mm.

In cats, the adrenals have been reported to have a maximum diameter 4.6 to 5.3 mm. The author considers normal a maximum diameter of up to 6 mm for the caudal pole of the adrenals in cats.

Both poles of the adrenals should be similar, but not necessarily identical, in size.

Table 1. Appearance of the adrenals and possible causes.

Adrenal appearance	Consider
Normal adrenals	Normal gland Pituitary dependent hyperadrenocorticism
Uniformly, bilaterally enlarged adrenals	Pituitary dependent hyperadrenocorticism
Mass in one on both adrenals	Adrenal neoplasia
Adrenal mineralisation	Adrenal neoplasia Incidental finding in cats
Small or difficult to find or having a maximum diameter of less than 3.2 mm	Addison's disease Exogenous steroid administration
Adrenals not visible	Scanning technique Addison's disease Exogenous steroid administration

Variations from normal

- A normal appearance and size of the adrenals do not exclude the possibility of pituitary-dependent hyperadrenocorticism (PDH).

- Bilaterally enlarged adrenals, with symmetrical enlargement of both the cranial and caudal poles, are indicative of pituitary-dependent hyperadrenocorticism. Pituitary-dependent hyperadrenocorticism accounts for approximately 80 % of dogs with hyperadrenocorticism (Fig. 12).

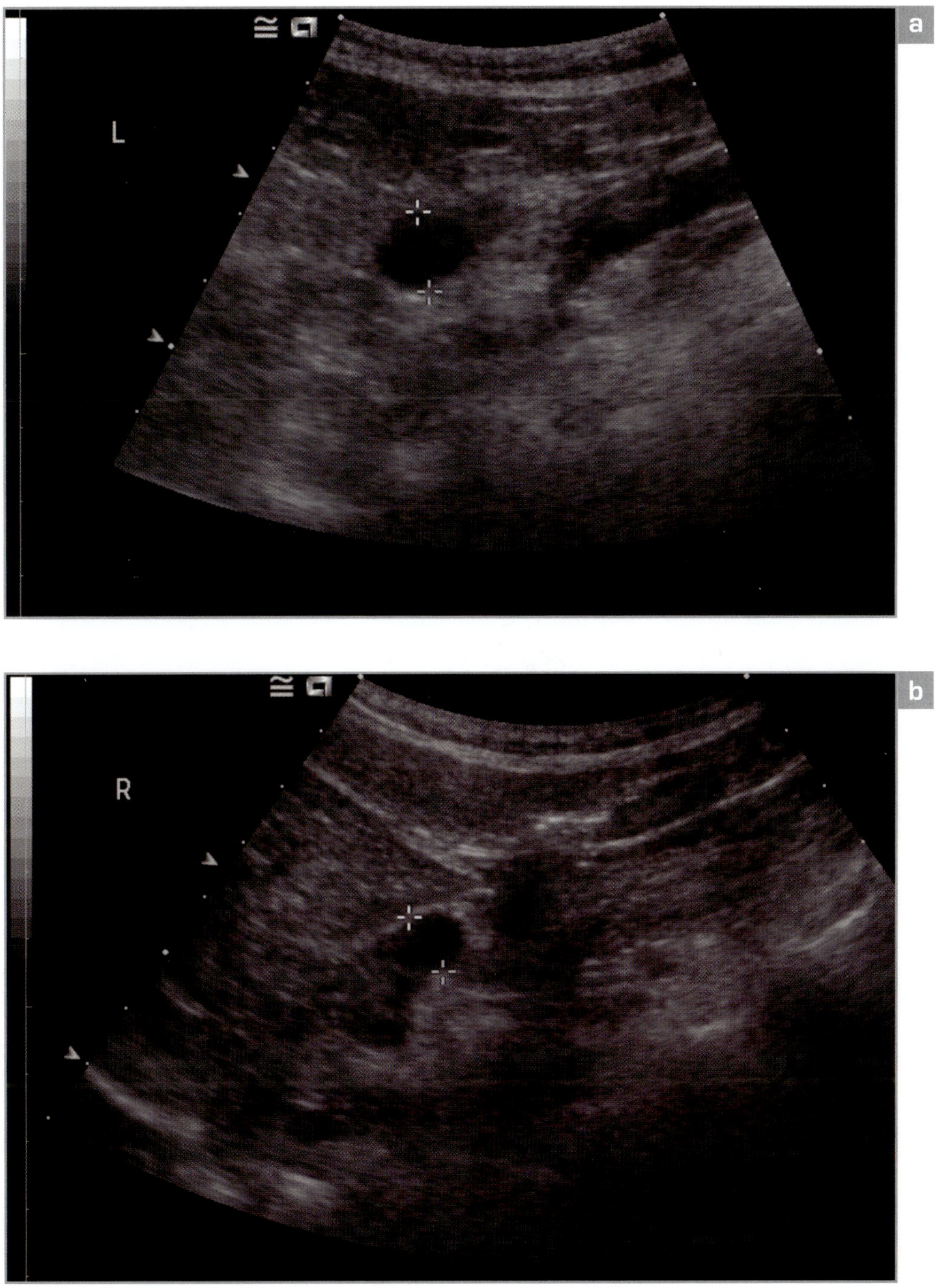

Figure 12. The caudal pole of a symmetrically enlarged left **(a)** and enlarged right **(b)** adrenal in a dog with pituitary-dependent hyperadreno- corticism. Both adrenal glands are enlarged; however, they have maintained their shape.

- If one adrenal is enlarged or contains a nodule or mass, and the contralateral adrenal is difficult to identify or it appears small or normal in size, this is suggestive of adrenal neoplasia (Fig. 13). Hyperadrenocorticism caused by a functional adrenal tumour accounts for approximately 20 % of dogs with naturally occurring hyperadrenocorticism. In some cases, a nodule or mass can be identified in both adrenals. This can be compatible with bilateral adrenal neoplasia. In the cases of adrenal neoplasia the invasion into the surrounding vessels is possible, especially the aorta for the left adrenal and the caudal vena cava for the right adrenal (Fig. 14) and should be assessed. Solid lesions with diameter more than 2 cm generally indicate neoplasia (benign or malignant). Lesions more than 4 cm in diameter usually indicate malignant neoplasia

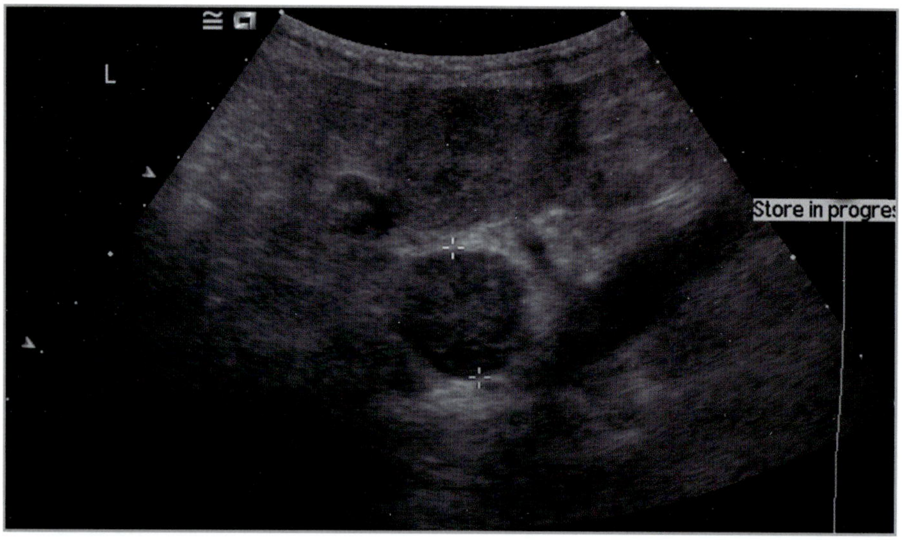

Figure 13. Left adrenal pheochromocytoma in a dog. A large, mixed echogenicity mass has replaced the left adrenal.

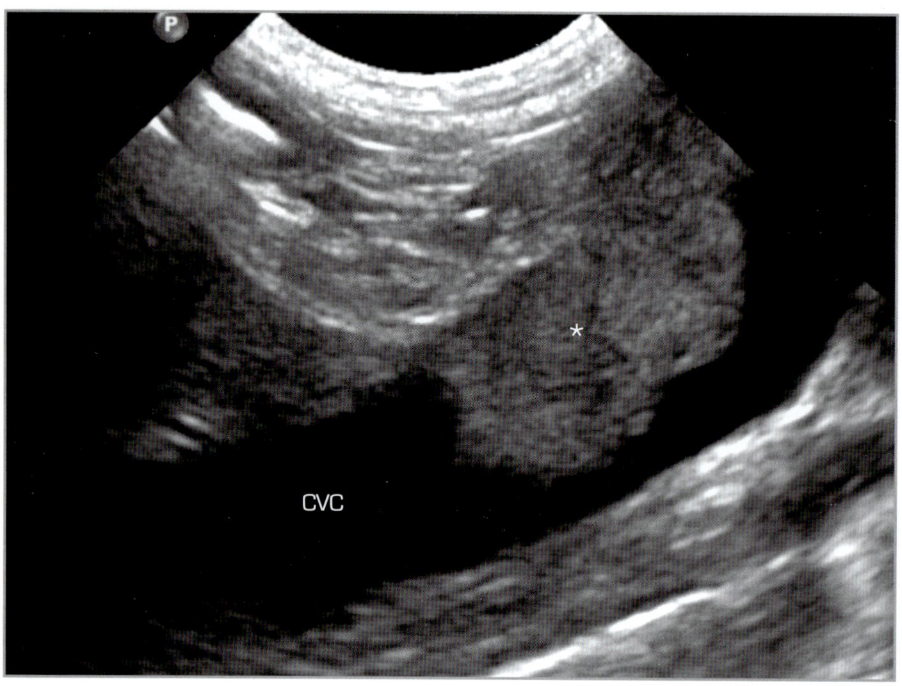

Figure 14. Right adrenal mass invading (*) the Cauda Vena Cava (CVC) in a 15-year-old English Springer Spaniel.

- Adrenal nodules and masses can be found unexpectedly and create a diagnostic dilemma. Some call them "incidentalomas". Reported diagnoses with "incidentalomas" include normal adrenal, cortical tumor (non-functioning), granulomas, adrenal cysts, myelolipoma (Fig. 15), haemorrhage, metastatic tumour, and phaeochromocytoma.

- In dogs with hyperadrenocorticism secondary to exogenous steroid administration, the adrenal glands may be difficult to identify, not visible, or smaller than normal.

- Adrenal mineralisation (hyperechoic shadowing area within the adrenal gland) is suggestive of neoplasia in the dog, although it may also be seen associated with benign lesions. Adrenal mineralisation is an incidental finding in cats (Fig. 16).

- Addison's disease cannot be diagnosed ultrasonographically. A reduction in the thickness and length of the adrenal glands compared with those of normal dogs has been shown. In a dog with clinical and laboratory findings compatible with Addison's disease, difficulty in identifying the adrenals and/or the adrenals having a maximum diameter of less than 3.2 mm should be considered suggestive of Addison's disease (Fig. 17). In cats with clinical suspicion, normal appearing adrenals on ultrasound examination do not exclude hypoadrenocorticism.

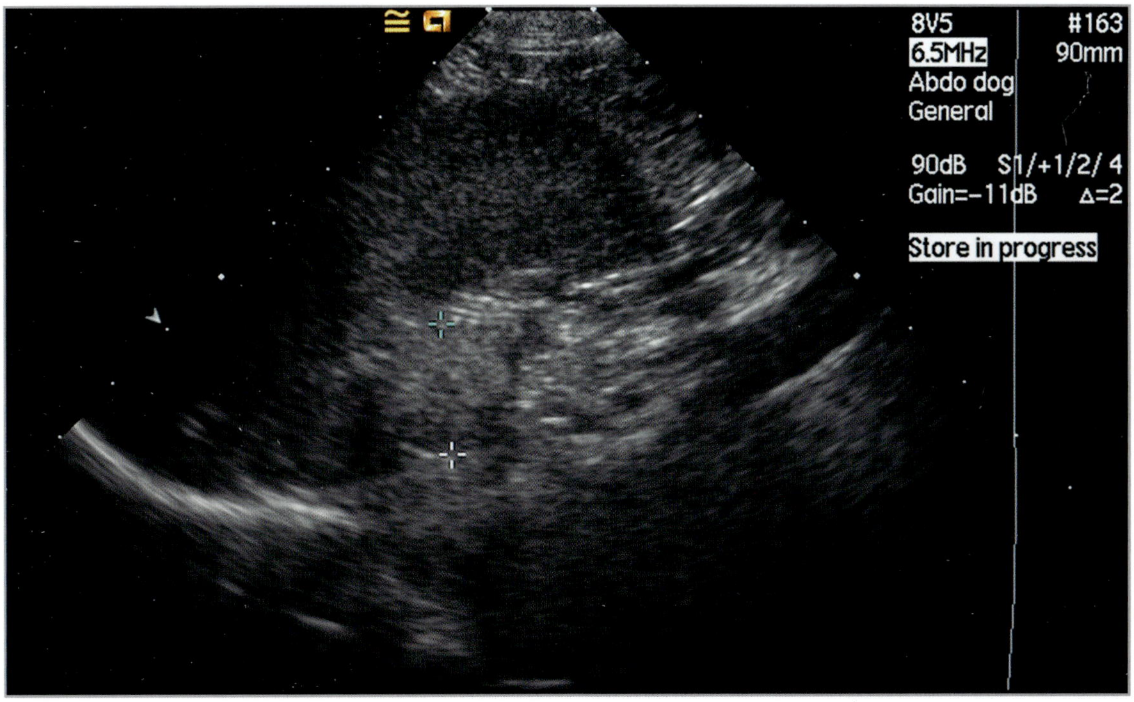

Figure 15. Confirmed myelolipoma in the cranial pole of the left adrenal for a 10-year-old Cocker Spaniel.

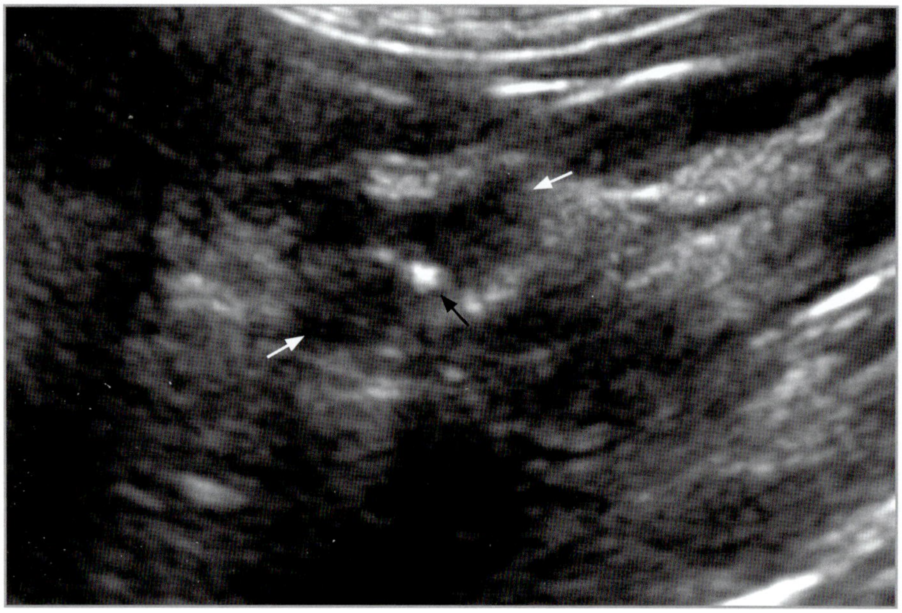

Figure 16. Incidental mineralised focus (black arrow) in the right adrenal (white arrows) of a cat.

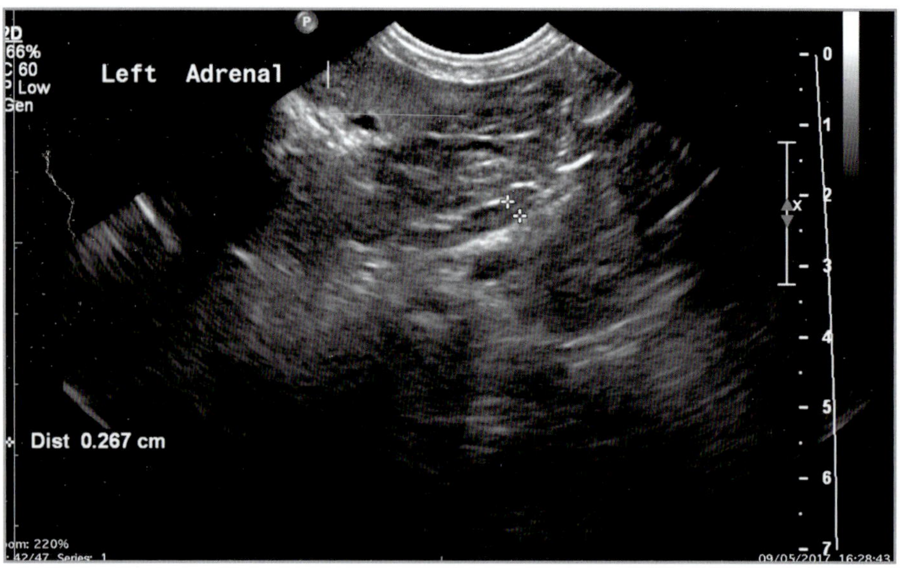

Figure 17. Reduced thickness (less than 3.2 mm thick) of the left adrenal in a 13-year-old terrier with Addison's disease.

10

CHAPTER

URINARY BLADDER AND URETHRA

Scanning technique

A high-frequency transducer is required to examine the urinary bladder. Usually, a 7–10 MHz transducer is adequate for dogs and cats.

1. Position the animal in right lateral recumbency with the head towards the ultrasound machine and the limbs towards the examiner.

2. Ask the assistant to lift the left hind limb towards him/her, after flexing the stifle joint (Fig. 1).

3. To locate the urinary bladder, place the transducer on the caudal abdomen with the marker towards the head of the animal (Fig. 2). A small or intrapelvic bladder may not be visible. If the urinary bladder cannot be identified, slide the transducer caudally, fanning and rocking the transducer until it is located.

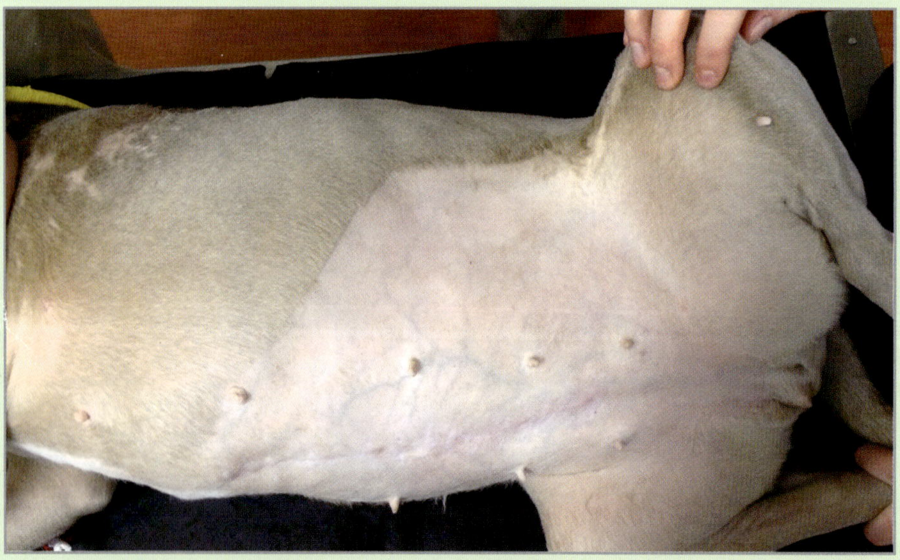

Figure 1. Positioning for the examination of the urinary bladder. The animal is in right lateral recumbency. Lifting of the non-recumbent hind limb, after flexing the stifle joint, helps with the placement of the transducer.

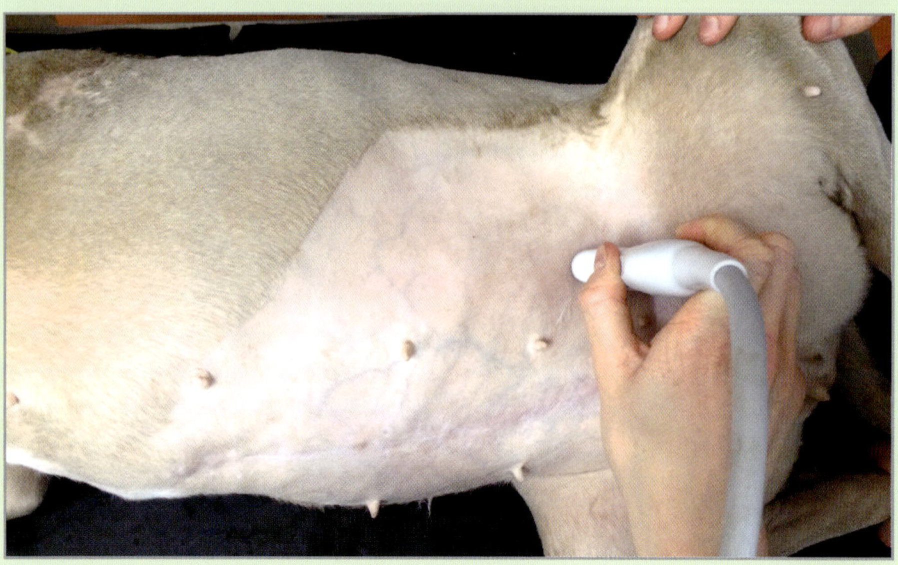

Figure 2. Initial transducer placement for the assessment of the urinary bladder. The marker of the transducer is pointing to the head of the animal.

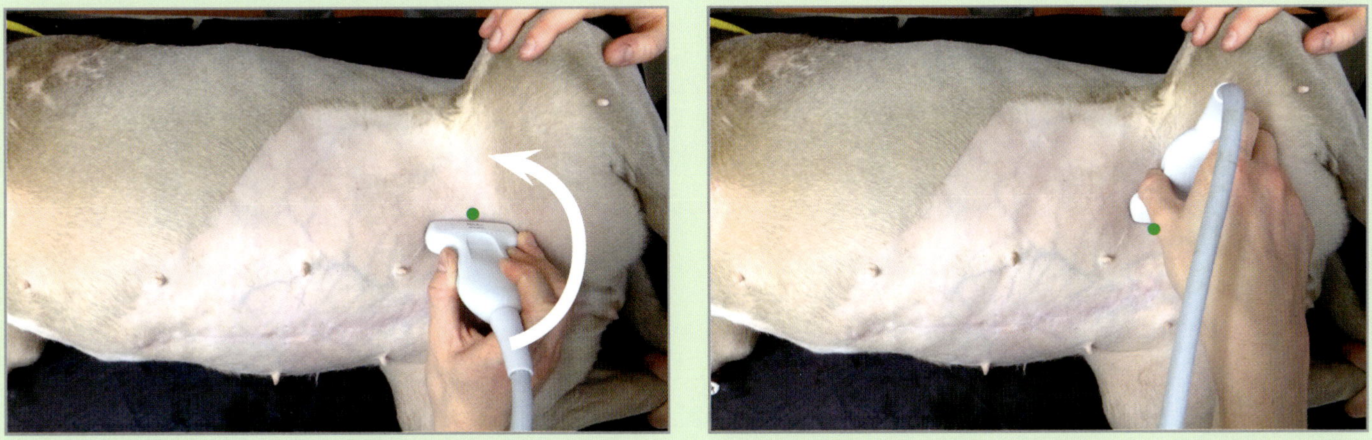

Figure 3. Fanning motion for the evaluation of the urinary bladder in a longitudinal plane. The transducer is fanned to the left and right until the urinary bladder is seen all the way through.

4. After identifying the urinary bladder, fan the transducer dorsally and then ventrally until the entire bladder has been examined (Fig. 3).

A side-lobe artefact (Fig. 4) is commonly seen and should not be confused with sediment.

5. Rotate the transducer 90° clockwise and fan it cranially and caudally until the entire bladder has been examined (Fig. 5).

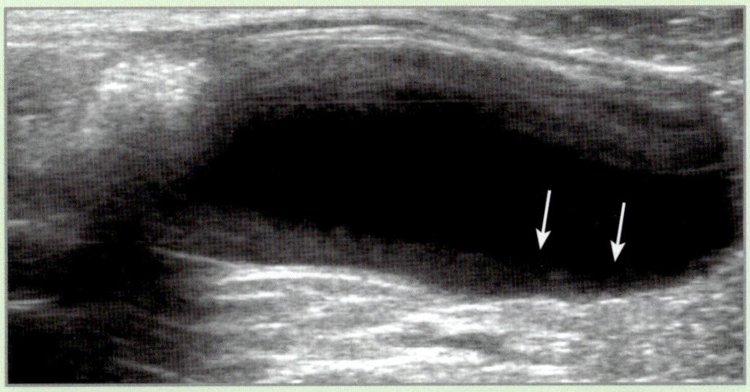

Figure 4. A side-lobe artefact (arrows) is visible in the urinary bladder. This artefact should not be confused with sediment (pseudosludge). Note how the artefact extends to the whole ventral urinary bladder.

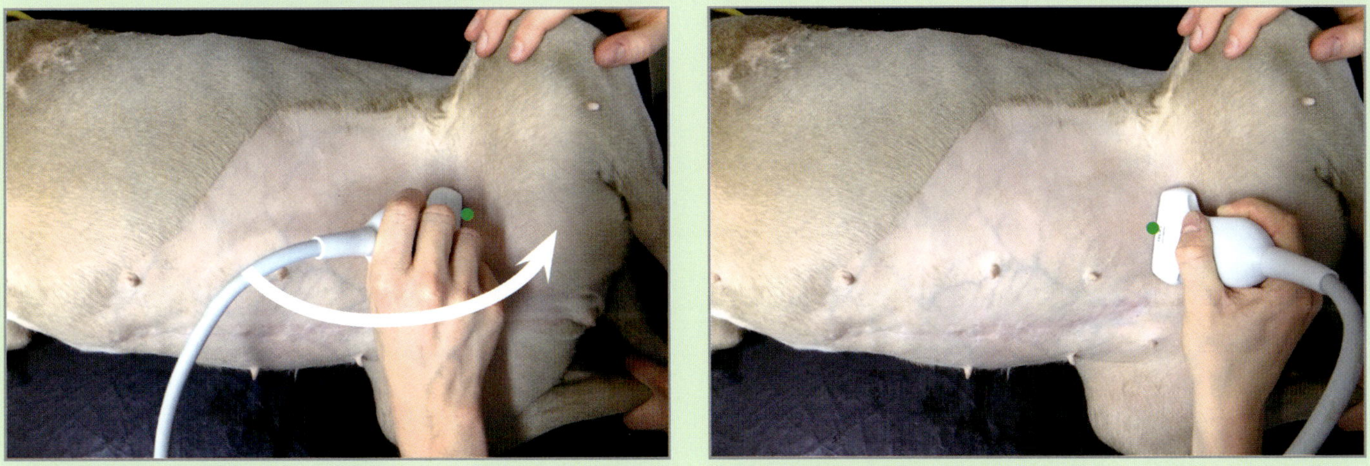

Figure 5. The urinary bladder is assessed in a transverse plane by rotating the transducer 90° clockwise and fanning cranially and caudally.

6. As you move the transducer, assess its lumen and wall, measuring the wall thickness (Fig. 6).

7. Orient your transducer in a vertical plane (perpendicular to the tabletop) with the marker pointing to the head of the animal. Place the transducer on the left lateral wall of the urinary bladder and evaluate its most dependent aspect (Fig. 7). Small dorsal and ventral sliding movements ensure comprehensive examination of the dependent aspect of the urinary bladder lumen.

8. If it is unclear as to whether a structure within the lumen is attached to the wall or floating within the lumen, turn the dog over into left lateral recumbency. Place the transducer perpendicular to the tabletop to assess the dependent aspect of the urinary bladder on the opposite side (Fig. 8). If the structure is free in the lumen, it will move to the dependent aspect.

Agitating the urine by applying external pressure to the urinary bladder can help demonstrate movement of the structure(s) visible in the lumen.

9. Slide the transducer caudally to examine the trigone of the urinary bladder and the cranial urethra. Try to follow the urethra caudally to the pelvis by sliding and/or rocking the transducer.

10. In male dogs, the penile urethra can also be examined. This is best achieved by using a linear transducer (Fig. 9) and a standoff pad (though light touch and a lot of gel is usually adequate).

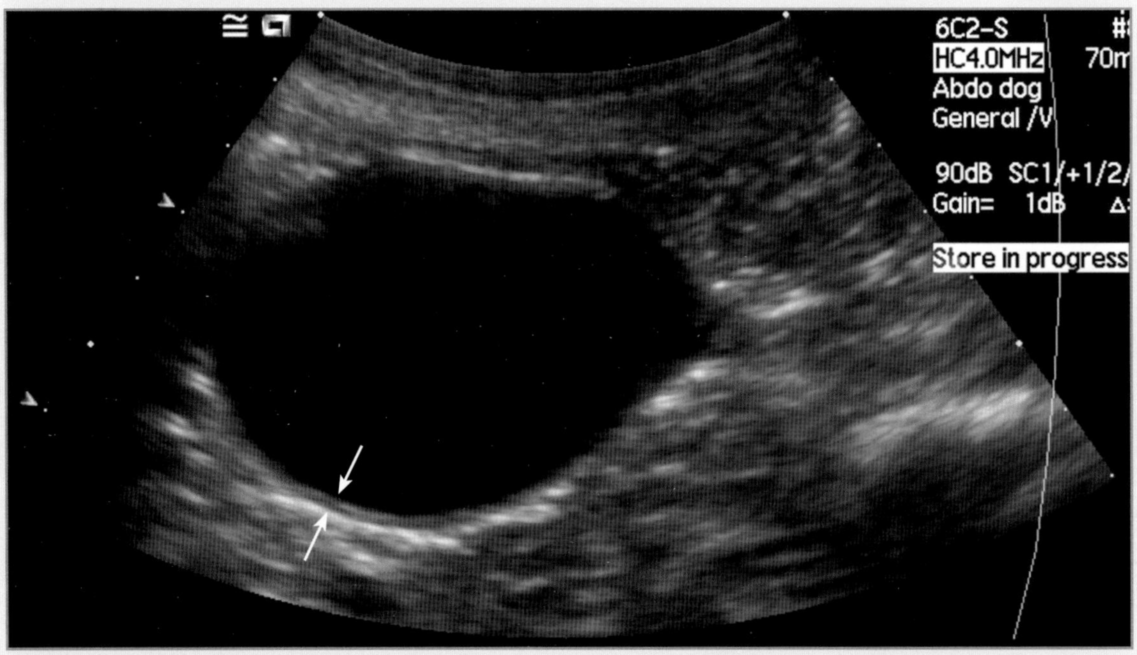

Figure 6. Normal ultrasonographic appearance of a canine urinary bladder. The urinary bladder wall (between arrows) has a normal thickness and uniform echogenicity. The wall layers are visible.

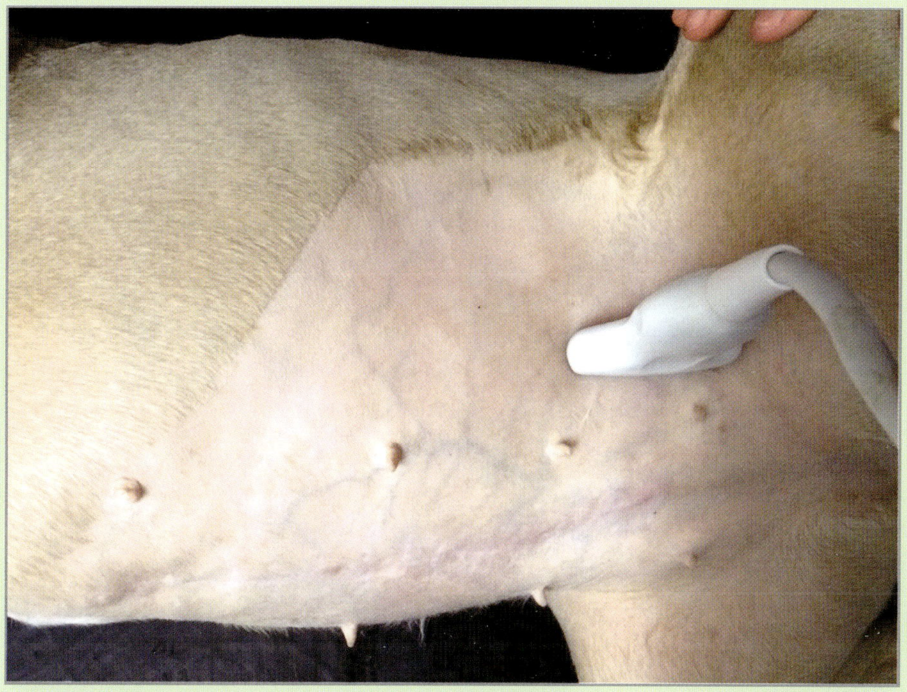

Figure 7. By orienting your transducer perpendicular to the table and placing it at the level of the urinary bladder, you can examine its dependent aspect. Sliding your transducer dorsally and ventrally allows assessment of the whole dependent aspect of the urinary bladder.

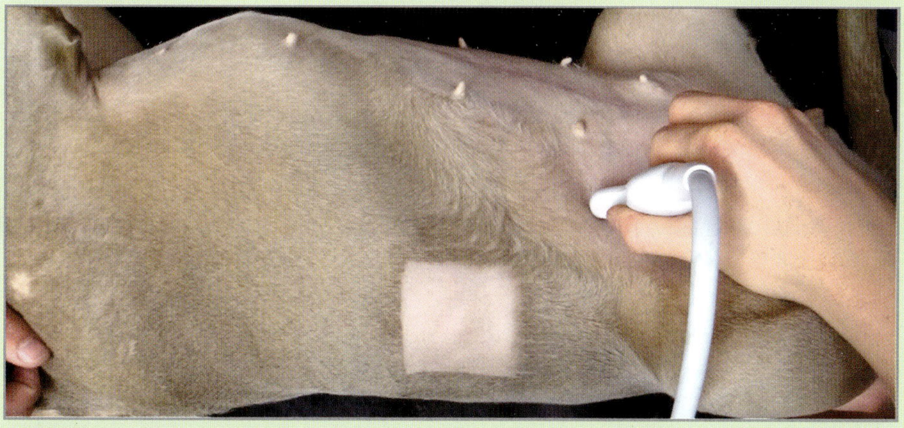

Figure 8. By turning the dog in left lateral recumbency you can evaluate if a structure is in the lumen of the urinary bladder or attached to the wall. If the structure is within the lumen it will drop to the dependent aspect; otherwise, it will stay in the same location.

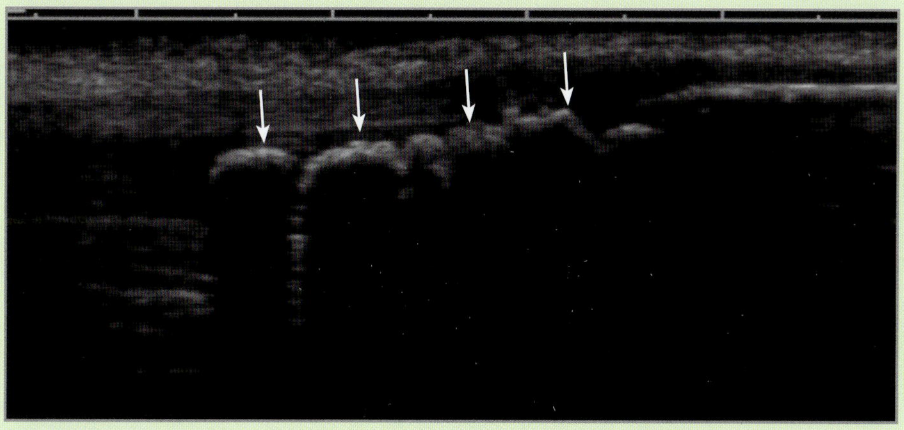

Figure 9. Ultrasound image of the penile urethra in a dog presenting with urethral calculi (arrows). Observe the distal acoustic shadowing below the calculi.

Normal appearance

The urinary bladder contains urine, which is normally anechoic.

The layers of the urinary bladder wall are difficult to identify; however, they may be distinguished according to their echogenicity (see Fig. 6): hypoechoic mucosa, hyperechoic submucosa, hypoechoic smooth muscle layers and hyperechoic serosa.

Although the layers of the urinary bladder wall are difficult to identify, the margins of the bladder wall are usually clearly visible.

The thickness of the urinary bladder wall varies depending on the degree of distension caused by urine and the weight of the patient. In dogs, the bladder wall has been reported to have an average thickness of approximately 1.4 to 2.3 mm in a moderately- to minimally- -distended urinary bladder, respectively. In cats, the urinary bladder wall has an average thickness of between 1.3 and 1.7 mm.

In the clinical setting, the author considers a uniform wall thickness of up to 2 mm to be normal in a full urinary bladder and up to 5 mm in an empty bladder (in both dogs and cats).

The distal ureters are usually difficult to identify unless they are dilated. The ureterovesicular junctions may be seen as small triangular projections in the caudal aspect of the urinary bladder (Fig. 10).

The ureteral jets of urine (expulsion of urine from the ureters into the urinary bladder) can sometimes be seen exiting the ureterovesicular junctions as "bubbles" or "smoke" within the lumen of the urinary bladder (Fig. 11). Doppler ultrasound may be useful to identify these ureteral jets (Fig. 12).

Visualising the ureteral jets requires patience as it may take some time to see them. If not contraindicated, administration of an intravenous diuretic can aid in their identification.

The colon is dorsal to the urinary bladder, so care should be taken not to confuse the shadowing faeces in the colon with calculi in the urinary bladder (pseudocalculi) (Fig. 13).

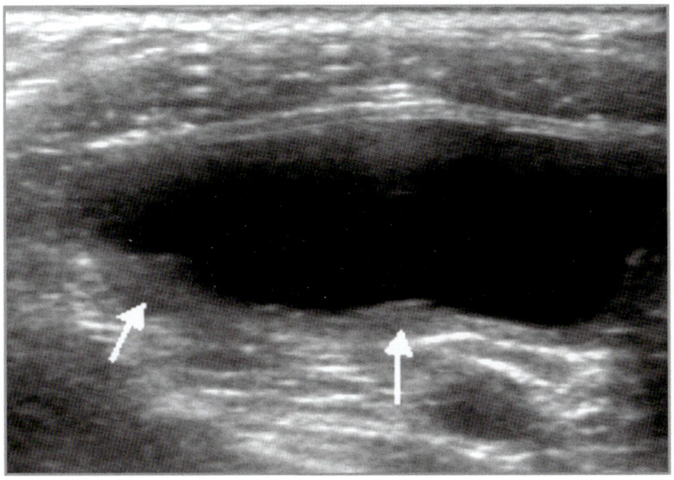

Figure 10. In dogs, the ureterovesicular junctions can be identified as small triangular projections (arrows) in the caudal aspect of the urinary bladder. Once identified, confirmation by visualisation of the ureteral jets is required.

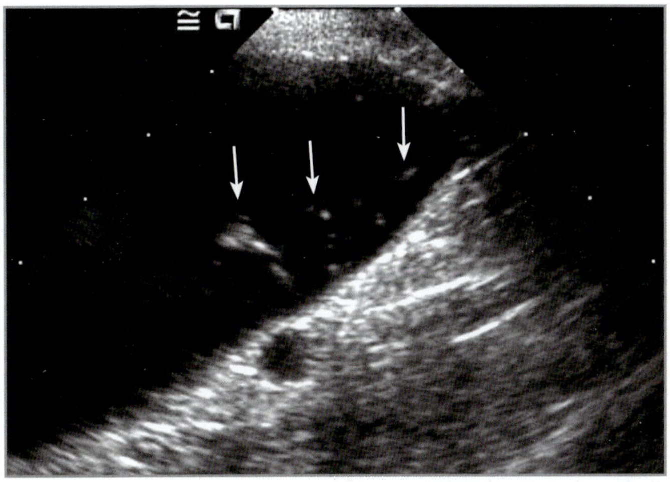

Figure 11. Ureterales jets appearing as echogenic "smoke" (arrows) in the caudal aspect of the urinary bladder in a dog.

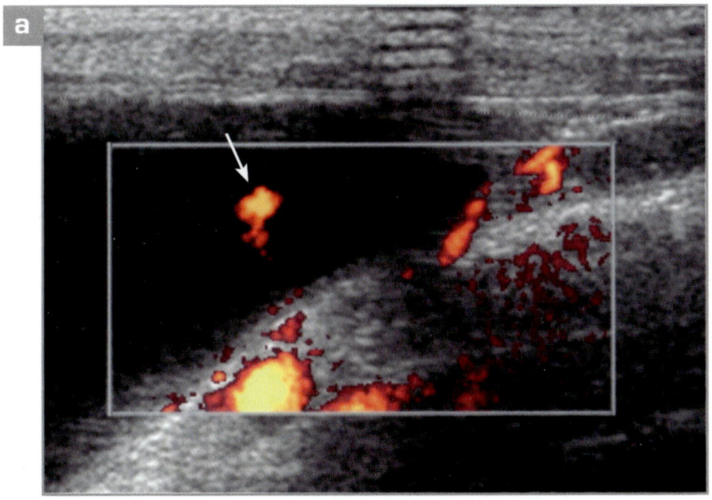

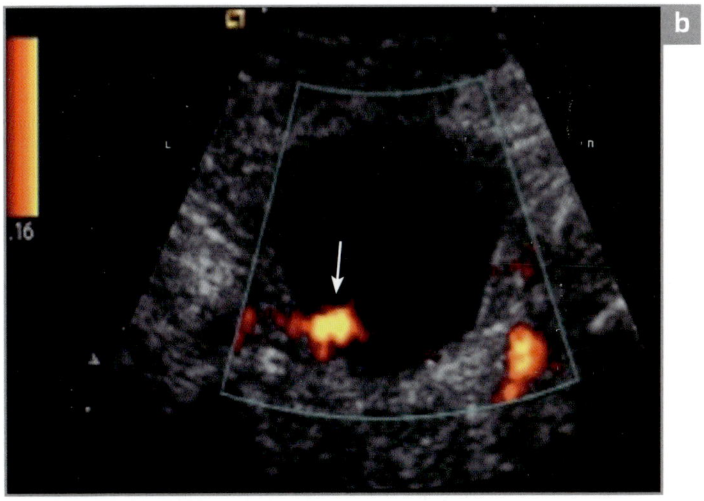

Figure 12. **(a)** Sagittal view of the urinary bladder in a dog. One ureteral jet (arrow) is visible within the bladder using power Doppler. **(b)** Transverse view of a canine urinary bladder at the level of the trigone area. Power Doppler has been used to identify the left ureteral jet (arrow).

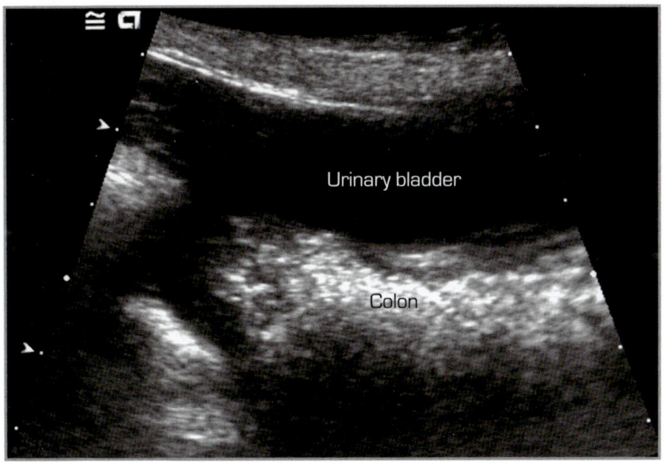

Figure 13. Faeces in the descending colon may be confused with calculi in the urinary bladder, especially when the transducer is placed in the ventral midline and the urinary bladder is not filled with urine.

Variations from normal

Cystitis typically appears as irregular thickening of the urinary bladder wall, more evident in its cranioventral region (Fig. 14). In polypoid cystitis, a pedunculated cauliflower-like mass or masses protrude from a thickened bladder wall into the lumen (Fig. 15). Emphysematous cystitis usually appears as multifocal hyperechoic interfaces with reverberation artefacts within the wall of the urinary bladder (Fig. 16).

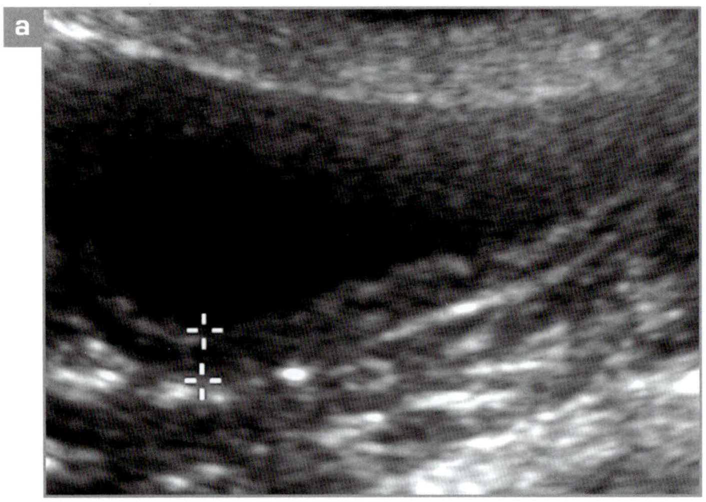

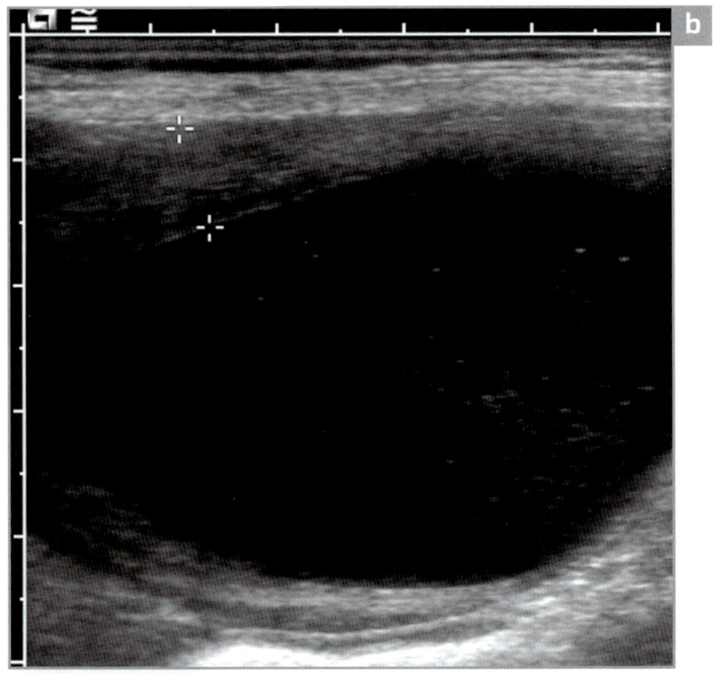

Figure 14. Thickened urinary bladder wall in a cat [a] and a dog [b] with cystitis. The urinary bladder wall (between callipers) is uneven and thick.

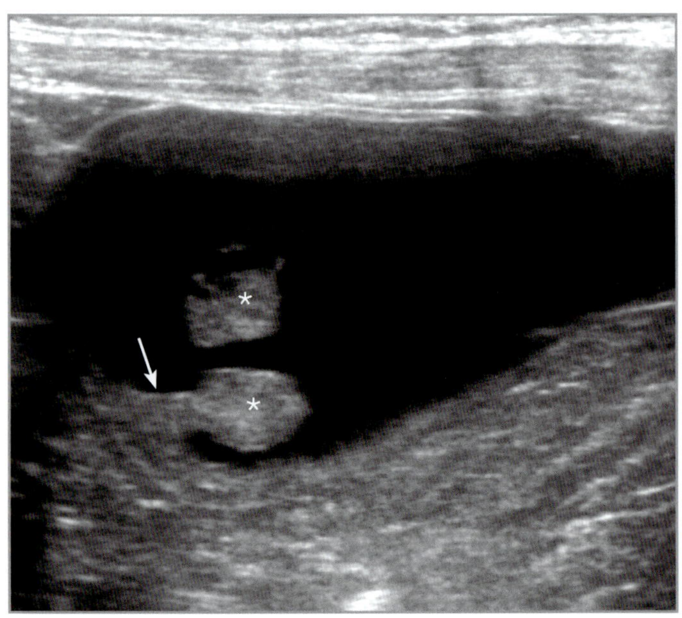

Figure 15. Pedunculated masses (*) in the urinary bladder of a dog with polypoid cystitis. Note the neck of the mass (arrow) which connects the pedunculated mass to the wall.

Calculi are commonly seen in the dependent aspect of the urinary bladder and the urethra. Ultrasonographically, they appear as hyperechoic interfaces with distal acoustic shadowing, regardless of their composition (Figs. 9 and 17). The faeces in the descending colon may be confused with calculi (pseudocalculi), especially if the transducer is placed on the ventral midline and/or the urinary bladder is relatively empty (see Fig. 13). Moving the transducer towards the lateral aspect usually helps to differentiate them from true calculi.

Repositioning the animal or letting the animal stand up can also help to differentiate faeces in the colon from calculi in the urinary bladder

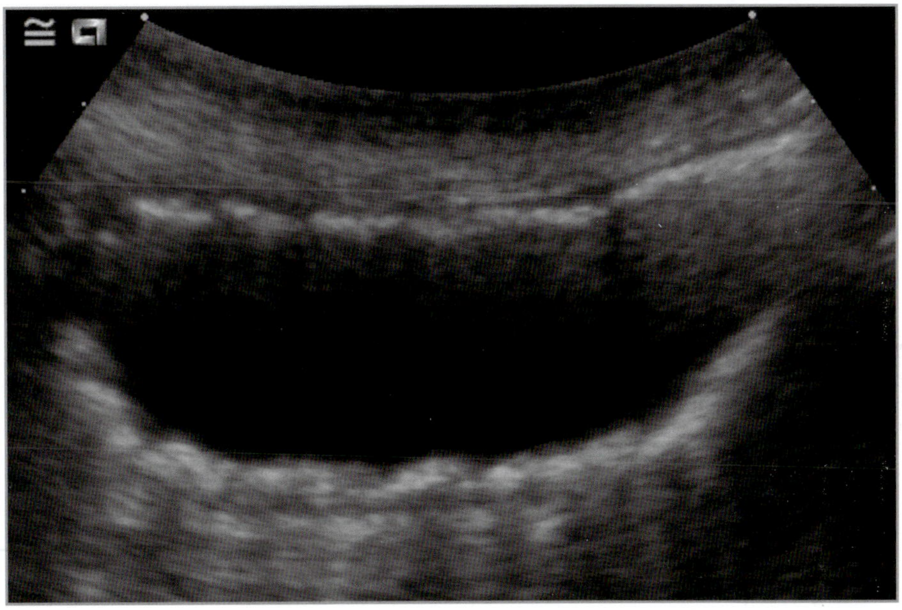

Figure 16. Emphysematous cystitis in a dog. Multifocal hyperechoic interfaces with reverberation artefacts are visible in the urinary bladder wall.

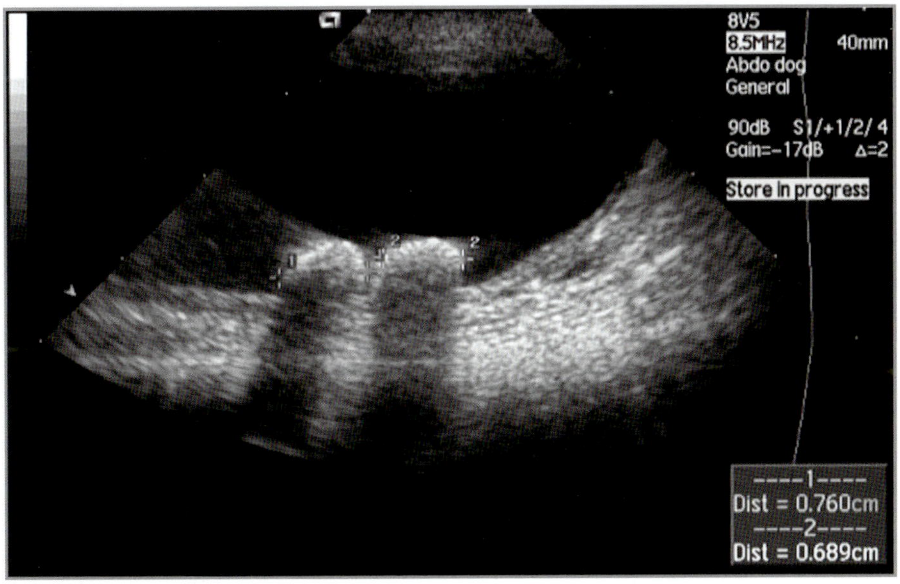

Figure 17. Two urinary calculi (between callipers) are visible on the dependent aspect of the urinary bladder in a dog. Note the distal acoustic shadowing.

Blood clots in the lumen of the urinary bladder are generally hyperechoic to the urinary bladder wall and can have variable shapes (Fig. 18). If attached to the wall, Doppler ultrasound can help to differentiate blood clots from bladder wall masses. Foreign bodies, like retained catheters, may be found in the urinary bladder. Catheters appear as parallel echogenic lines.

Ectopic ureters (Fig. 19; see Fig. 24 in Chapter 8), urachal diverticulum, patent urachus, urachal cysts and ureterocoeles (Fig. 20; see Fig. 25 in Chapter 8) can also be identified using ultrasonography.

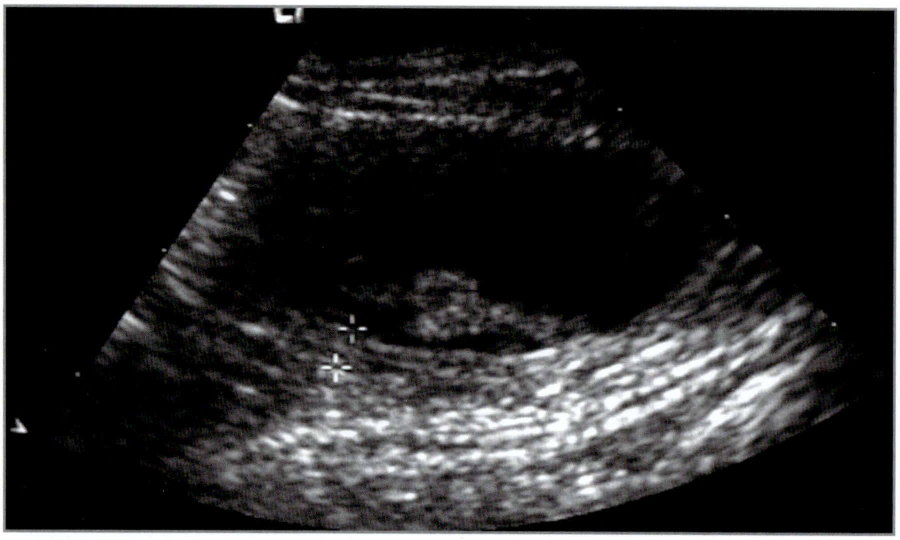

Figure 18. Cystitis in a cat. The urinary bladder wall (between callipers) is thick. An irregular echogenic blood clot is visible in the lumen.

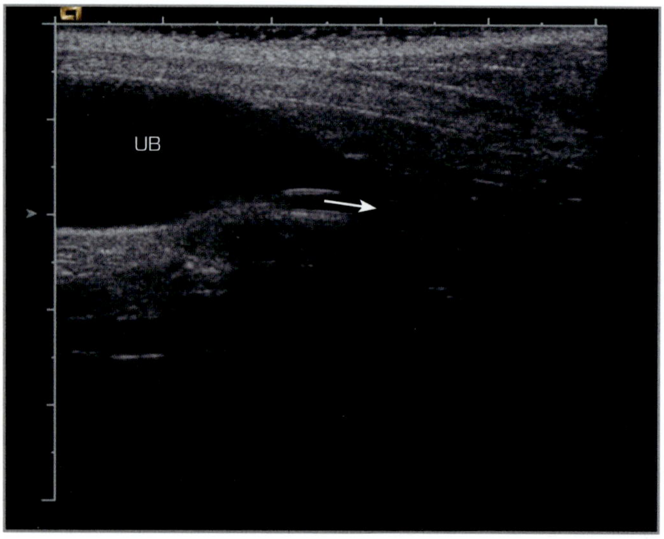

Figure 19. Ectopic ureter in a dog. The ureter (arrow) appears to bypass the urinary bladder (UB) terminating in the beginning of the urethra.

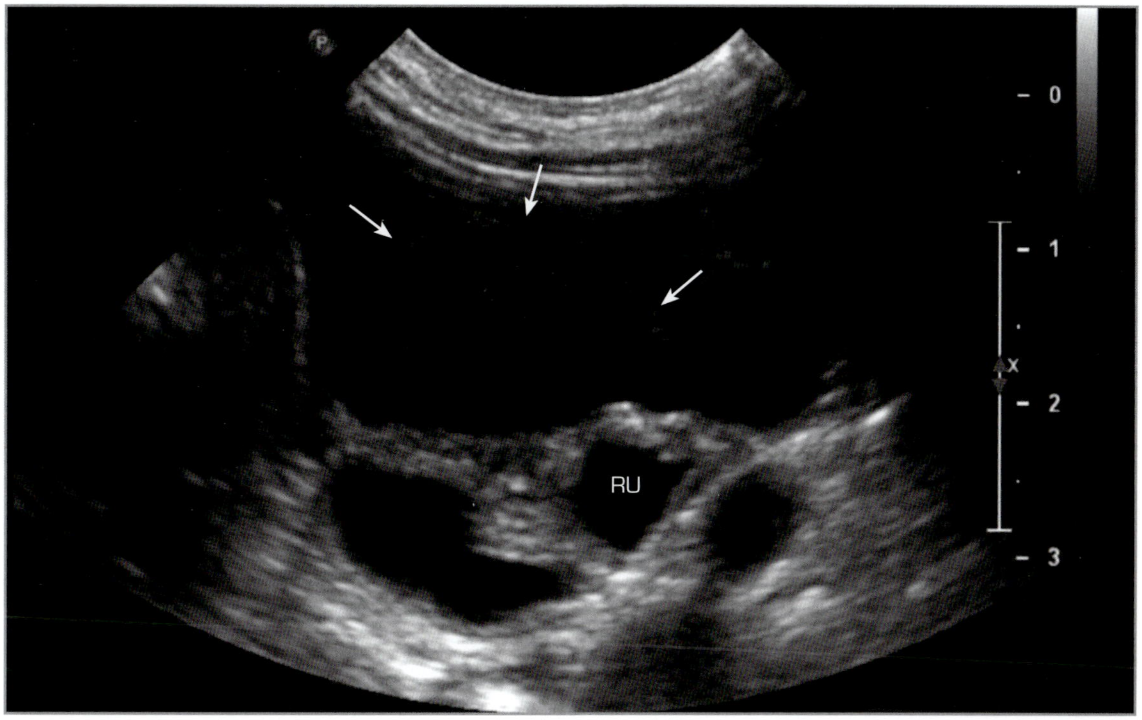

Figure 20. Ureterocoele in an 8-month-old, female, golden retriever associated with a dilated ectopic right ureter (RU). A thin linear structure (arrows) is visible dorsally within the urinary bladder lumen near the bladder neck.

Transitional cell carcinoma commonly appears as an irregular mass of mixed echogenicity (it may also be hypoechoic or hyperechoic to the bladder wall) within the wall of the bladder trigone (Fig. 21). The mass can extend into the proximal urethra. Transitional cell carcinomas may obstruct ureteral flow, resulting in hydroureter (unilateral or bilateral). Other tumours such as squamous cell carcinoma may also be identified. Urinary bladder tumours rarely affect the whole bladder wall. Urethral tumours, such as transitional cell carcinomas, adenocarcinomas and squamous cell carcinomas, may also extend into the urinary bladder (Fig. 22) and/or prostate.

A ruptured urinary bladder wall may be suspected especially in animals with ascites and interruption of the urinary bladder wall. A ruptured urinary bladder is best diagnosed with positive contrast cystography. On ultrasound an interrupted urinary bladder wall, especially when the urinary bladder appears full, may be secondary to refraction artefact.

> The type of many bladder or urethral tumour cannot be determined based solely on its ultrasonographic appearance.

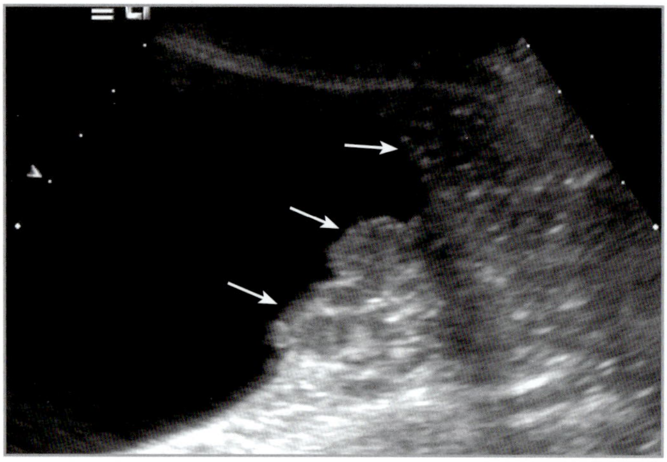

Figure 21. Transitional cell carcinoma in the urinary bladder in a dog (arrows). The urinary bladder wall is thick and irregular in the area of the mass.

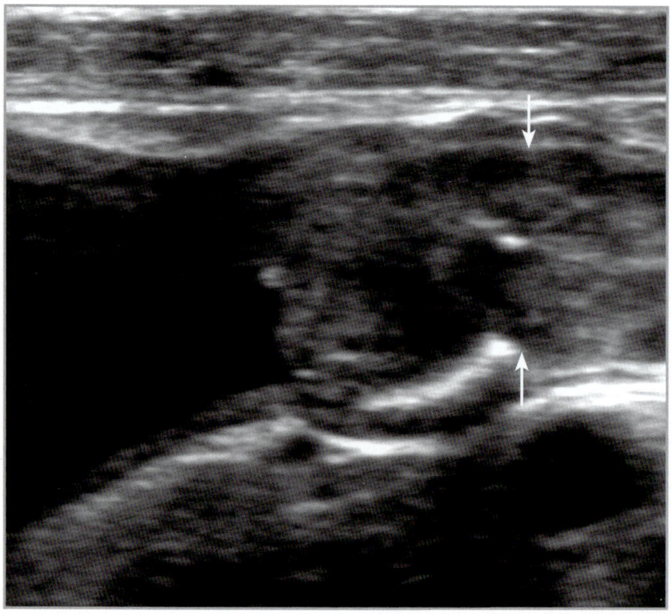

Figure 22. Transitional cell carcinoma (between arrows) in a dog originating from the urethra and extending to the urinary bladder.

11

CHAPTER

PERITONEAL CAVITY, LYMPH NODES AND MAJOR ABDOMINAL VESSELS

Scanning technique

The examination of the peritoneal cavity and lymph nodes is usually performed along with the gastrointestinal tract. Thus, the visible mesentery and any lymph nodes identified are assessed while scanning across the abdomen in a "castle" pattern (Fig. 1).

A 7–10 MHz transducer is adequate for small dogs and cats. For larger dogs, frequencies between 5–7 MHz should be used. A lower-frequency transducer is also appropriate for patients with peritonitis, due to the increased attenuation of the ultrasound beam.

As many of the lymph nodes are small-sized and, therefore, difficult to identify, the following assumptions are usually made:

- If lymph nodes are seen during the routine examination of the gastrointestinal tract, then they are evaluated.
- If lymph nodes are not identified during the routine examination, they are considered within normal limits.

The only lymph nodes that are regularly identified and evaluated during a routine abdominal examination are the medial iliac lymph nodes at the aortic bifurcation.

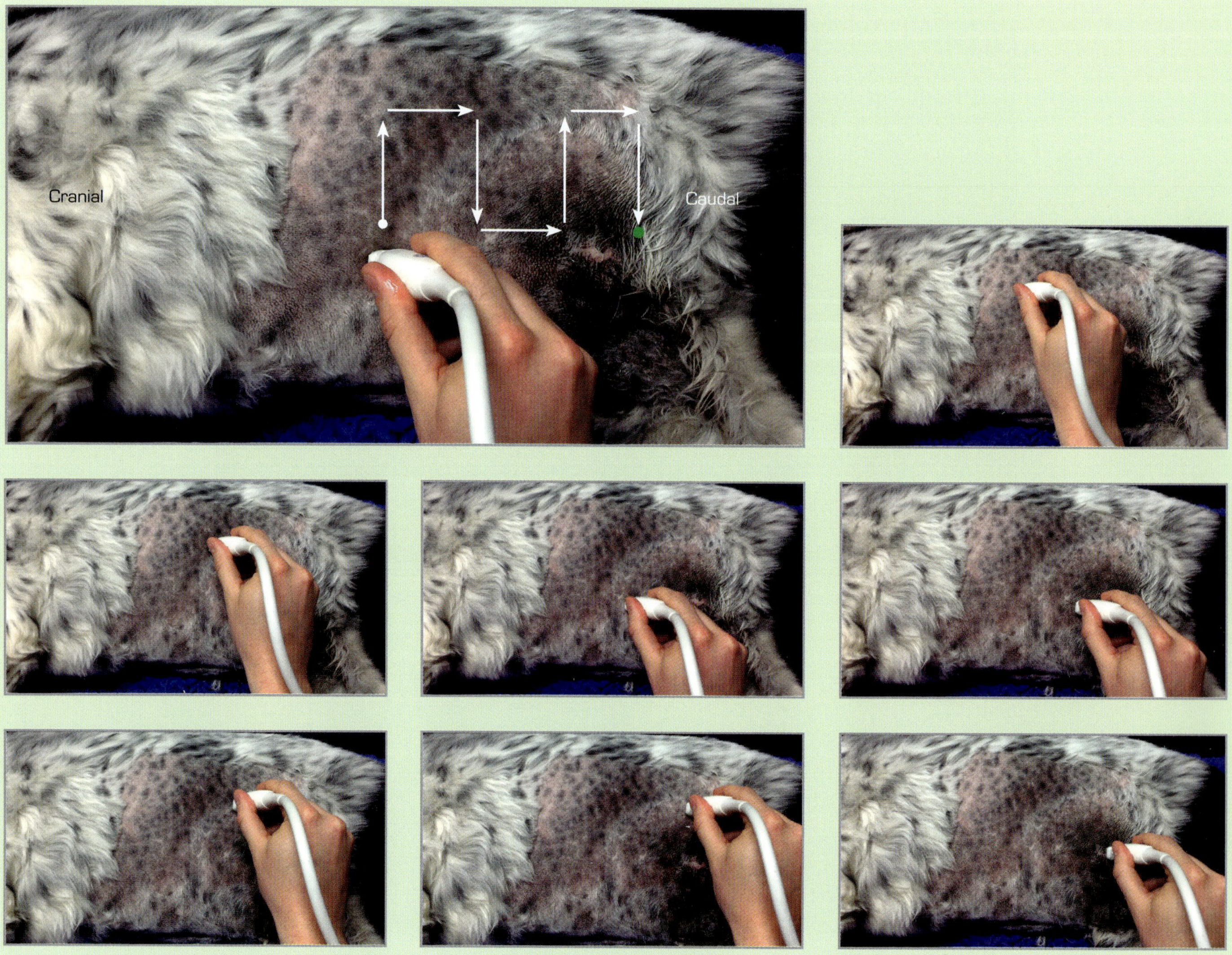

Figure 1. The "castle pattern" to evaluate the gastrointestinal tract is also used for the ultrasound examination of the peritoneum and lymph nodes.

Medial iliac lymph nodes

1. Position the animal in right lateral recumbency with the head towards the ultrasound machine and

2. Slide the transducer dorsally towards the spine (Fig. 2) to locate the aorta, which is the largest, most dorsal pulsating vessel visible on the screen. The caudal vena cava can be seen next to the aorta (Fig. 3a).

3. The medial iliac lymph nodes are seen at the level of the aortic bifurcation (Figs. 3b and 3c). They are often small and difficult to see. However, when enlarged or abnormally shaped, they are much more conspicuous (Fig. 4) and are often clearly visible.

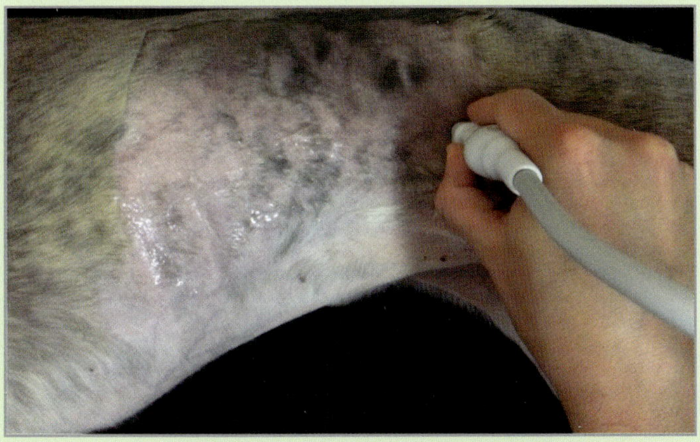

Figure 2. Transducer position for the assessment of the aortic bifurcation. From the urinary bladder, slide the transducer dorsally until the aorta and aortic bifurcation are identified below the lumbar spine.

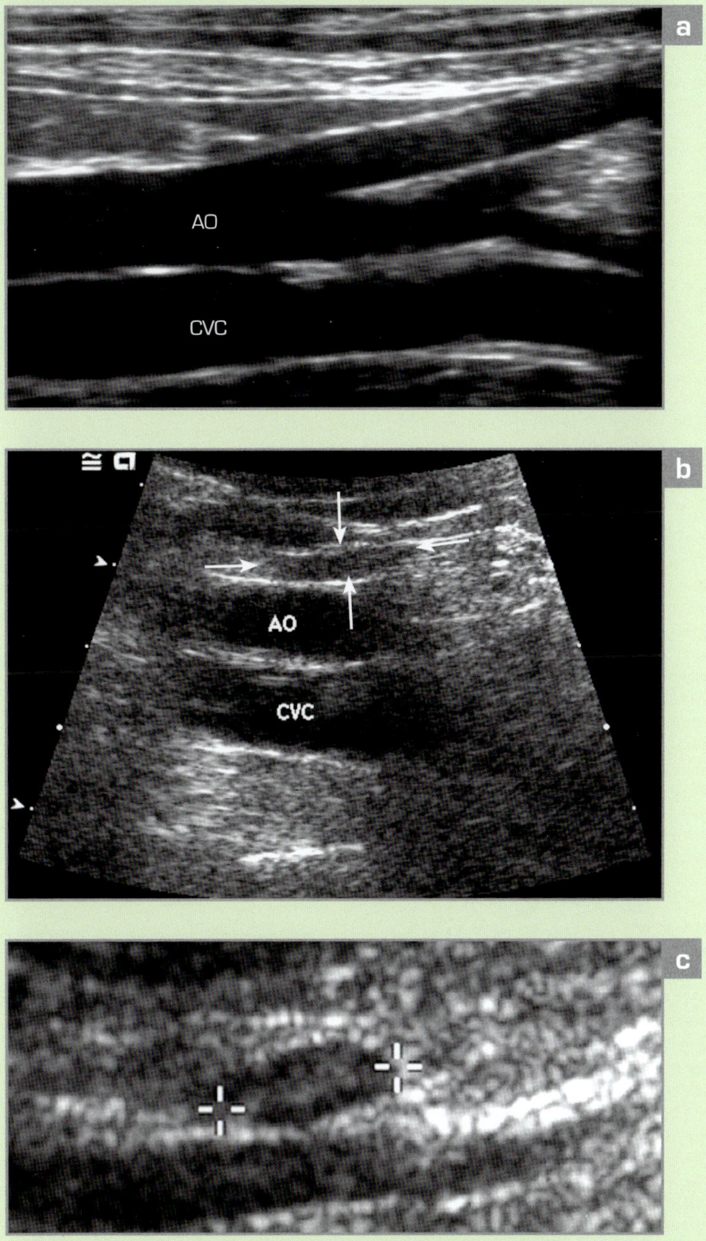

Figure 3. Aortic bifurcation. (a) The caudal vena cava (CVC) is visible near the aorta (AO). (b) A normal medial iliac lymph node (between arrows). (c) Close-up image of a normal lymph node. Note the hypoechoic cortex and the hyperechoic medulla.

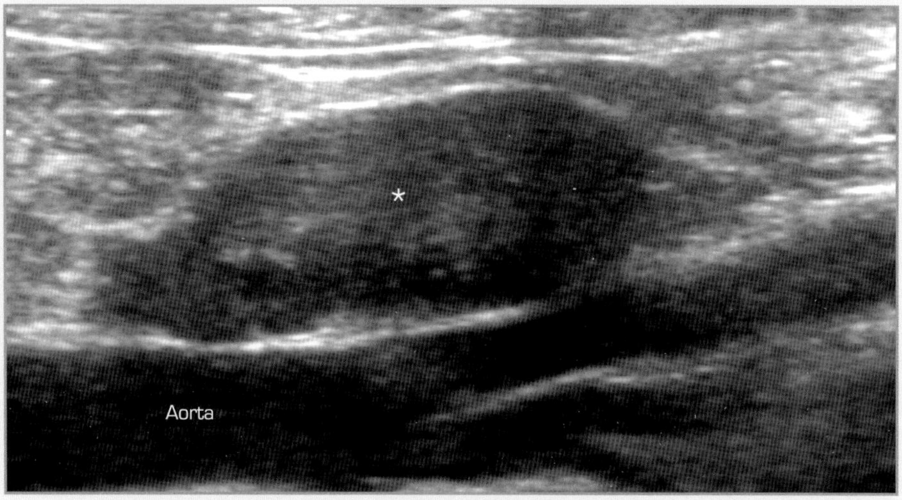

Figure 4. Medial iliac lymphadenopathy. The left medial iliac lymph node (*) (located at the level of the aortic bifurcation) is markedly enlarged.

Other lymph nodes

Apart from the medial iliac lymph nodes, other lymph nodes may be of interest in a routine ultrasound examination:

- The hepatic lymph nodes are small and commonly seen at the level of the hepatic hilum, near the portal vein.
- The splenic lymph nodes are located along the splenic artery and vein.
- The gastric lymph nodes are adjacent to the lesser curvature of the stomach and pylorus.
- The pancreaticoduodenal lymph node is located between the pylorus and the right pancreatic lobe.
- The jejunal lymph nodes are embedded in the mesentery.
- The colic lymph nodes are often multiple and located close to the colon.
- The internal iliac (hypogastric) lymph nodes are located caudal to the medial iliac lymph nodes.
- The aortic, renal and lumbar lymph nodes are small and located along the aorta and caudal vena cava.

Major abdominal vessels

The aorta and caudal vena cava are the two largest vessels in the abdomen. They can usually be followed to their bifurcation. They are the most accessible vessels in the caudal abdomen, where they are easier to evaluate.

The aorta is pulsatile and less compressible than the caudal vena cava. However, the caudal vena cava may appear pulsatile due to the referred motion from the aorta.

The coeliac, cranial mesenteric and renal arteries and portal vein can also be evaluated. The portal vein is found ventral to the caudal vena cava, near the hepatic hilum.

Normal appearance

The peritoneum has normally a uniform echogenicity, best appreciated when there is ascites (Fig. 5). The mesenteric fat appears hyperechoic to isoechoic to the liver with a coarse echotexture (Fig. 6).

Normal lymph nodes are isoechoic to hypoechoic to the surrounding mesenteric fat and have an oval, sometimes elongated, shape (see Fig. 3b). A hypoechoic cortex and a hyperechoic (in relation to the cortex) medulla is occasionally seen (Fig. 3c).

Normal canine lymph nodes may be up to 5 mm thick. Based on the author's experience, this is true for most dogs; however, some very large dogs may have lymph nodes up to 7 mm thick. Young animals tend to have larger more obvious lymph nodes. A short-to-long axis ratio of less than 0.5 is considered normal.

The aorta, caudal vena cava and other abdominal vessels normally have anechoic contents (see Fig. 3a). The Doppler flow signal of the aorta is pulsatile (Fig. 7). Pulsatile flow is not present in the caudal vena cava.

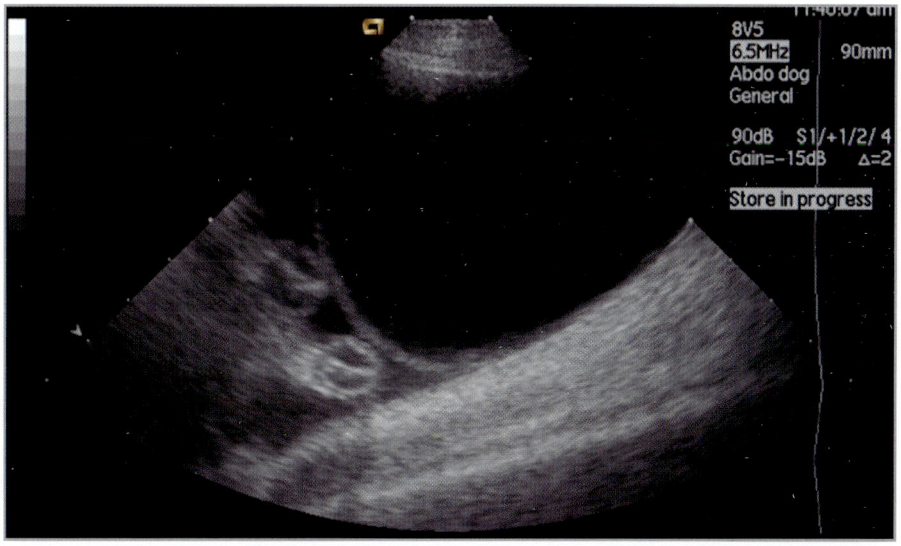

Figure 5. The transducer has been positioned for the evaluation of the dependent aspect of the urinary bladder. Anechoic free peritoneal fluid is present.

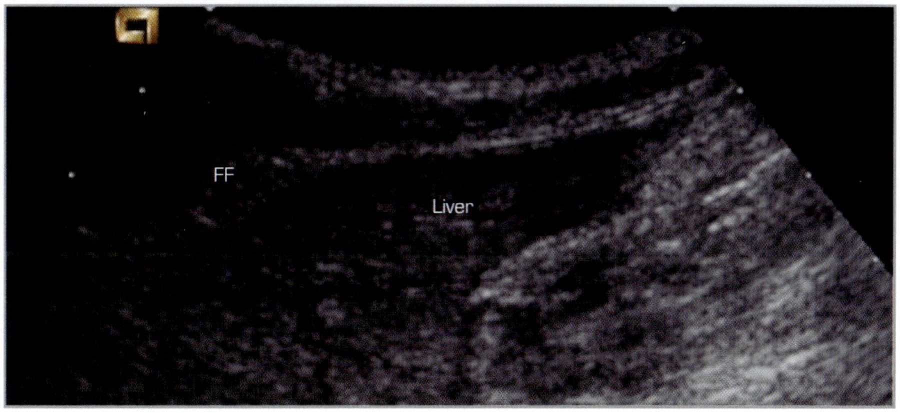

Figure 6. The falciform fat (FF) is hyperechoic to the liver and has a coarse echotexture.

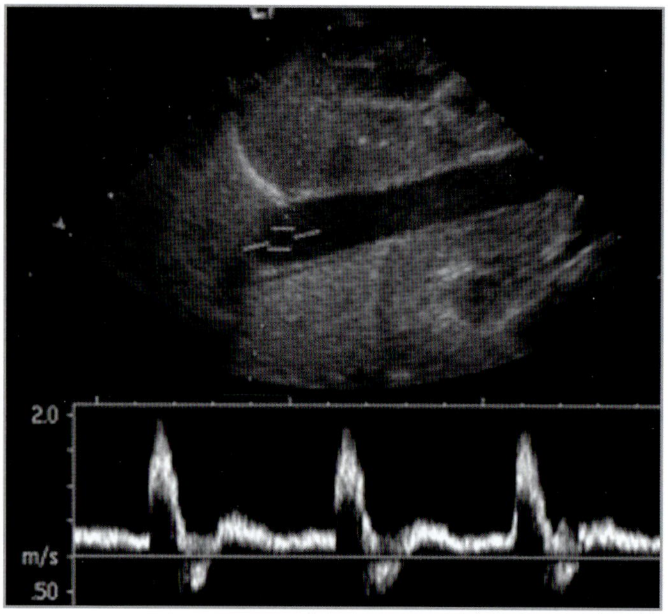

Figure 7. Pulsatile flow recorded using pulsed-wave Doppler to assess the aorta.

Variations from normal

Lymphadenopathy

The lymph nodes appear enlarged (see Fig. 4), homogeneously hypoechoic and smoothly marginated (Fig. 8). They may also have a mixed echogenicity and contain cavities or not. Enlarged lymph nodes may have an irregular outline and/or be abnormally shaped. It is not possible to reliably distinguish reactive from neoplastic lymph nodes on the basis of their ultrasonographic appearance alone.

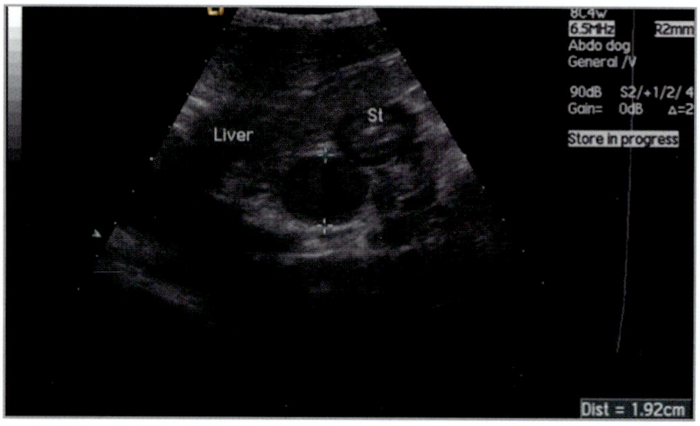

Figure 8. Enlarged, rounded and hypoechoic hepatic lymph node (between callipers). St: stomach.

Free peritoneal and retroperitoneal fluid

Free peritoneal fluid may be generalised or localised and appears as single or multiple anechoic areas separating the intraperitoneal structures. Small amounts of fluid can commonly be identified between the liver lobes or between the diaphragm and the liver (Fig. 9), and also between the urinary bladder wall and the abdominal wall (see Fig. 5). Ultrasonography alone cannot reliably distinguish the type of fluid (transudate, modified transudate, exudate). Suspended echogenic foci may indicate exudate or modified transudate but it is not a reliable test. In any case, an ultrasound-guided aspiration should always be performed to identify the type of fluid present.

Retroperitoneal fluid can be detected as anechoic areas around the kidneys. In some cases, it may be difficult to distinguish retroperitoneal from peritoneal fluid. Evaluation of the fluid accumulated from multiple angles, during the abdominal ultrasound examination, can help to distinguish peritoneal from retroperitoneal effusion.

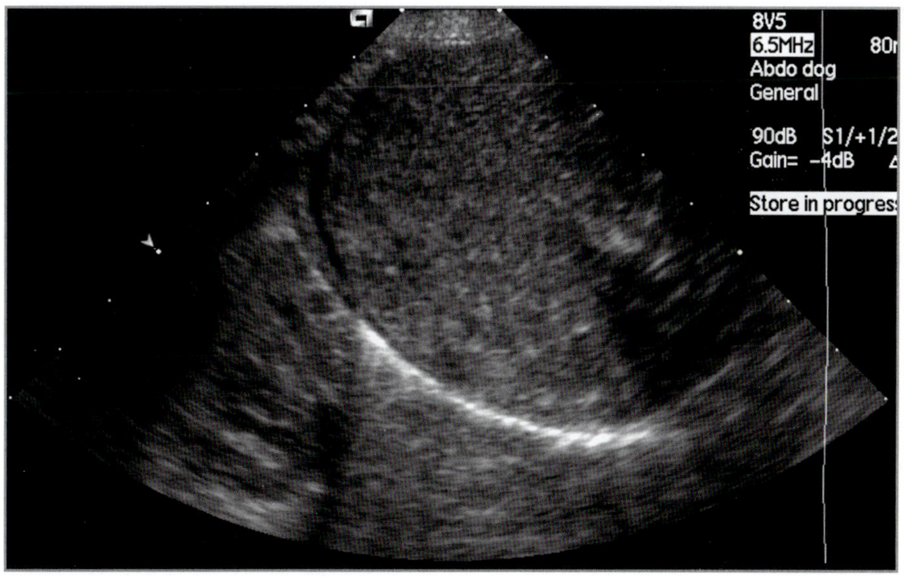

Figure 9. A small amount of free peritoneal fluid is visible as an anechoic linear crescent between the diaphragm and liver.

Peritonitis

The peritoneum, omentum and mesentery usually appear markedly hyperechoic in peritonitis; however, they can also have a mixed echogenicity with significant ultrasound beam attenuation (Fig. 10). Peritonitis can be focal or general, with or without concurrent peritoneal effusion.

Peritoneal carcinomatosis may appear similar to peritonitis.

a
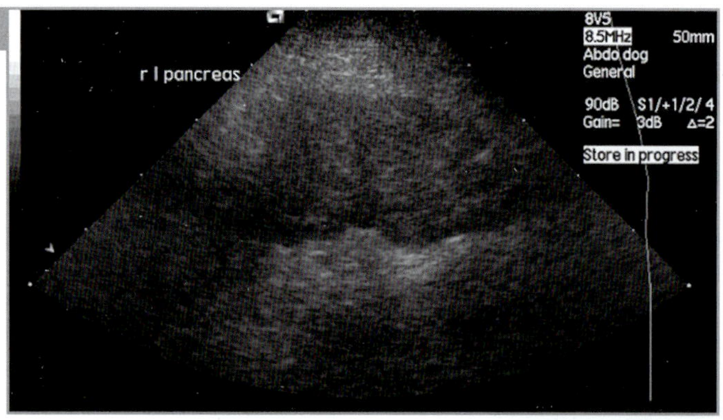

b
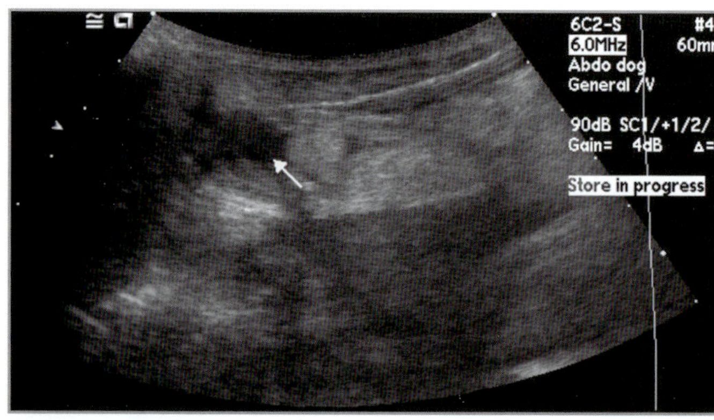

c
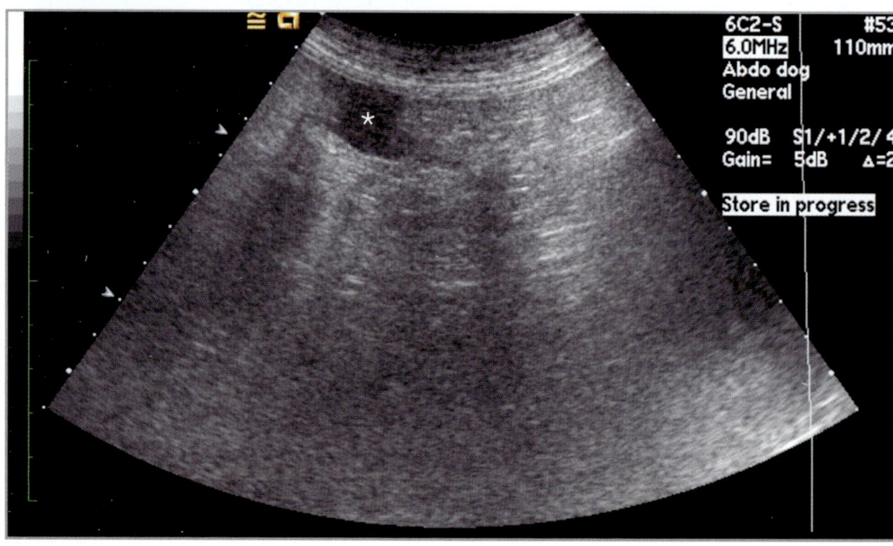

Figure 10. (a) Hyperechoic mesentery surrounding an inflamed pancreas in a dog. This is compatible with peripancreatic inflammation (focal peritonitis). (b) Peritonitis and mild ascites (arrow) in a dog. Note the hyperechoic mesentery. (c) Markedly hyperechoic mesentery secondary to inflammation. Note how the image appears darker in the deeper parts due to beam attenuation. A small amount of free peritoneal fluid is also visible (*).

Pneumoperitoneum and pneumoretroperitoneum

Free intraperitoneal gas (pneumoperitoneum) appears as echogenic foci or lines with a reverberation artefact between the abdominal structures and the non-dependent wall of the abdomen (Fig. 11).

When free air in the peritoneum is detected during the evaluation of the gastrointestinal tract, intestinal rupture should be suspected. This should prompt a thorough evaluation of the patient's history. Pertinent details such as a previous traumatic episode or chronic use of non-steroidal anti-inflammatory drugs are of the utmost importance.

Peritoneal air can take several days before being completely resorbed following abdominal surgery. Postoperative pneumoperitoneum is a common finding and should be interpreted with caution.

Pneumoretroperitoneum has a similar appearance to pneumoperitoneum, but with the gas located in the retroperitoneal space.

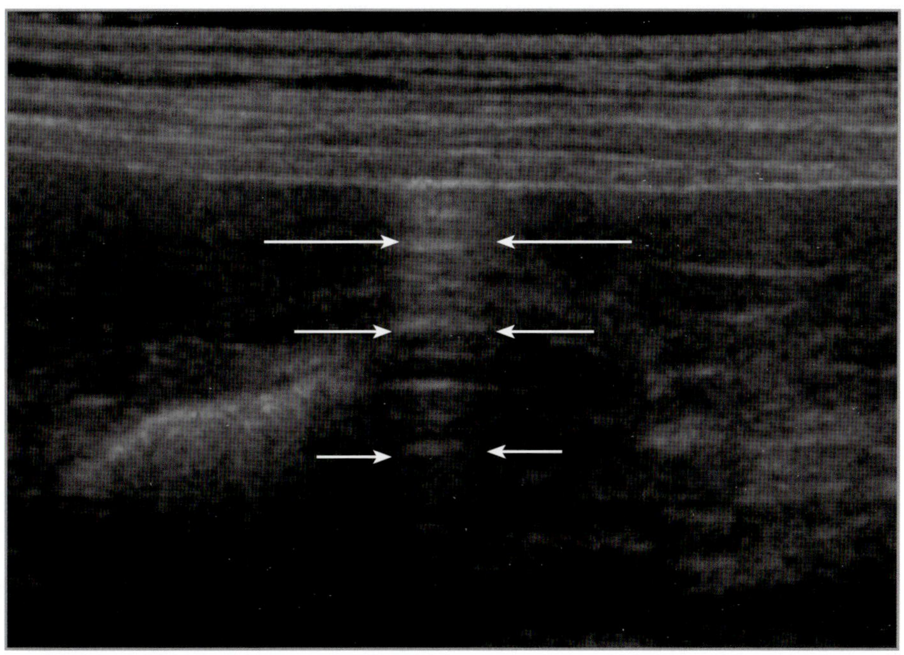

Figure 11. Free intraperitoneal gas after a major abdominal surgery in a dog. The gas appears as an echogenic line with a reverberation artefact (arrows) between the abdominal structures and the non-dependent abdominal wall.

Peritoneal and retroperitoneal masses

If an abdominal mass does not appear to be continuous with an organ, it may be peritoneal in origin. However, depending on the location, pancreatic masses and/or masses originating from lymph nodes should also be considered in the differential diagnosis.

Abscesses (Fig. 12) are typically septated with thick walls; however, their appearance can be variable with a complex internal architecture. Distal acoustic enhancement may also be present depending on the volume of fluid contained within the abscess.

Granulomas are commonly associated with a peritoneal foreign body (that may or may not be identified in the granuloma). Ultrasonographically, granulomas can appear as masses or even have a similar appearance to peritoneal abscesses. Retained surgical sponges appear as hypoechoic masses with irregular hyperechoic centres.

Haematomas vary in appearance depending on their age. They commonly appear as cavitary masses of mixed echogenicity. Doppler evaluation helps to distinguish avascular haematomas from other more vascular masses in the abdomen.

Lipomas (Fig. 13) appear on ultrasound as well-defined masses with the same echogenicity and echotexture as adipose tissue.

Retroperitoneal masses (Fig. 14) commonly have mixed echogenicity and may invade major vessels such as the aorta and caudal vena cava. It may be difficult to differentiate a large retroperitoneal mass from a peritoneal mass, and, as previously explained, scanning from multiple angles may be beneficial. In any case, definitive diagnosis requires an ultrasound-guided fine-needle aspiration or biopsy.

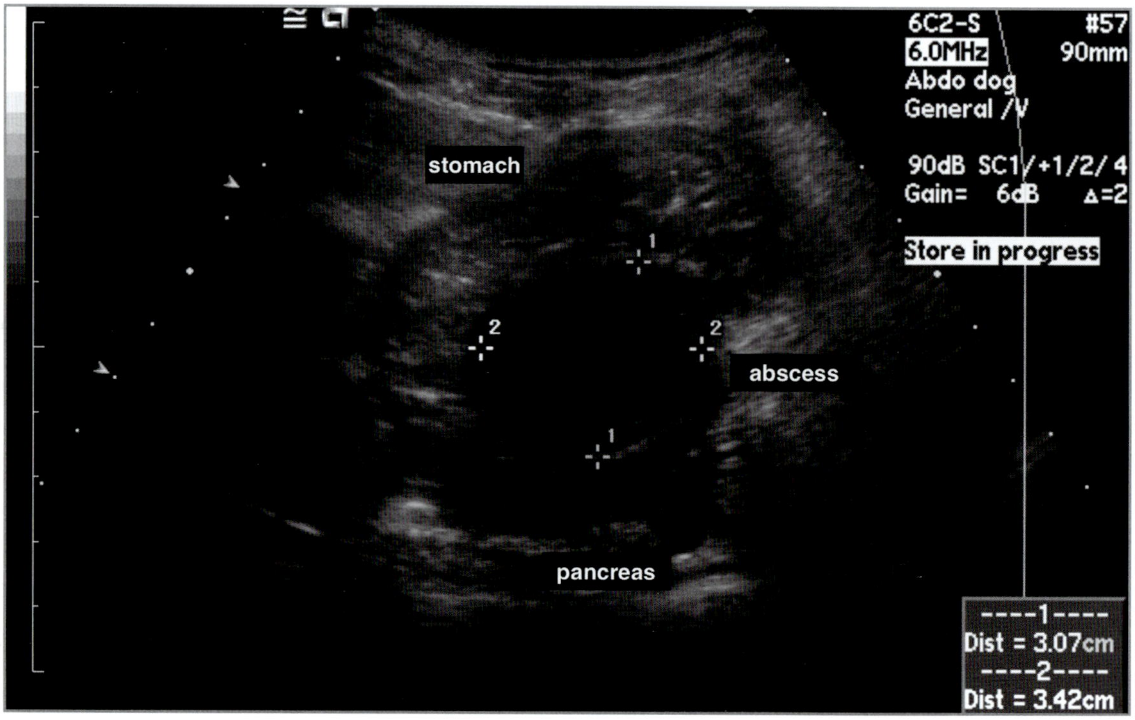

Figure 12. Peritoneal abscess in a dog (between callipers). The abscess was attached to the stomach and was removed surgically.

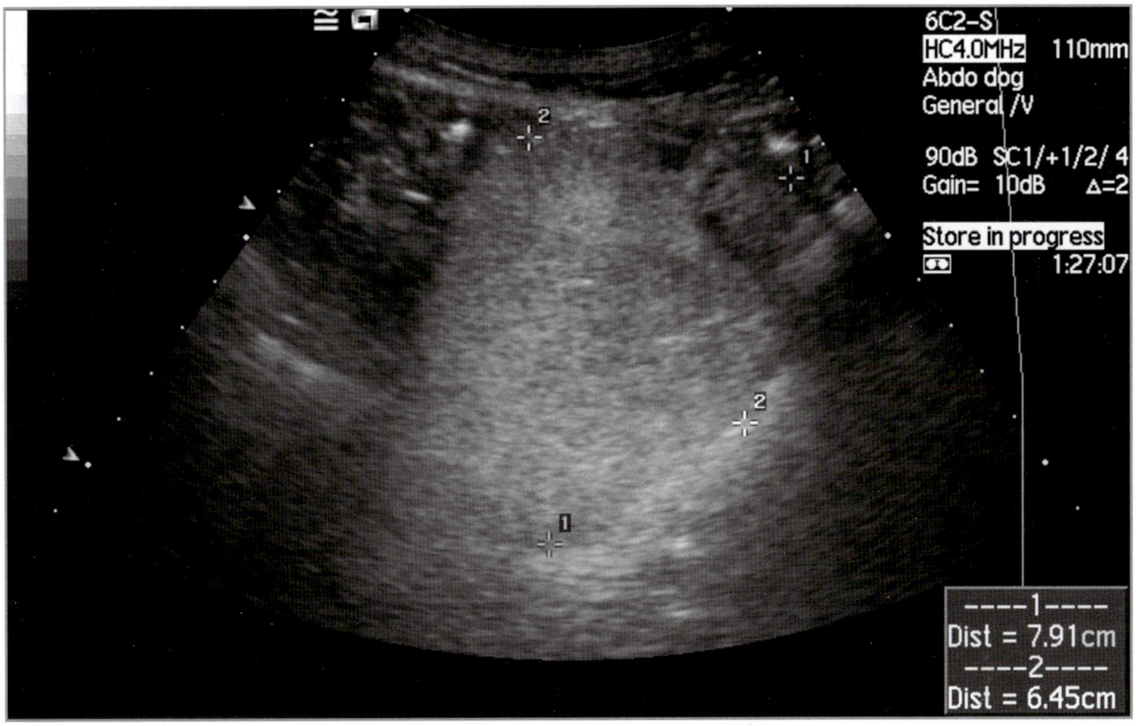

Figure 13. Peritoneal lipoma (between callipers). The mass is well marginated and has the same echogenicity and echotexture as the surrounding mesenteric fat.

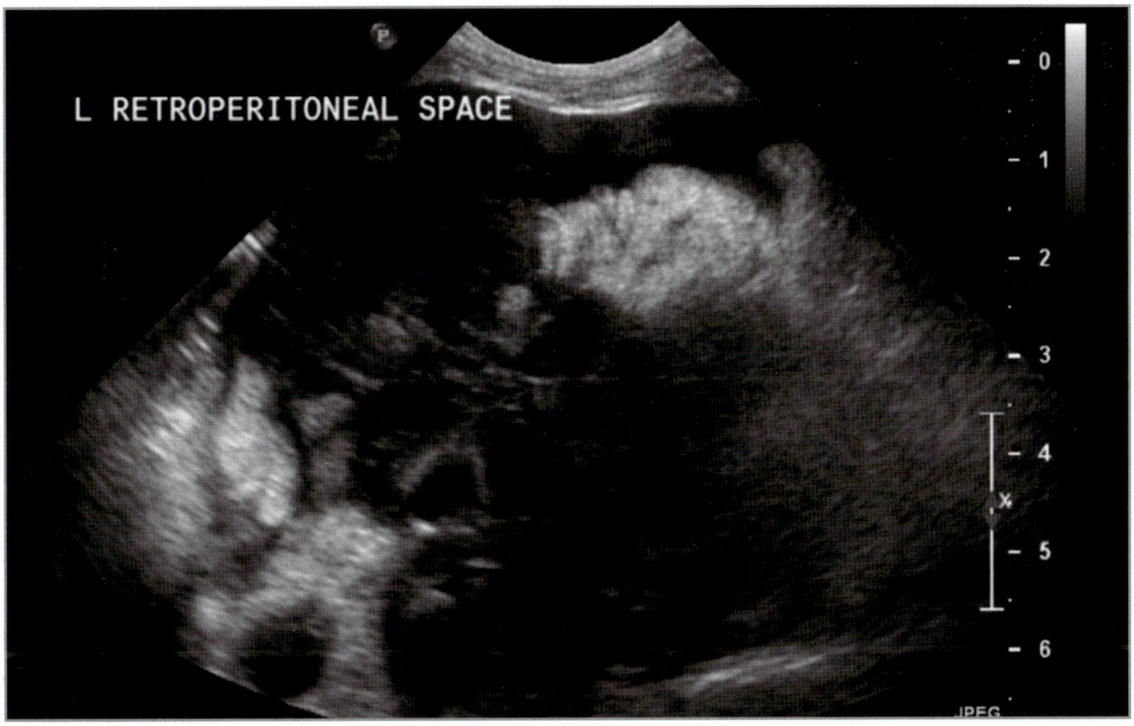

Figure 14. Large, irregular, mixed echogenicity mass extending from the left kidney to the pelvic inlet in the left, mainly, retroperitoneal space of a 12-year-old Patterdale terrier. The mass obstructed the left ureter. More caudally the mass extended more to the midline and right and appeared to envelop the aorta. The fine needle aspirates of the mass confirmed lymphoma.

Nodular fat necrosis

Nodular fat necrosis is an incidental finding in dogs and cats (Fig. 15). It commonly appears as a solitary mass or multiple masses partially mineralised in the abdominal fat. They present distal acoustic shadowing and may have a hypoechoic centre.

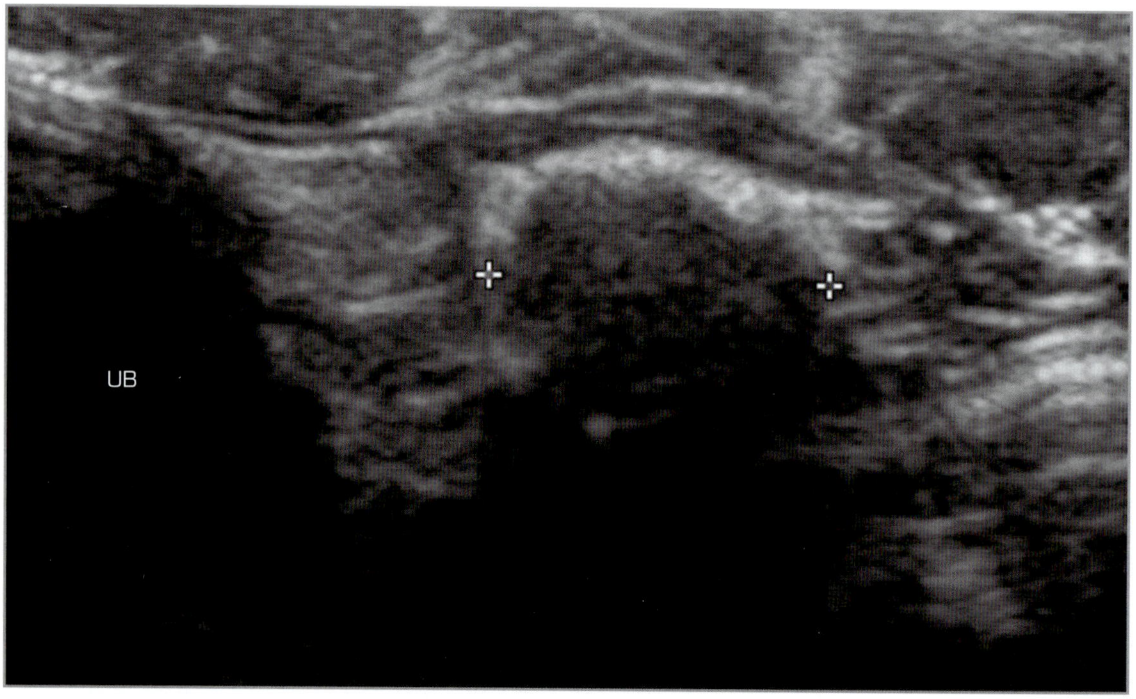

Figure 15. Nodular fat necrosis in a 9-year-old, male neutered cat. A well-defined, ovoid heterogeneous lesion (between callipers) with a hyperechoic rim and acoustic shadowing structure is visible next to the urinary bladder (UB).

Vascular lesions

The ultrasonographic appearance of vascular thrombosis varies with chronicity. In early stages, the thrombus can be hypoechoic and difficult to identify. As it becomes more chronic, an echogenic structure, commonly attached to the vessel wall, can often be identified within the lumen of the affected vessel (Fig. 16). Thrombi may have homogeneous or heterogeneous echogenicity.

> Doppler evaluation of the blood vessels (power or colour-flow Doppler) may aid the identification of an early, hypoechoic thrombus.

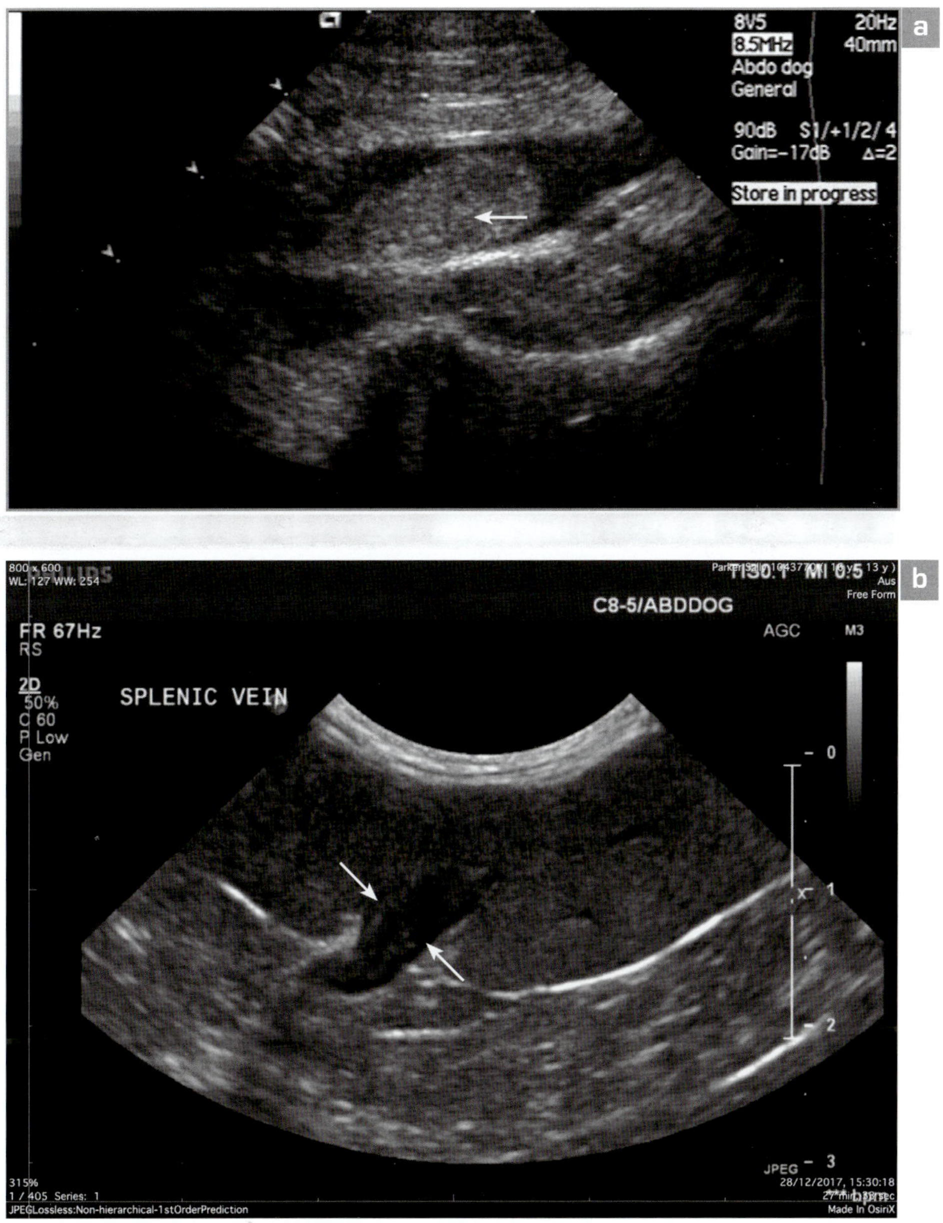

Figure 16. **(a)** Thrombus in the aorta (arrow), just cranial to the aortic bifurcation. **(b)** Thrombus in the splenic vein of a 13-year-old spaniel (between arrows).

12

CHAPTER

PROSTATE GLAND AND TESTES

Scanning technique

Prostate gland

High-frequency transducers are used to examine the prostate. Frequencies between 8 and 10 MHz are recommended, although in larger dogs' frequencies as low as 3.5-5 MHz may be used. The prostate is not routinely evaluated in cats due to its small size.

- The prostate gland is normally located caudal to the urinary bladder. Digital manipulation may aid in the identification of an intrapelvic prostate.

Transrectal transducers may also be used to evaluate the prostate. Transrectal ultrasonography is superior to transabdominal ultrasonography for prostatic examination, although it is rarely employed in small animals. A transabdominal approach is preferred, and the techniques are described below.

In neutered animals, especially in those neutered at a very young age, the prostate gland is very small and more difficult to identify.

Technique 1 to identify the prostate

1. Position the animal in right lateral recumbency with the head towards the ultrasound machine and the limbs towards the examiner.
2. Ask an assistant to lift the left hind limb towards him/her with the stifle joint in flexion.
3. Place the transducer with the marker pointing to the head of the animal on the caudal abdomen to locate the urinary bladder.
4. Slide the transducer caudally to the trigone area and identify the beginning of the urethra (Fig. 1).
5. The prostate is identified caudal to the urinary bladder bisected by the urethra.

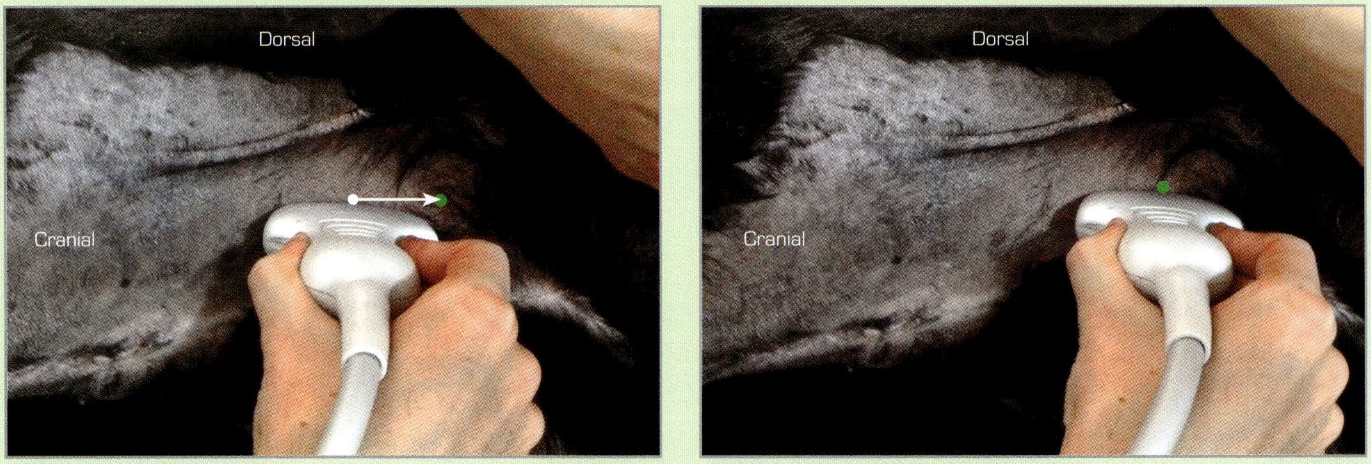

Figure 1. Transducer position and movement for the identification of the prostate gland. The transducer is placed with the marker pointing to the head (dorsal or dorsal-oblique plane) and then moved caudally to locate the prostate gland, caudal to the urinary bladder.

Technique 2 to identify the prostate

1. Position the animal in right lateral recumbency with the head towards the ultrasound machine and the limbs towards the examiner.

2. Ask an assistant to lift the left hind limb towards him/her with the stifle joint in flexion.

3. Obtain a transverse image of the urinary bladder.

4. Fix the image of the urinary bladder in the middle of the screen and slide and fan the transducer caudally towards the hip joints (Fig. 2).

5. Continue to slide and fan the transducer caudally until the urinary bladder disappears and the prostate appears on the screen.

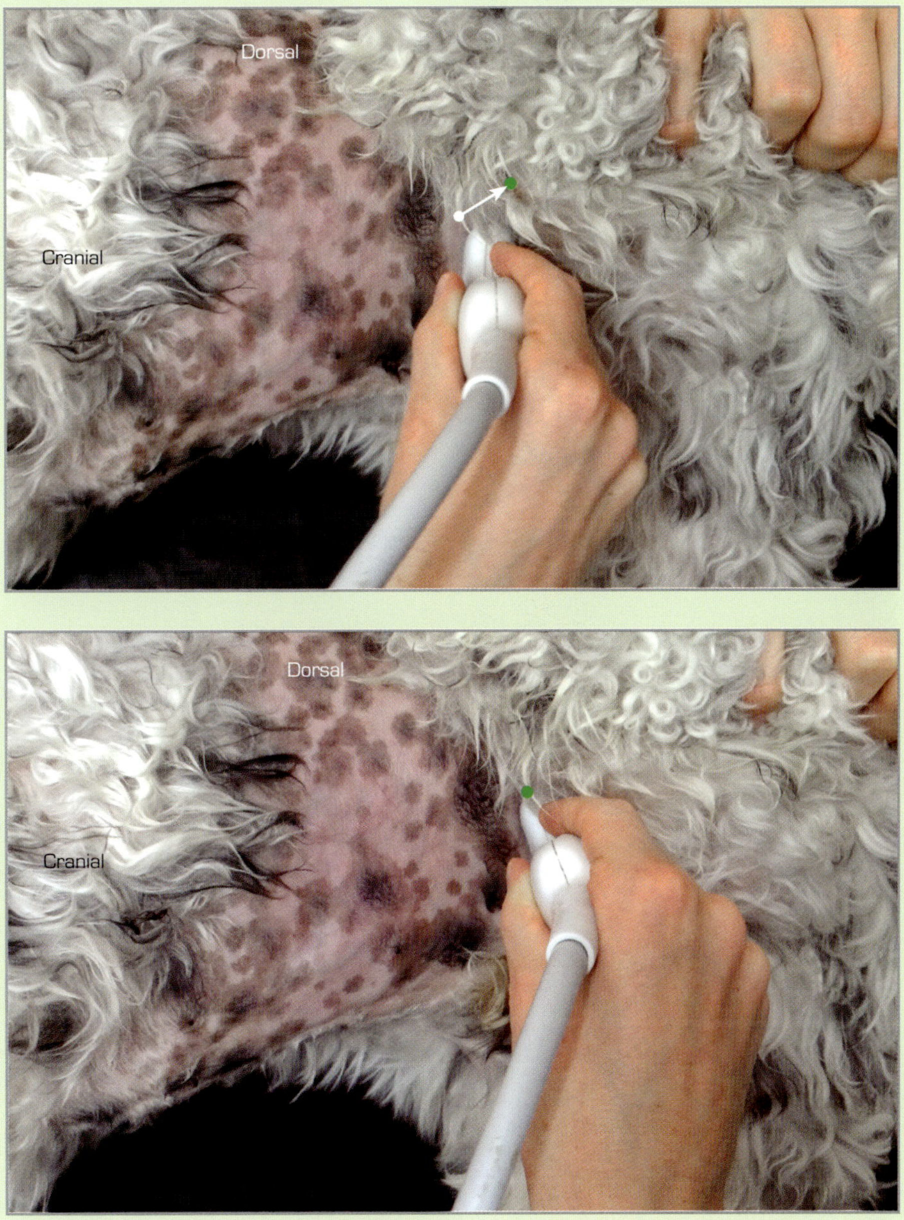

Figure 2. The prostate may also be identified in a transverse plane. Locate the urinary bladder and slide the transducer caudally towards the hip joints. Soon after the urinary bladder disappears, the prostate gland should appear.

Examination technique of the prostate

1. With the marker pointing to the head of the animal, fan the transducer dorsally and ventrally to examine the prostate in a longitudinal orientation (Fig. 3).

2. Rotate the transducer 90° clockwise and fan it cranially and caudally to examine the prostate in a transverse orientation (Fig. 4).

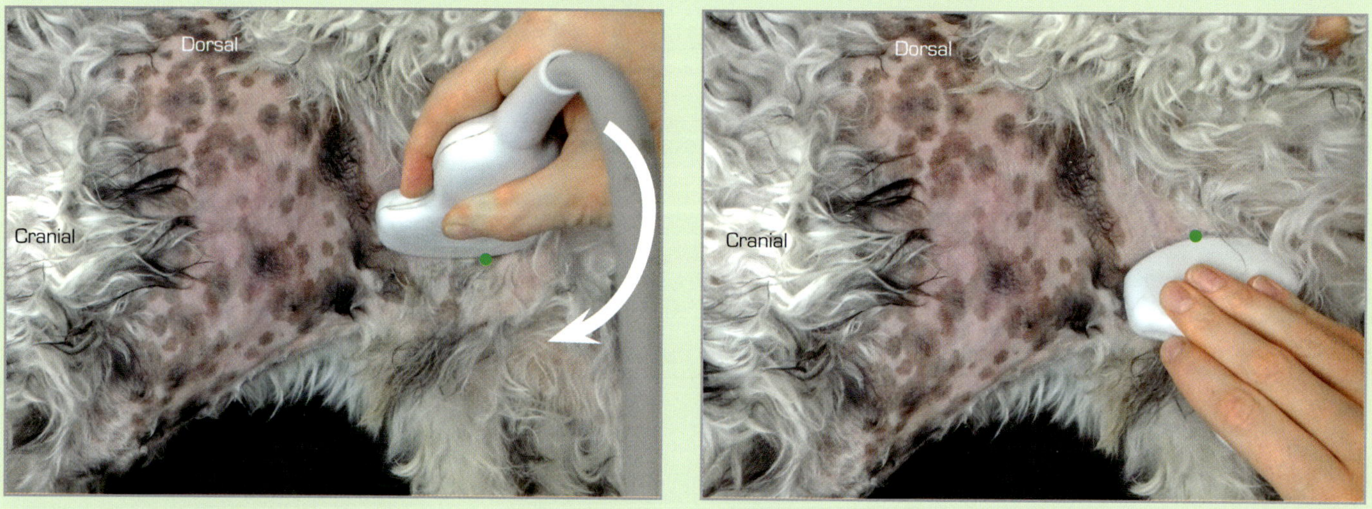

Figure 3. Fanning of the transducer to examine the prostate in a longitudinal plane.

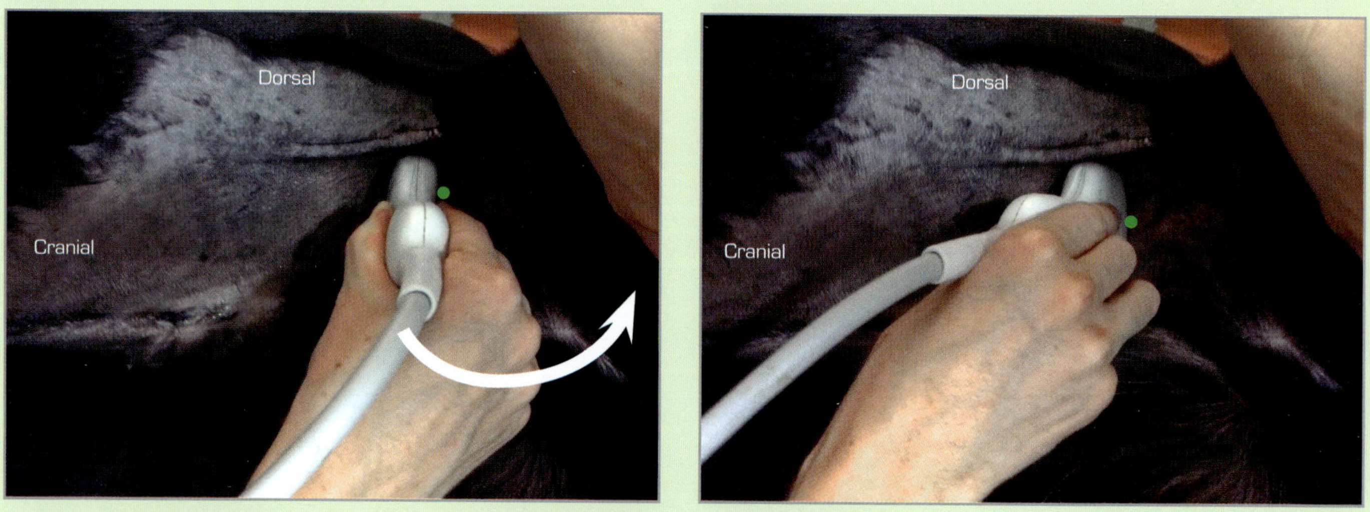

Figure 4. Transducer position and movement to examine the prostate gland in a transverse plane.

Testes

Examination of the descended testes is easy due to their superficial location.

Ultrasonographic examination of the testes can be performed in sagittal, transverse or dorsal orientation by fanning the transducer from one end of each testicle to the other in at least two orthogonal orientations (Fig. 5).

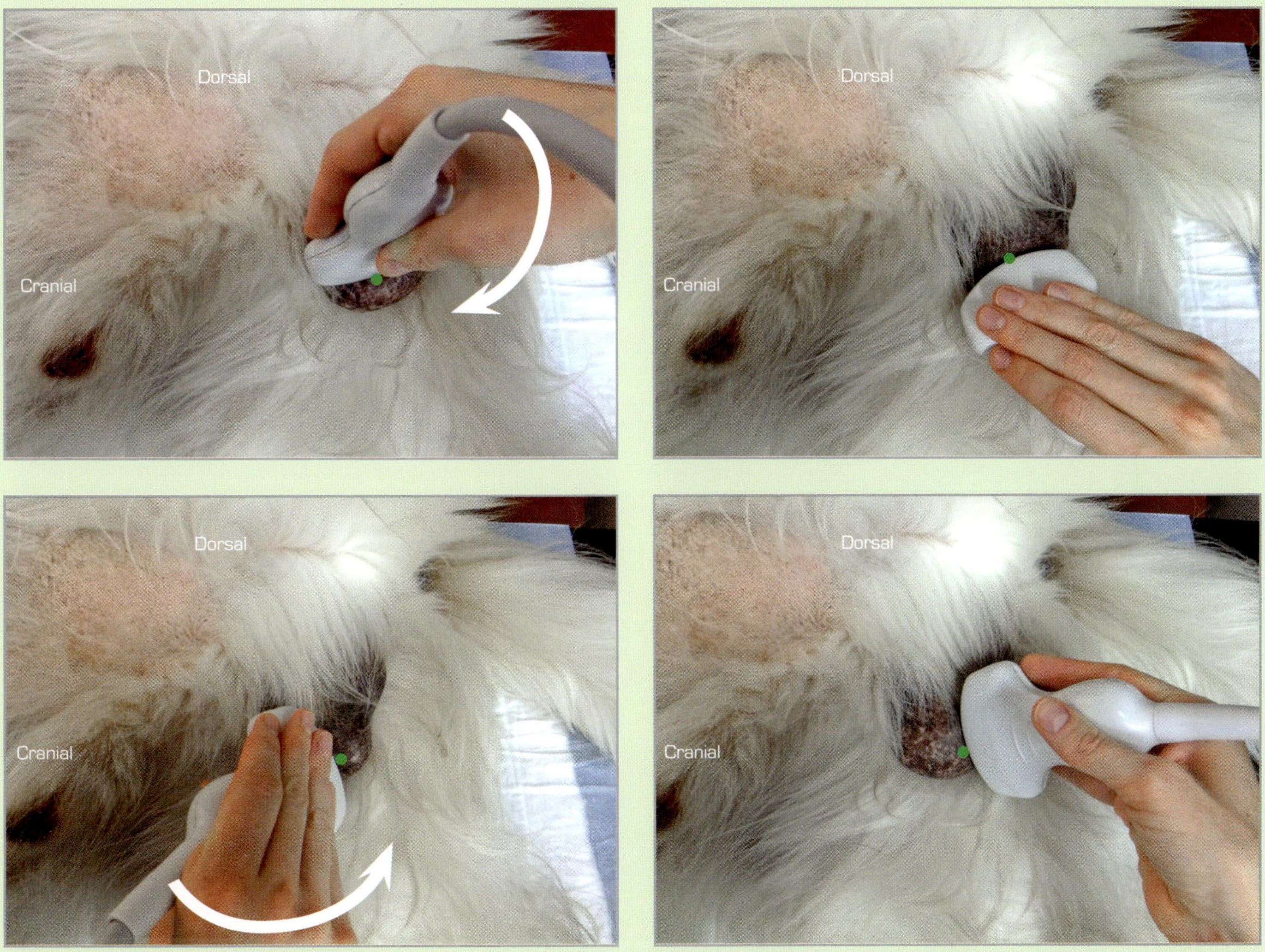

Figure 5. Transducer position and movement to evaluate the testes in two orthogonal planes. Normal appearance.

Normal appearance

Prostate gland

The normal appearance of the prostate gland in the dog varies depending on its age and neutering status.

The canine prostate is an oval, bilobed organ. It is hyperechoic relative to the surrounding structures and has a homogeneous echotexture (Fig. 6). In neutered animals, the prostate gland is smaller, more hypoechoic and more difficult to identify (Fig. 7).

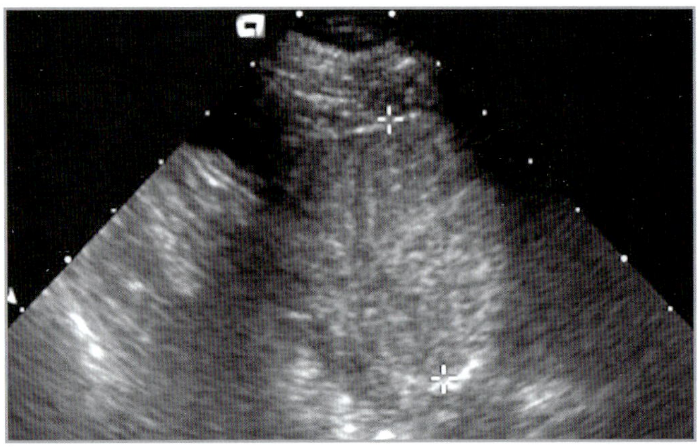

Figure 6. Normal prostate gland (between callipers) in an entire male dog. The prostatic parenchyma is homogeneously echogenic with a fine echotexture.

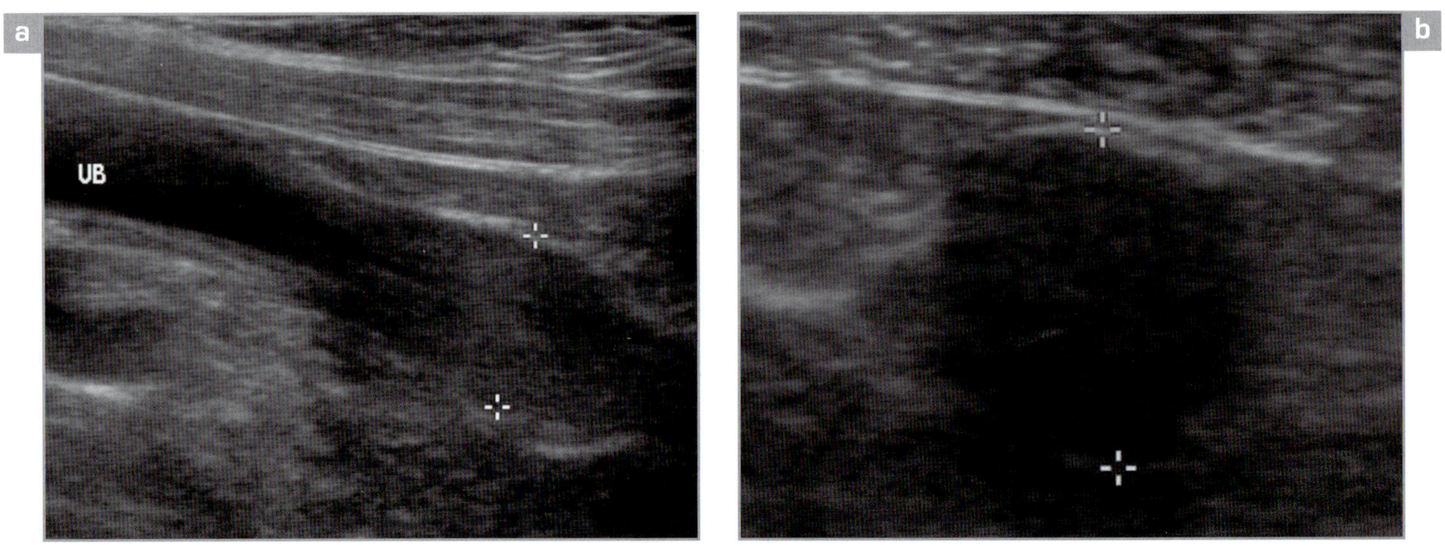

Figure 7. Longitudinal (a) and transverse (b) images of a normal canine prostate (between callipers) in a neutered dog. Compared to that of an entire male dog, the prostate gland is smaller and more hypoechoic, making it more difficult to identify. UB: urinary bladder.

The prostatic urethra bisects the prostate. In long axis, it appears as a hypoechoic to anechoic linear structure. In short axis, it appears as a hypoechoic to anechoic circular area in the centre of the prostate.

The size of the canine prostate varies with the breed and size of the animal. Although formulas to estimate the size of the prostate are available, it is easier for beginners to measure the prostatic size on abdominal radiographs. On a lateral radiograph of the abdomen, no dimension of the prostate should exceed 70 % the distance from the sacral promontory to the pubic rim; on a ventrodorsal radiograph of the abdomen, the prostate is rarely larger than two-thirds the width of the pelvic inlet.

Testes

In dogs, the testes are moderately echogenic and present a fine homogeneous echotexture (Fig. 8). Each testis consists of: a thin hyperechoic rim (created from the parietal and visceral tunics), the mediastinum testis (visible as a central echogenic line) and the epididymis (hypoechoic to the testicular parenchyma) (Fig. 9). The testes are not routinely checked in cats.

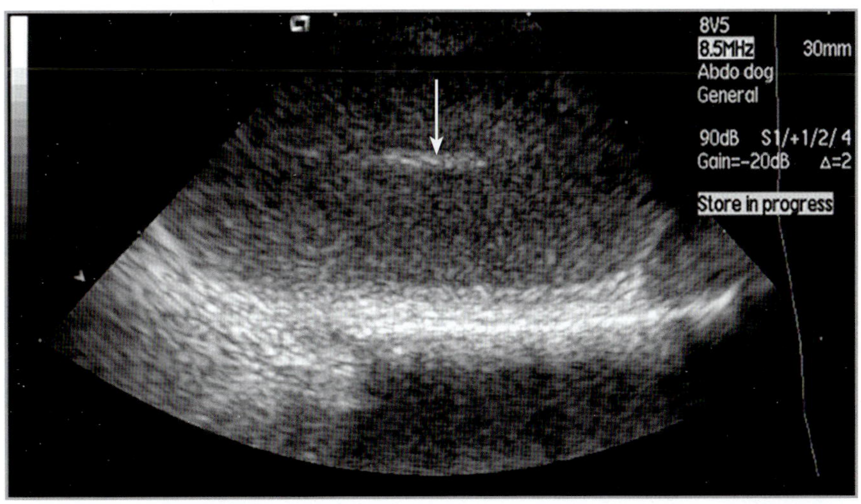

Figure 8. Normal canine testis. The testis is homogeneously echogenic with medium parenchymal echotexture. The echogenic linear structure in the central area of the testicle is the mediastinum testis (arrow).

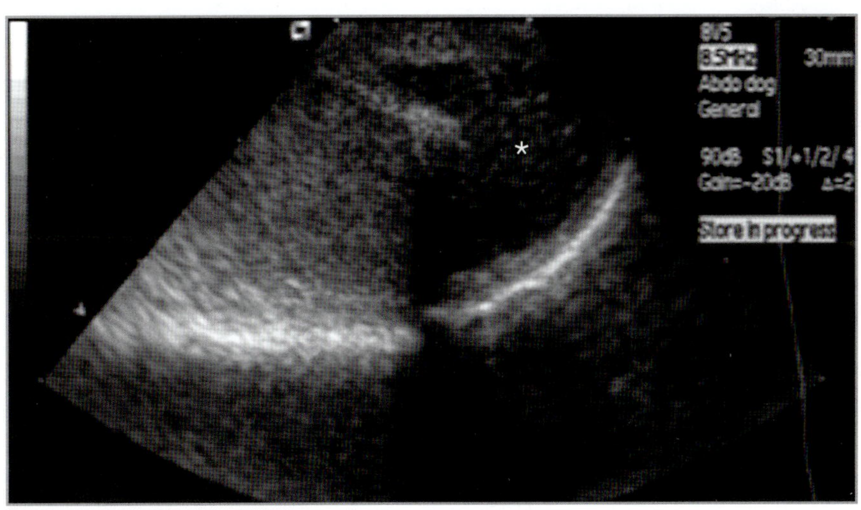

Figure 9. The head of the epididymis (*) is seen as a more hypoechoic structure to the right of the testicle.

Variations from normal

Prostate

The typical appearance of benign prostatic hyperplasia (BPH) is a symmetrically enlarged prostate of homogeneous echogenicity containing numerous small intraparenchymal cysts (Fig. 10). However, the appearance of BPH varies markedly. The prostatic enlargement may be either symmetrical or asymmetrical, the echotexture may be homogeneous or heterogeneous, and the echogenicity may be hypoechoic or hyperechoic. Benign prostatic hyperplasia does not disrupt the prostatic capsule and it does not cause medial iliac lymphadenopathy.

In patients with prostatitis, the prostate appears enlarged and has mixed echogenicity (Fig. 11). The enlargement is more often symmetrical, although asymmetrical enlargement also occurs depending on the presence or absence of cystic structures e.g. cysts or abscesses (Fig. 12). Prostatitis may look similar to BPH and both conditions can concurrently occur (Fig. 11). Fine-needle aspiration and/or biopsy of the prostatic parenchyma are required for a definitive diagnosis. In some dogs with prostatitis, hyperechoic fat (indicating inflammation) and a small amount of free fluid (periprostatic fluid) may be seen surrounding the prostate.

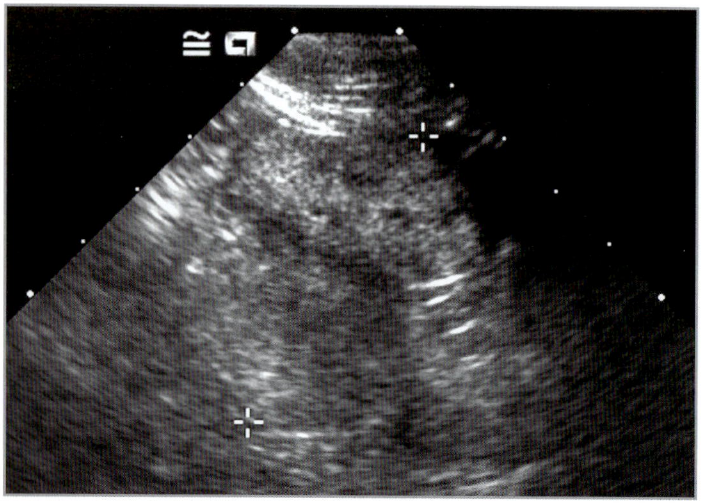

Figure 10. Benign prostatic hyperplasia. The prostate (between callipers) is enlarged, hyperechoic and contains multiple small intraparenchymal cysts. Its normal shape is maintained.

Prostatic cysts typically have a thin, hyperechoic wall and anechoic contents with distal acoustic enhancement. They can be either congenital or developmental and may be an incidental finding, although they are often associated with prostatic disease (e.g. BPH).

Paraprostatic cysts should be suspected when an additional structure resembling the urinary bladder is identified. These cysts are located near, and may communicate with, the prostate gland. They can become very large and occupy a large proportion of the caudal abdomen and pelvic canal. Ultrasonographically, they are anechoic with variable wall thickness (Fig. 13). The wall may be thin or thick and is sometimes irregular. Echogenic foci and septa are occasionally present. This type of cysts may become infected. Catheterisation allows confident differentiation between the urinary bladder and an adjacent paraprostatic cyst.

Adenocarcinomas and undifferentiated carcinomas are the most common type of canine prostatic tumours. Transitional cell carcinoma is the most common prostatic tumour in neutered male dogs. The ultrasonographic appearance of prostatic tumours varies. The prostate gland usually appears enlarged with an irregular shape and heterogeneous echotexture. Cyst-like structures and hyperechoic foci may also be present (Fig. 14). The presence of mineralisation in the canine prostatic parenchyma suggests malignancy (Fig. 15).

Table 1 includes a list of the most likely differential diagnoses when identifying prostatic lesions on ultrasound.

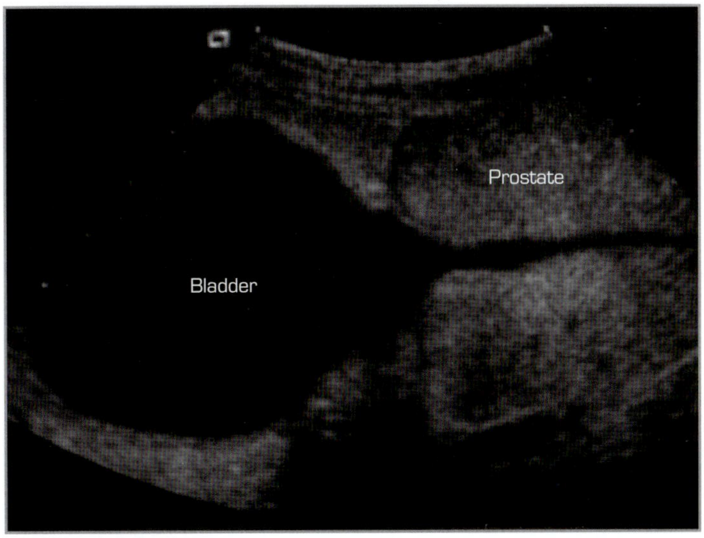

Figure 11. Benign prostatic hyperplasia and prostatitis in a dog. The prostate is uniformly enlarged, with a slightly mixed echogenicity and contains multiple intraparenchymal cysts. The prostatic urethra is visible as an anechoic tubular structure continuous with the urinary bladder.

a

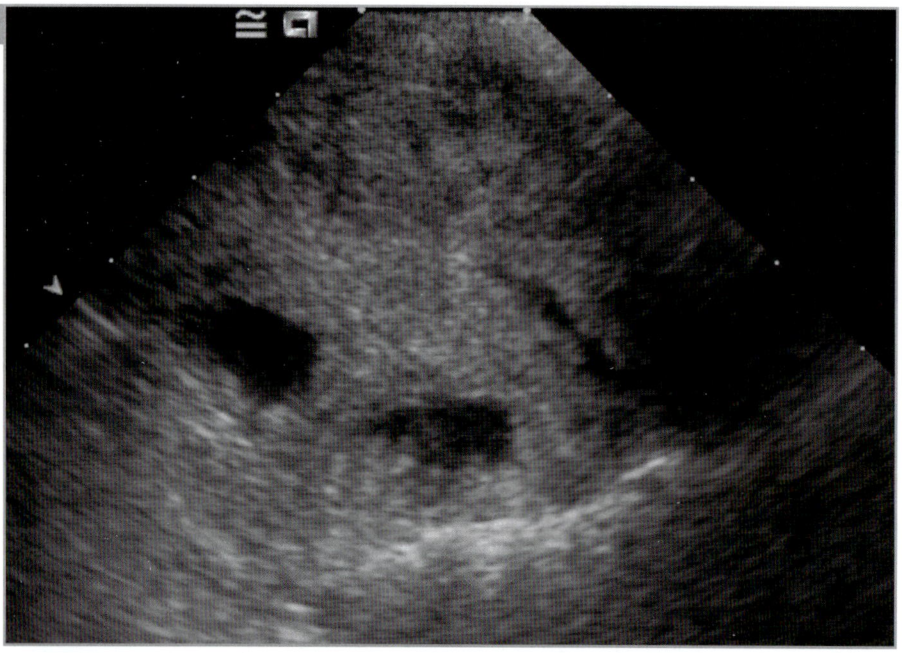

b

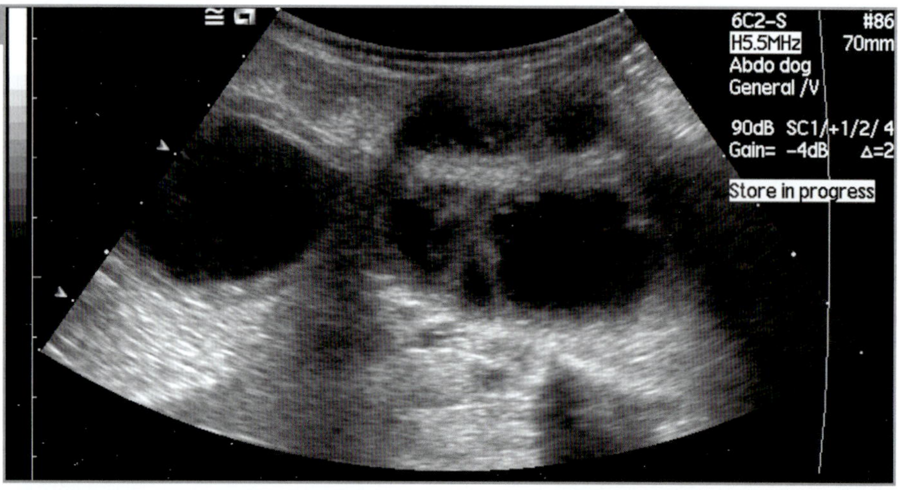

c

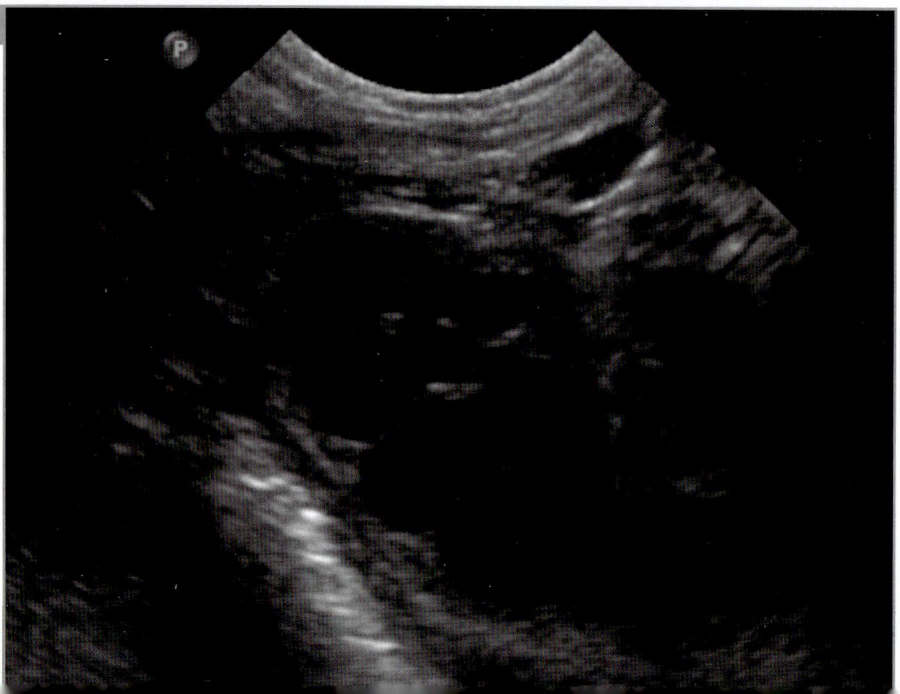

Figure 12. (a) Dog with bacterial prostatitis. The prostate gland is asymmetrically enlarged; it has a mixed parenchymal echogenicity and contains two large irregular cystic lesions in the right lobe compatible with prostatic abscessation. (b) Prostatic abscesses in a dog. The prostate is asymmetrically enlarged and contains large, septated cystic lesion. (c) Multi-cystic lesion in the prostate of an 11-year-old cocker spaniel that was proved to be prostatic abscess. In this dog the medial iliac lymph nodes were also enlarged and cystic.

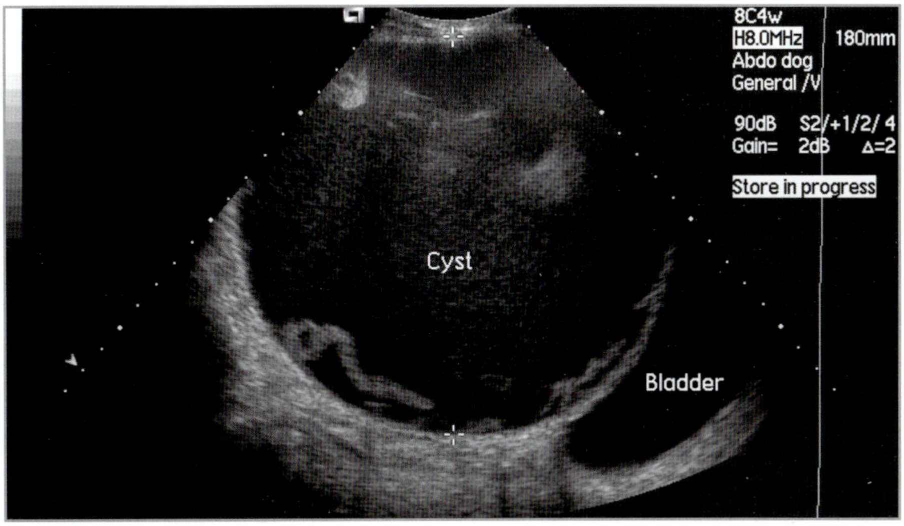

Figure 13. Large paraprostatic cyst occupying the caudal abdomen and compressing the urinary bladder.

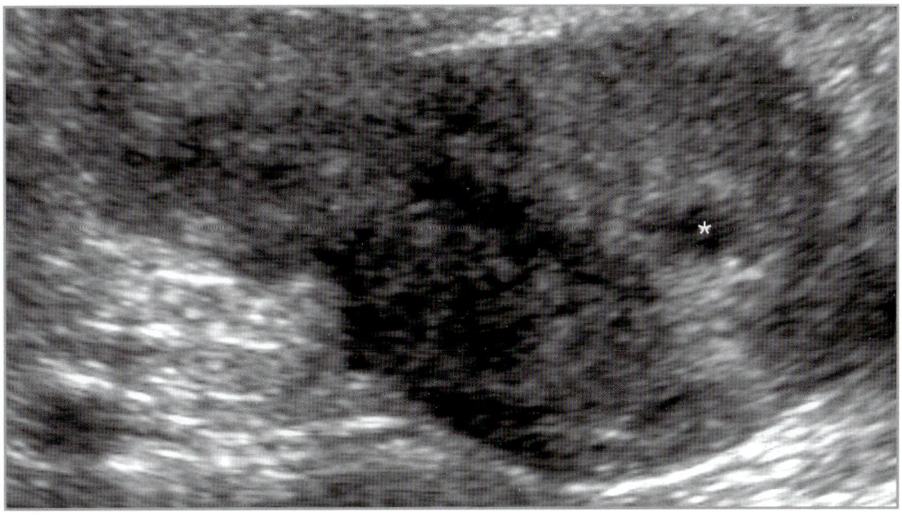

Figure 14. Prostatic carcinoma in a dog. The prostate appears enlarged with mixed parenchymal echogenicity and containing a small cystic lesion (*) in the left lobe. The appearance is very similar to prostatitis.

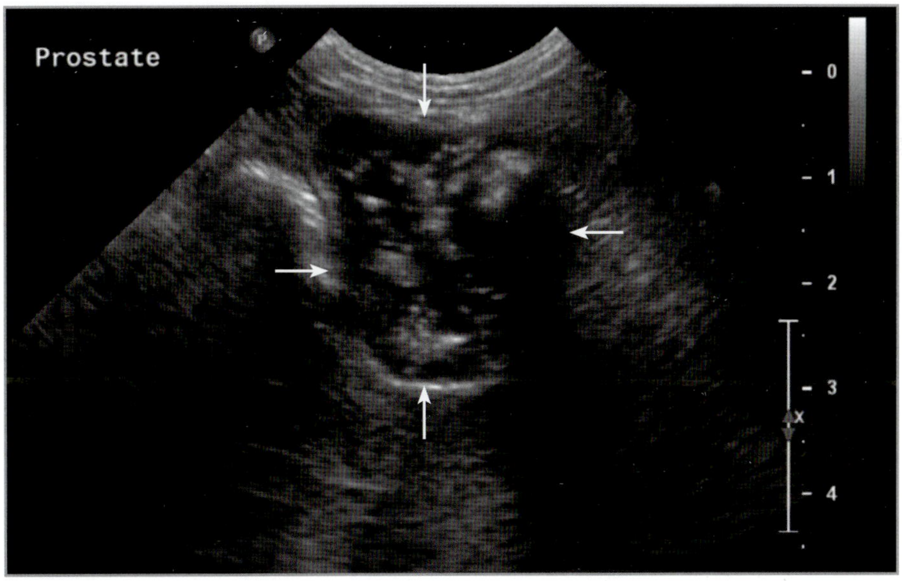

Figure 15. Prostatic carcinoma in an 11-year-old male neutered miniature Dachshund. The prostate (between arrows) is enlarged containing hyperechoic foci and hyperechoic areas, some with distal acoustic shadowing indicating mineralisation.

Table 1. Differential diagnosis of focal, multifocal and diffuse prostatic lesions.

Ultrasound appearance	Most likely differential diagnoses
Focal anechoic lesion	• Cyst (thin wall) • Abscess (thin or thick wall) • Necrosis
Focal hypoechoic nodules	• Neoplasia
Hyperechoic foci	• Calculi • Prostatic calcification • Gas
Normal prostatic appearance	• Normal • Benign prostatic hyperplasia
Increased echogenicity	• Benign prostatic hyperplasia • Prostatitis
Mixed echogenicity	• Prostatitis • Neoplasia

Testes

Orchitis is usually accompanied by epididymitis. The testicle is enlarged, and both the testicle and epididymis are of mixed echogenicity (Fig. 16). Anechoic areas may appear secondary to abscess formation. It is often difficult to differentiate orchitis from testicular neoplasia.

In testicular torsion, the testicle is enlarged with a hypoechoic parenchyma, the epididymis is enlarged and there is scrotal thickening. There is also absence of testicular blood flow, which can be demonstrated using Doppler ultrasonography.

Interstitial cell tumours, Sertoli cell tumours and seminomas are the most common testicular tumours. Sertoli cell tumours (Fig. 17) are associated with feminising syndrom. The ultrasonographic appearance of testicular tumours is variable. They may appear as nodules or more complex lesions of variable echogenicity and echotexture.

Cryptorchid (retained) testes may be located anywhere between the kidney and the inguinal canal and are generally small and hypoechoic. Identification of the central mediastinum testis allows differentiation of the retained testicle from a lymph node (Fig. 18). A neoplastic cryptorchid testicle has a mixed echogenicity, often resulting in loss of the mediastinum testis.

Atrophied testes are usually smaller than normal testes and either have the same or a reduced echogenicity.

Testicular or epididymal cysts are usually an incidental finding and appear as well-marginated anechoic areas with distal acoustic enhancement (Fig. 19).

Table 2 includes a list of the most likely differential diagnoses when identifying testicular lesions on ultrasound.

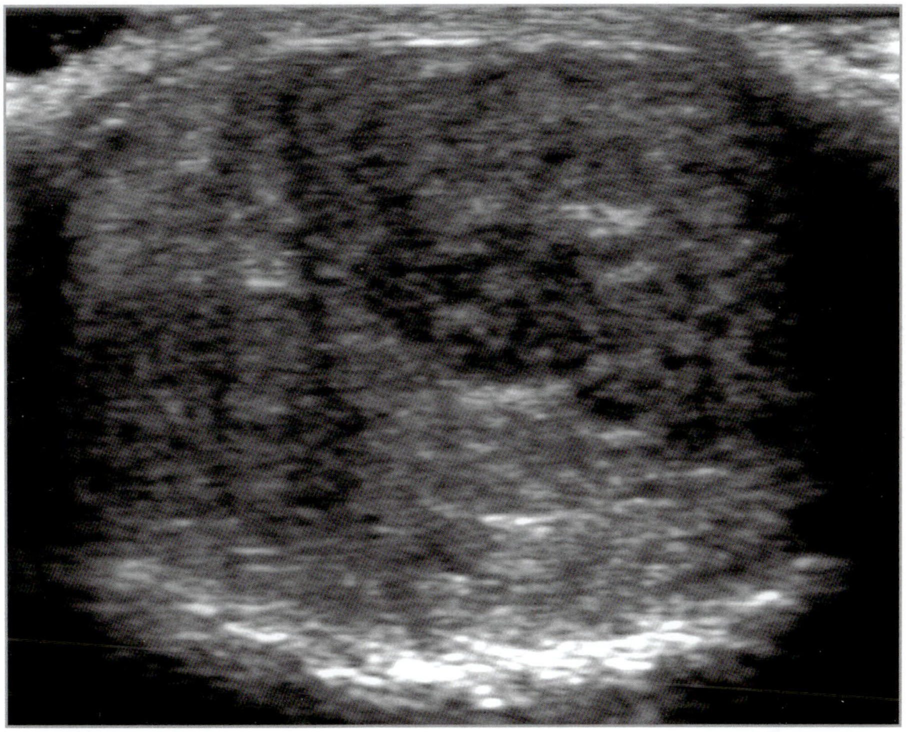

Figure 16. Canine orchitis. The testis appears markedly enlarged with mixed echogenicity.

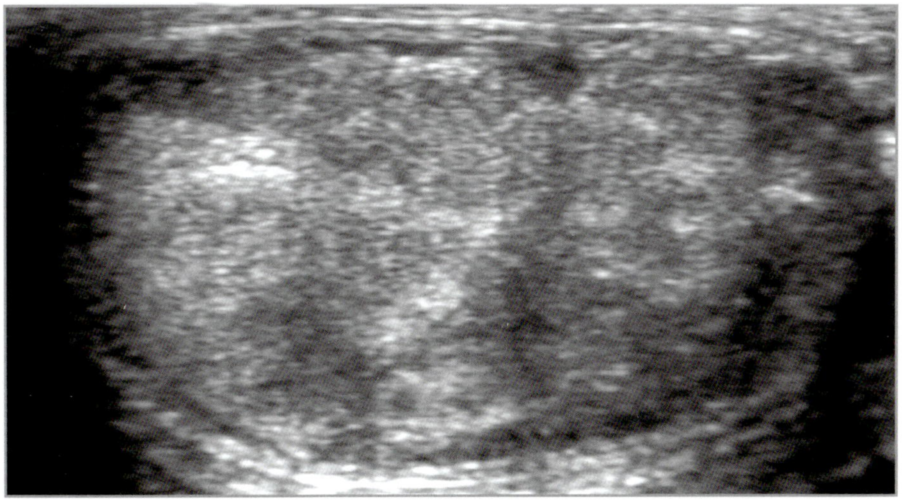

Figure 17. Sertoli cell tumour in a dog. The testis appears enlarged, with mixed echogenicity and loss of its normal architecture.

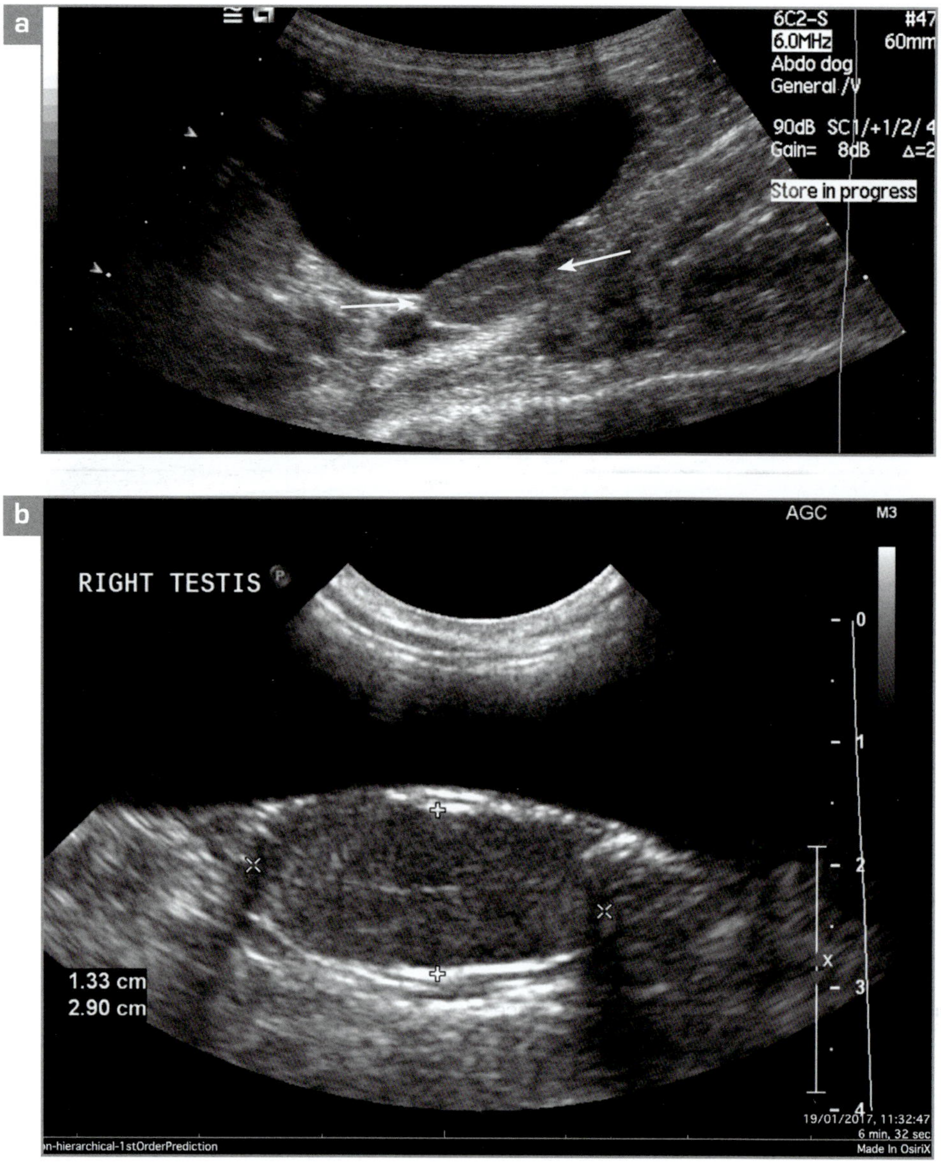

Figure 18. (a) A retained testicle (arrows) is identified next to the urinary bladder in a dog. The mediastinum testis distinguishes the retained testicle from a lymph node. (b) Close-up image of a retained testicle (between callipers) from a 5-year-old boxer. The retained testicle is next to the urinary bladder. The mediastinum testis is clearly visible.

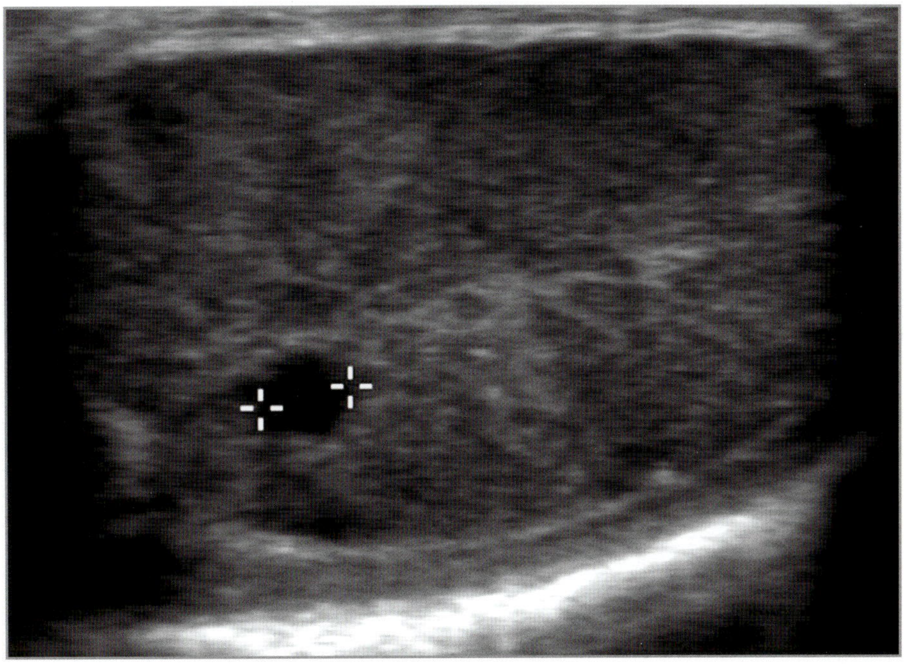

Figure 19. Testicular cyst (between callipers) in a dog. Testicular cysts are often an incidental finding

Table 2. Differential diagnosis of focal, multifocal and diffuse testicular lesions.

Ultrasound appearance	Most likely differential diagnoses
Anechoic focal lesion	• Cyst • Abscess
Hypoechoic focal lesion	• Abscess • Neoplasia • Infarct
Mixed focal lesions	• Neoplasia • Orchitis
Diffusely hypoechoic testes	• Atrophy • Torsion
Diffusely mixed echogenicity testes	• Orchitis • Neoplasia

13

CHAPTER

OVARIES, UTERUS AND MAMMARY GLANDS

Scanning technique

A 7–10 MHz transducer is required to evaluate the ovaries and uterus in dogs and cats. In pregnant females or large-sized dog breeds, a 5 MHz transducer is sufficient for the evaluation of the uterus.

Ovaries

1. The animal may be positioned in dorsal or lateral recumbency (right lateral recumbency for the left ovary and left lateral recumbency for the right ovary). The examination may also be performed with the patient in standing position, which is preferable for large and giant dog breeds. The author's preference is to perform the examination with the animal in lateral recumbency.

2. With the animal in lateral recumbency, place the transducer over the kidney (left or right) with the marker pointing to the head (Fig. 1).

3. Once the kidney is identified, scan the area up to 2 cm caudally, fanning the transducer dorsoventrally to identify the ovary (Fig. 2).

4. Each ovary is then evaluated in both longitudinal and transverse planes by fanning the transducer along the whole length and width of the organ.

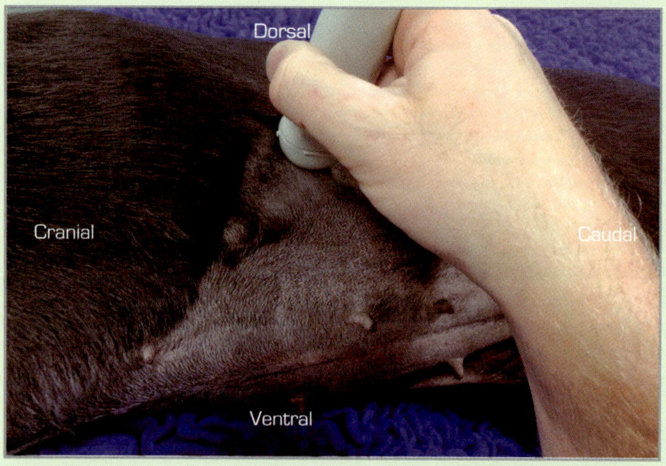

Figure 1. Placement of the transducer for the identification of the left kidney. The transducer is moved up to 2 cm caudally and fanned dorsoventrally to identify the left ovary. The technique is similar for the right kidney, with the animal in left lateral recumbency.

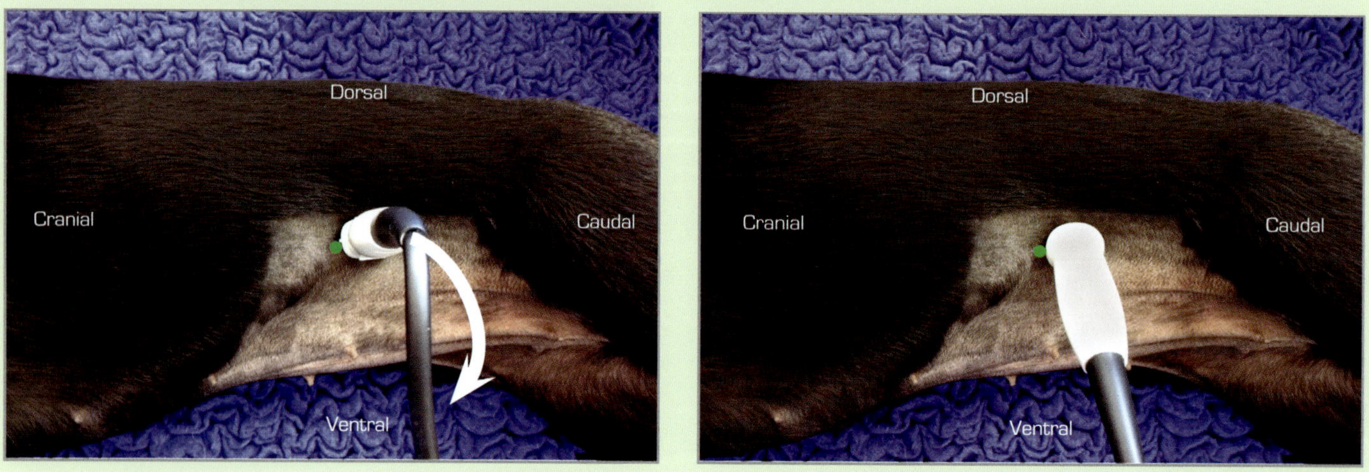

Figure 2. The transducer is fanned in a dorsal-to-ventral direction, 2 cm caudal to the left kidney in order to identify the left ovary.

Uterus

1. The animal may be positioned in dorsal or lateral recumbency, or in standing position. The technique is similar regardless of position.

2. With the animal in right lateral recumbency, the left hind limb is lifted and the transducer is placed onto the midline, at the level of the urinary bladder, in a transverse orientation and parallel to the tabletop with the marker pointing towards the tabletop (Fig. 3).

A standing examination is beneficial when performing pregnancy diagnosis or when searching for fluid in the uterus (e.g. pyometra). It may also be beneficial in large and giants breeds of dogs that are heavy and difficult to position and manipulate on a table.

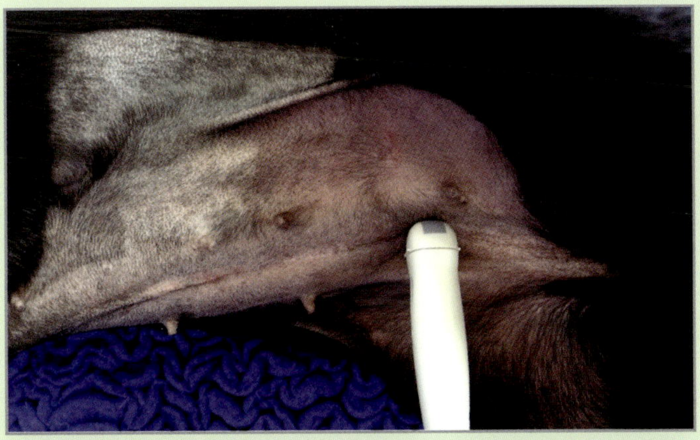

3. Identify the urinary bladder and colon and slide the transducer caudally (Fig. 4). The uterus (or uterine stump if the female has been neutered) is located between the urinary bladder and the colon (Figs. 5 and 6).

Figure 3. The transducer is placed on the midline and parallel to the tabletop for the identification of the uterus. For correct image orientation on the screen, the marker points to the tabletop (if the marker is on the left of the screen).

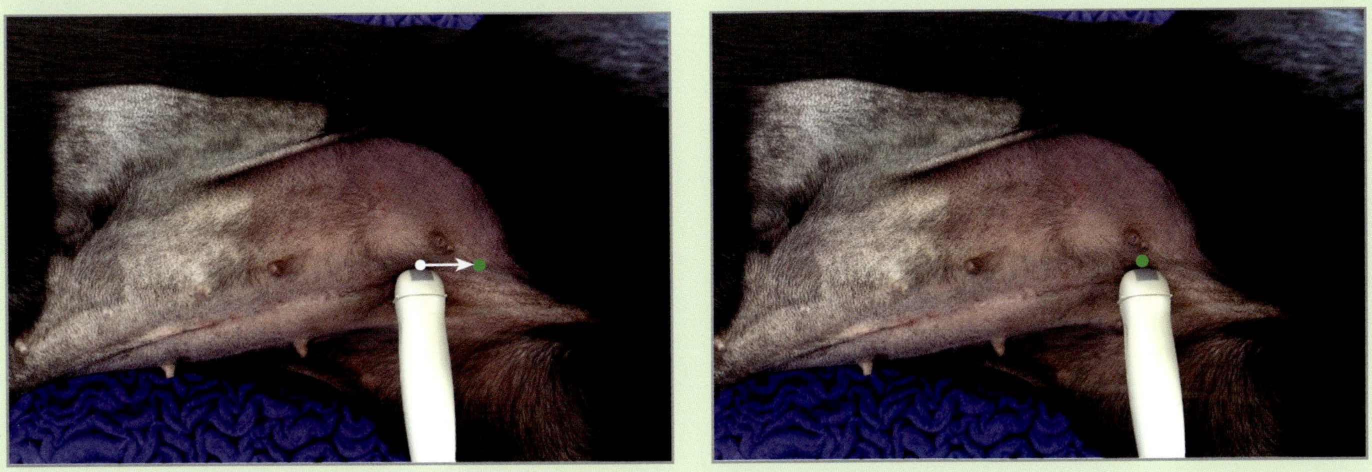

Figure 4. After identification of the urinary bladder and colon, the transducer is moved caudally to identify the uterus or uterine stump which lies between the urinary bladder and colon.

4. Once the uterus has been located, the transducer is rotated 90° clockwise to evaluate the organ longitudinally (Fig. 6a).

5. The uterus (or uterine stump if the female has been neutered) is examined in both transverse and longitudinal orientations by sliding the transducer cranially and caudally.

Uterine horns are not always clearly visible and it may not be possible to examine each horn entirely, especially during anoestrus.

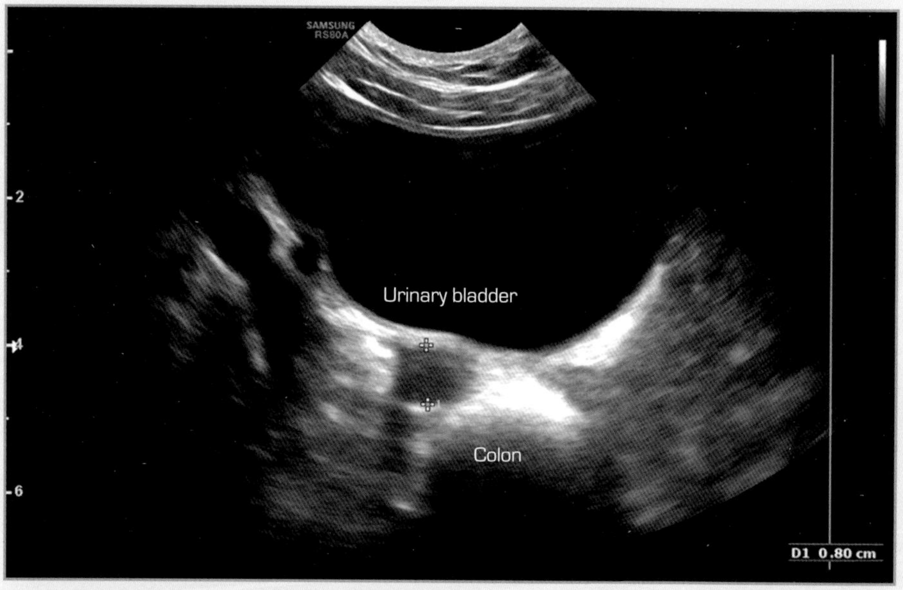

Figure 5. Transverse image of the uterus in a Great Dane. The hypoechoic uterine body (between callipers) is seen between the urinary bladder and the descending colon.

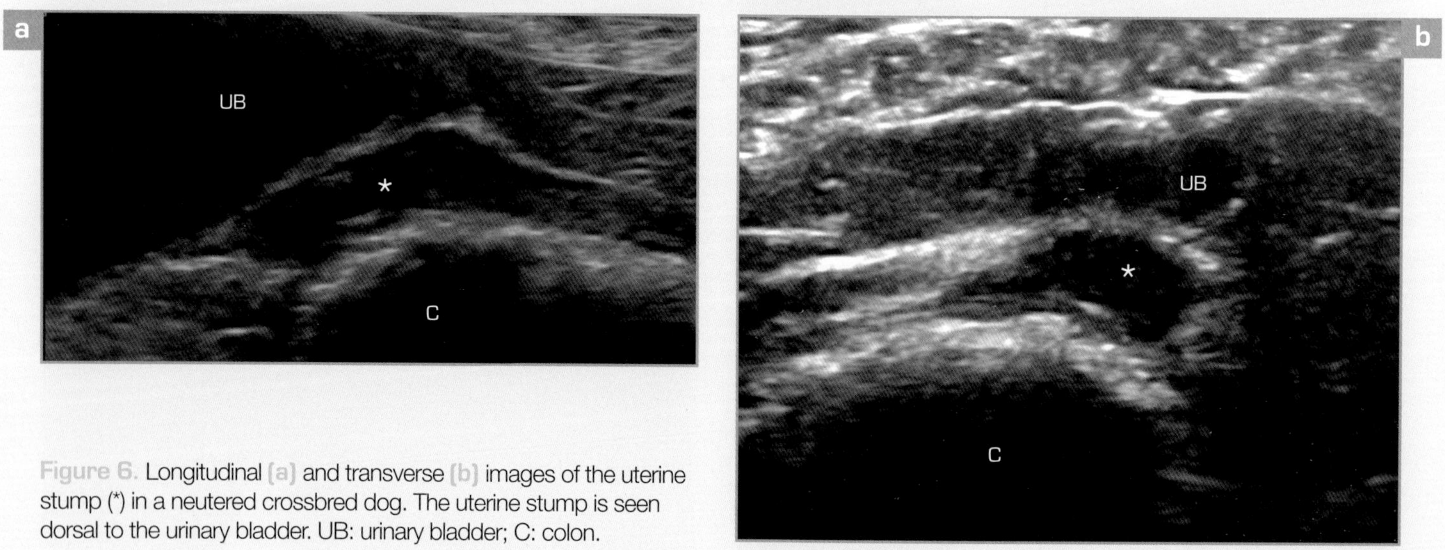

Figure 6. Longitudinal (a) and transverse (b) images of the uterine stump (*) in a neutered crossbred dog. The uterine stump is seen dorsal to the urinary bladder. UB: urinary bladder; C: colon.

Normal appearance

Ovaries

The ultrasonographic appearance of the ovaries varies throughout the oestrus cycle:

- In anoestrus and early proestrus, the ovaries are roughly oval, mildly hypoechoic and difficult to distinguish from the surrounding tissues (Fig. 7). The cortex and the medulla cannot be differentiated ultrasonographically.
- Follicular cysts can be identified between days 1 and 7 in proestrus and appear as thin-walled, anechoic cystic structures with distal acoustic enhancement (Fig. 8). Numerous small follicular cysts may not be identified individually, and the ovaries may appear diffusely hyperechoic.
- Follicular cysts grow until ovulation. Daily scanning is required to detect this phase.
- Ovulation leads to the development of a corpus haemorrhagicum, which is subsequently resorbed, forming a hypoechoic corpus luteum.

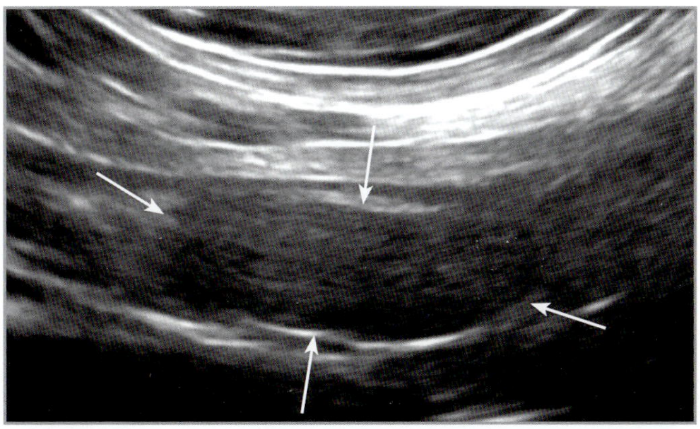

Figure 7. Normal right ovary (between arrows) of a Great Dane in anoestrus. The ovary is mildly hypoechoic to the surrounding mesentery.

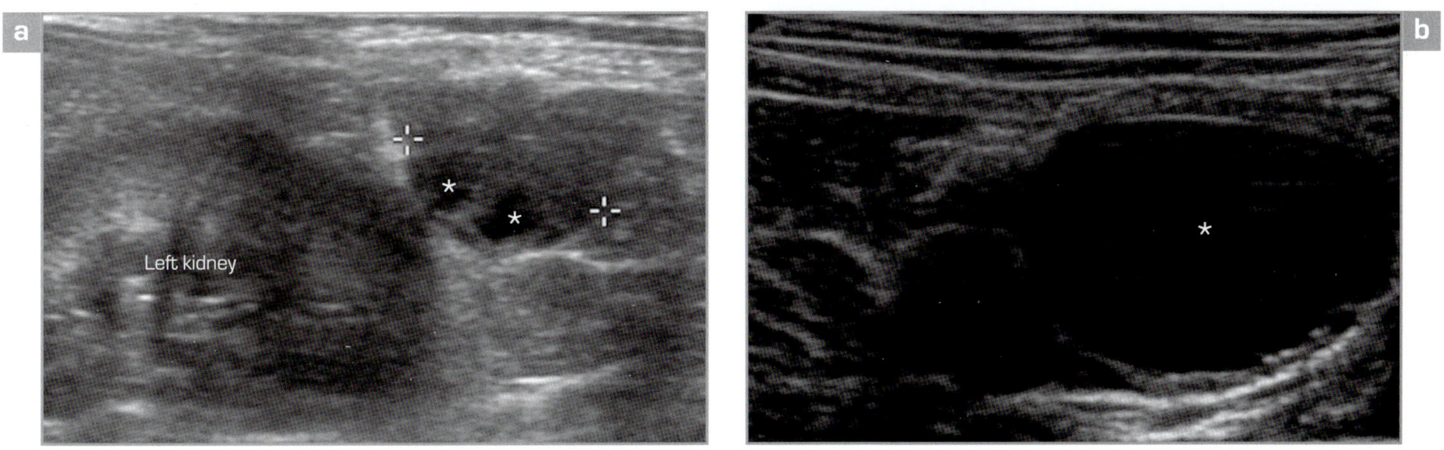

Figure 8. (a) Two small anechoic follicular cysts (*) are visible within the left ovary (between callipers) of a Chihuahua. **(b)** Large follicular cyst (*) in the left ovary of an 8-year-old Maltese Terrier.

Uterus

The normal non-gravid uterus appears as a small hypoechoic structure (see Figs. 5 and 6).

- The endometrium and myometrium cannot be differentiated ultrasonographically.
- The uterine lumen is normally empty or contains a small amount of mucus that appears as a small hyperechoic line. In oestrus, the uterine lumen may contain a very small amount of fluid.
- The uterine horns can be identified cranial to the bifurcation of the uterine body (Fig. 9). Examination from the bifurcation to each respective ovary can be challenging.

The uterus can be differentiated from a loop of small intestine because there is no wall layering or peristaltic movement. In addition, there is no gas or fluid present in the normal uterine lumen.

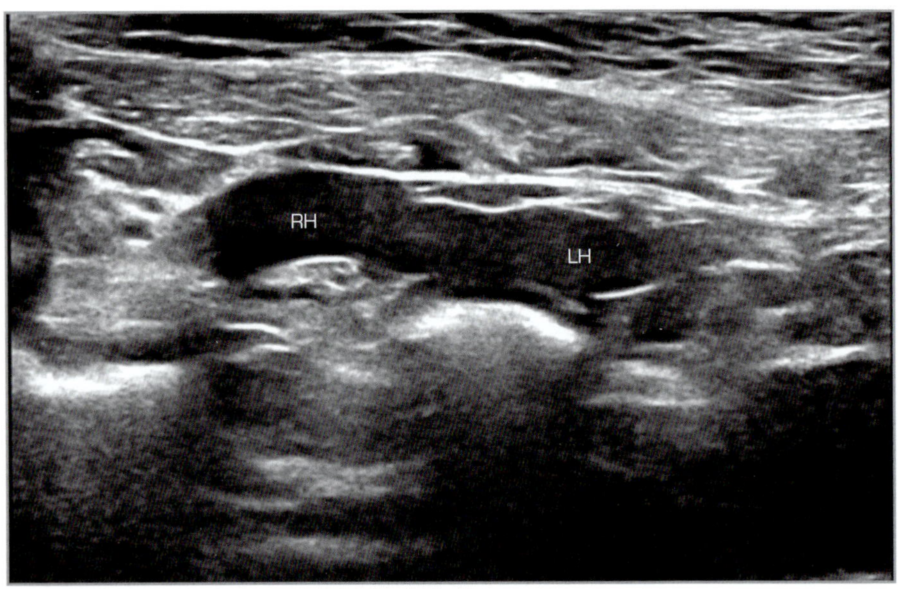

Figure 9. Appearance of the uterus from the uterine bifurcation to the two uterine horns, from the same Great Dane as in Fig. 7. The beginning of the right (RH) and the left horn (LH) are visible.

Variations from normal

Ovaries

Cystic ovarian disease appears as cystic lesions in the ovaries with anechoic contents and distal acoustic enhancement. It can be difficult to distinguish cystic ovarian disease from follicular cysts.

Ovarian neoplasms (Fig. 10) can be identified as masses in the area of one or both ovaries. They may be solid, cystic, or a combination. Large ovarian masses can appear in the mid-abdomen and may even be found lying in the ventral abdomen. Upon discovery of an intra-abdominal mass, an ovarian origin should be considered based on the location of the mass and the lack of association with other visible organs. It is not possible to distinguish the type of ovarian tumour ultrasonographically.

Ovarian stump granuloma may develop following ligature of the ovarian pedicle. It appears as a mass with a variable size, shape and echotexture. Patients with ovarian stump granuloma should be evaluated for concurrent ureteral occlusion.

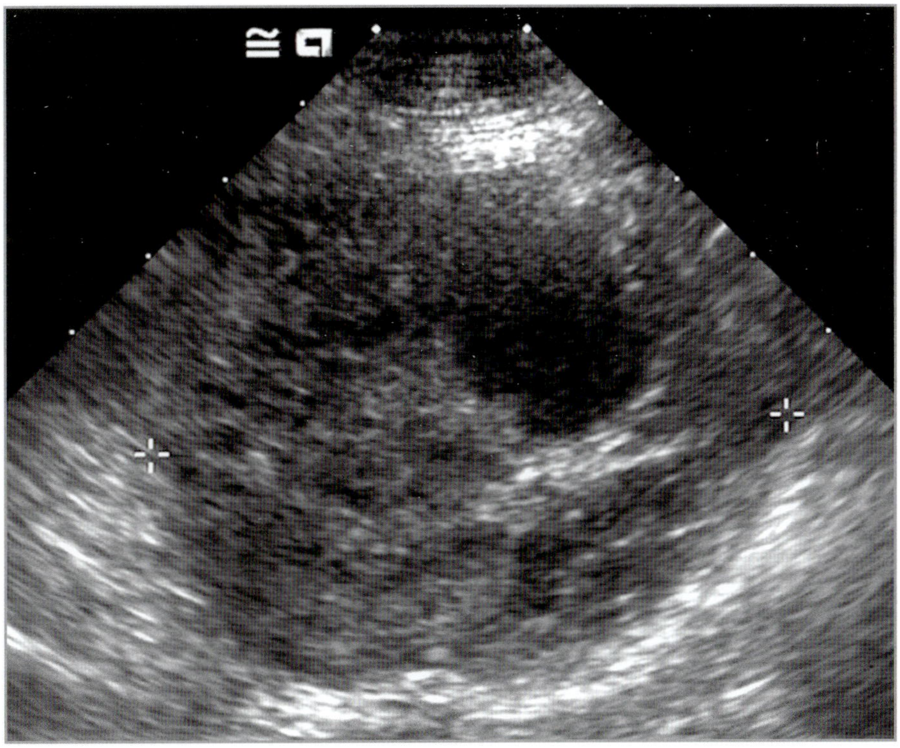

Figure 10. Ovarian carcinoma in an Irish Setter. The left ovary is rounded, has mixed echogenicity and contains anechoic cystic areas.

Uterus

Cystic endometrial hyperplasia (CEH) usually precedes pyometra and appears ultrasonographically as a thickened endometrium containing anechoic cystic structures (Fig. 11).

When pyometra is present, the uterus and uterine horns are enlarged and fluid-filled (Fig. 12). This enlargement is usually symmetrical, although focal or segmental changes can also be identified. The uterine contents may be anechoic or echogenic. Pyometra has to be differentiated from mucometra, haemometra and hydrometra, which have a similar ultrasonographic appearance (Table 1).

Table 1. Ultrasonographic features of the fluid in pyometra, hydrometra, mucometra and haemometra.

Ultrasonographic appearance of fluid in uterus	Suspected condition
Anechoic content	• Hydrometra • Mucometra • Pyometra • Haemometra
Hyperechoic content	• Pyometra • Haemometra • Mucometra

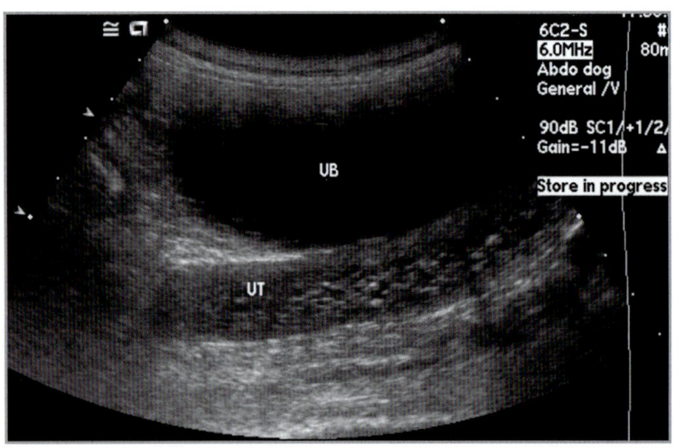

Figure 11. Cystic endometrial hyperplasia in a Dogue de Bordeaux. The uterine body (UT) is visible dorsal to the urinary bladder (UB). It is enlarged in diameter and the uterine wall contains multiple small anechoic cysts.

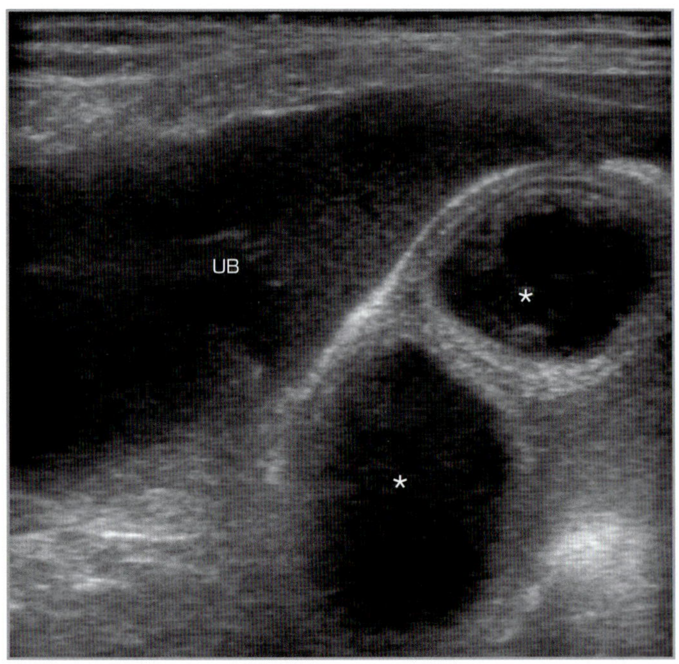

Figure 12. Pyometra in a dog. The uterus (*) appears dilated and fluid-filled. UB: urinary bladder.

> Differentiation between pyometra, mucometra, haemometra and hydrometra is not possible based on the ultrasonographic appearance of the uterine luminal fluid alone.

Uterine neoplasms (Fig. 13) are rare in dogs and cats. However, adenomas, adenocarcinomas, leiomyomas and leiomyosarcomas are the most commonly seen. They appear as masses or nodules of variable size, echogenicity and echotexture. Fluid within the uterine lumen may also be present.

> Differentiation between neoplastic and non-neoplastic lesions is not possible based on their ultrasonographic appearance alone.

In neutered females, uterine stump granuloma appears as a large mass associated with the uterine stump (Fig. 14).

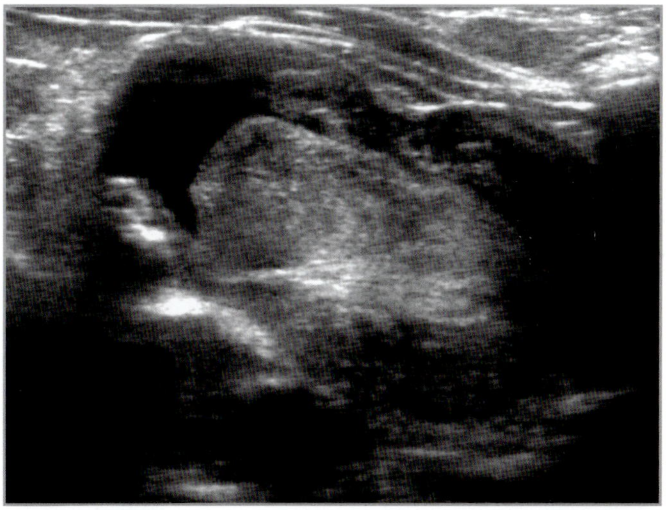

Figure 13. Uterine carcinoma in a Ragdoll cat. A mixed-echogenicity mass is visible surrounded by focal intraluminal fluid. Metastases were identified in the liver and the spleen.

a

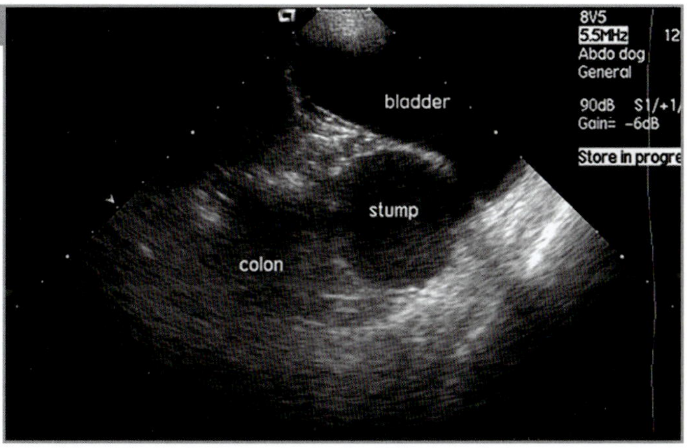

b

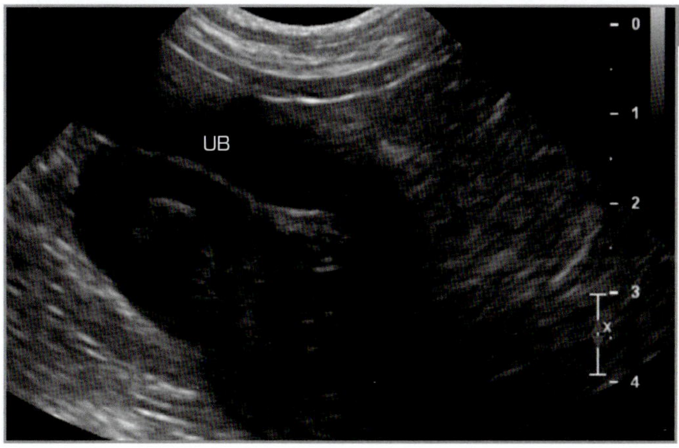

Figure 14. (a) Transverse image of a uterine stump granuloma (pyometra) in a Doberman. The uterine stump is visible between the urinary bladder and the descending colon. It appears thickened with mixed echogenicity. **(b)** Sagittal oblique image of a stump pyometra from an 11-year-old German Shepherd dog. The uterine stump appears as a mixed echogenicity cavitary mass dorsal to the urinary bladder (UB).

Pregnancy

Pregnancy can be diagnosed as early as 10–11 days after fertilisation; however, pregnancy diagnosis is most reliable 30 days after the last mating in dogs and 15–20 days after the last mating in cats.

Earlier detection may be difficult due to the small size of the uterus and gestational sac (Fig. 15). The gestational sac can be detected 18–19 days after the luteinising hormone (LH) peak.

Cardiac activity in dogs is detected as early as 23 days after the LH peak, while in cats it is detected 18–25 days post-breeding.

The normal heart rate in the foetus is approximately twice the maternal heart rate. A reduced heart rate is an indication of foetal stress.

In dogs (Yeager et al., 1992; Mattoon and Nyland, 1995; Sridevi, 2013), the foetal head and body may be seen by day 28, the limbs and foetal movement by day 35–36, and the foetal skeleton by day 33–39 (Fig. 16). The urinary bladder and stomach are identified by day 35–39. The kidneys are seen by day 39–47 and the four cardiac chambers can be distinguished by day 40. In the foetus, the lungs have the same echogenicity as the liver until day 38–42. After day 42, the lungs become hyperechoic to the liver. The intestines can be recognised at about 60 days (+/- 3 days).

In cats (Topie et al., 2015), the head and body may be seen by day 19–20, the heart can be observed by day 18, the stomach by day 27 while the front and hind limbs by day 24.

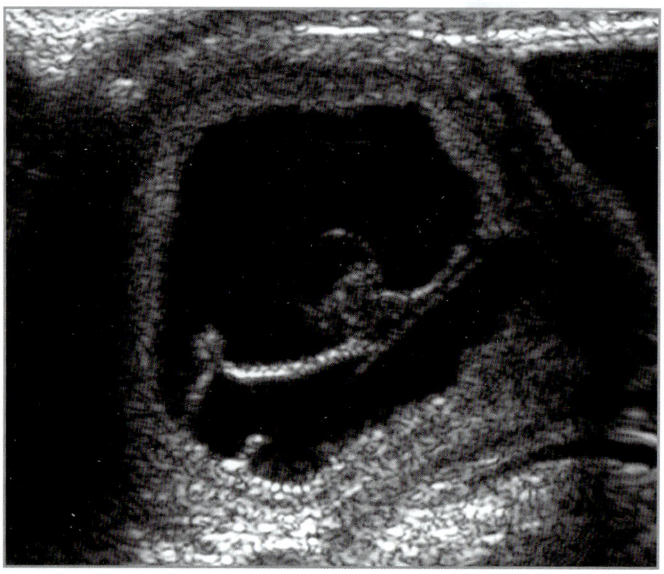

Figure 15. Three-week pregnancy in a cat. The embryo is visible in the centre.

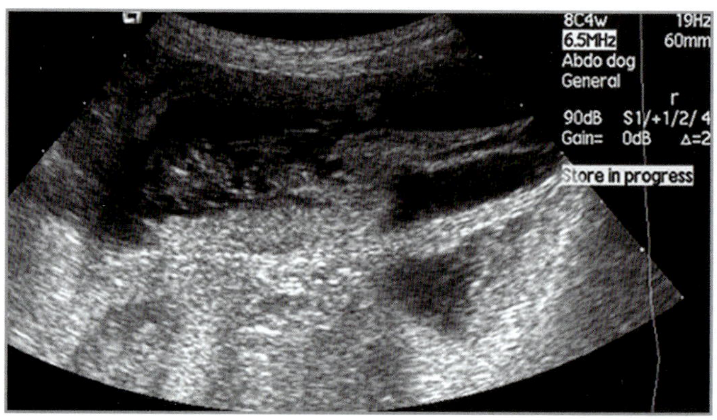

Figure 16. Five-week pregnancy in a dog. The limbs can be seen and there was movement in real time.

Foetal measurements for estimation of the foetal age

The most appropriate measurements depend on the stage of the gestation. Early in pregnancy, the gestational sac diameter is commonly used. The foetal crown-rump length can be measured and used if a long-axis view of the foetus can be obtained. Later in the gestation, the head diameter and the body diameter are used.

Estimation of foetal age in dogs

In dogs, the crown-rump length and the diameter of the gestational sac are used for estimating the gestational age until around day 40 (Fig. 17). The following formula has been used successfully by the author (as modified and adapted by Mattoon and Nyland, 1995):

6 × GESTATIONAL SAC DIAMETER + 20 = GESTATIONAL AGE +/– 3 DAYS

After about day 40, the transverse dimension of the skull (head diameter) and the transverse dimension of the body at the level of the liver are used. The author has used the following for dogs (as modified and adapted by Mattoon and Nyland, 1995):

15 × HEAD DIAMETER + 20 = GESTATIONAL AGE +/– 3 DAYS

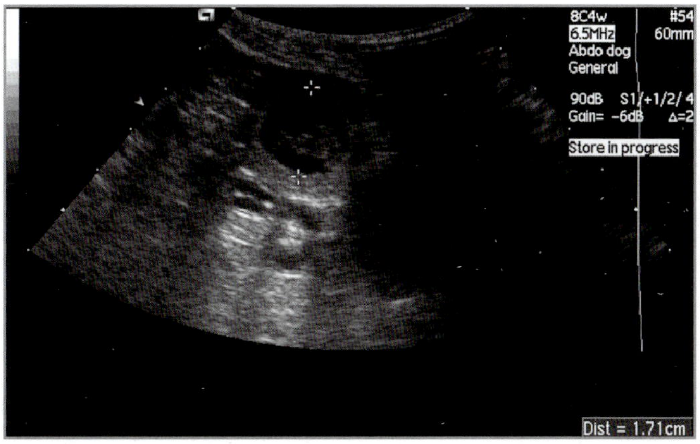

Figure 17. Gestational sac in a dog. Estimated gestational age: 30 +/– 3 days (6 × 1.7 + 20). Days before parturition: 35 +/– 3 days (65 – 30).

Estimation of foetal age in cats

In cats, both the gestational sac diameter and the crown-rump length can be used for the evaluation of the early gestational age (prior to 30 days). After 40 days, the head diameter and body diameter are commonly used. The author has used the head diameter for pregnancies of more than 40 days (as modified and adapted by Mattoon and Nyland, 1995):

25 × HEAD DIAMETER + 3 = GESTATIONAL AGE +/– 2 DAYS

More information about measurements for estimation of gestational age can be found in the recommended further reading list at the end of this book.

Days before parturition can also be calculated by subtracting the gestational age from 65 in the dog and 61 in the cat.

Although ultrasonography is sensitive for pregnancy diagnosis, it is not accurate for determining litter size because it is easy to miscount, for example, by including a foetus more than once. When it is considered necessary to accurately determine the litter size, abdominal radiography is recommended.

Involution of the postpartum period appears as gradual reduction of the uterine wall thickness and intraluminal fluid volume. It normally takes up to 28 days in dogs and 24 days in cats.

Abnormal pregnancy

If embryonic death occurs in early pregnancy, there is complete resorption of the embryo. In more advanced pregnancy, the dead embryo appears smaller than the others, with no heartbeat and echogenic amniotic fluid.

Foetal death later in pregnancy can be recognised by an absent heartbeat, lack of foetal movement, abnormal foetal posture, increased echogenicity of foetal fluid and gas accumulation.

Uterine torsion is characterised by increased thickness of the uterine wall, increased echogenicity of the uterine wall and foetal fluids, and signs of foetal death.

Congenital defects can also be diagnosed ultrasonographically.

Mammary glands

In non-lactating bitches, the mammary glands appear hypoechoic with a coarse echotexture.

Mammary tumours (Fig. 18) are variable in size and usually appear as masses with mixed echogenicity. The type of mammary tumour cannot be determined on the basis of the ultrasonographic signs alone. The regional lymph nodes should always be evaluated for signs of metastasis.

Mastitis (Fig. 19) appears as hypoechoic and enlarged mammary tissue, which can be heterogeneous in echogenicity. Abscesses may also be seen.

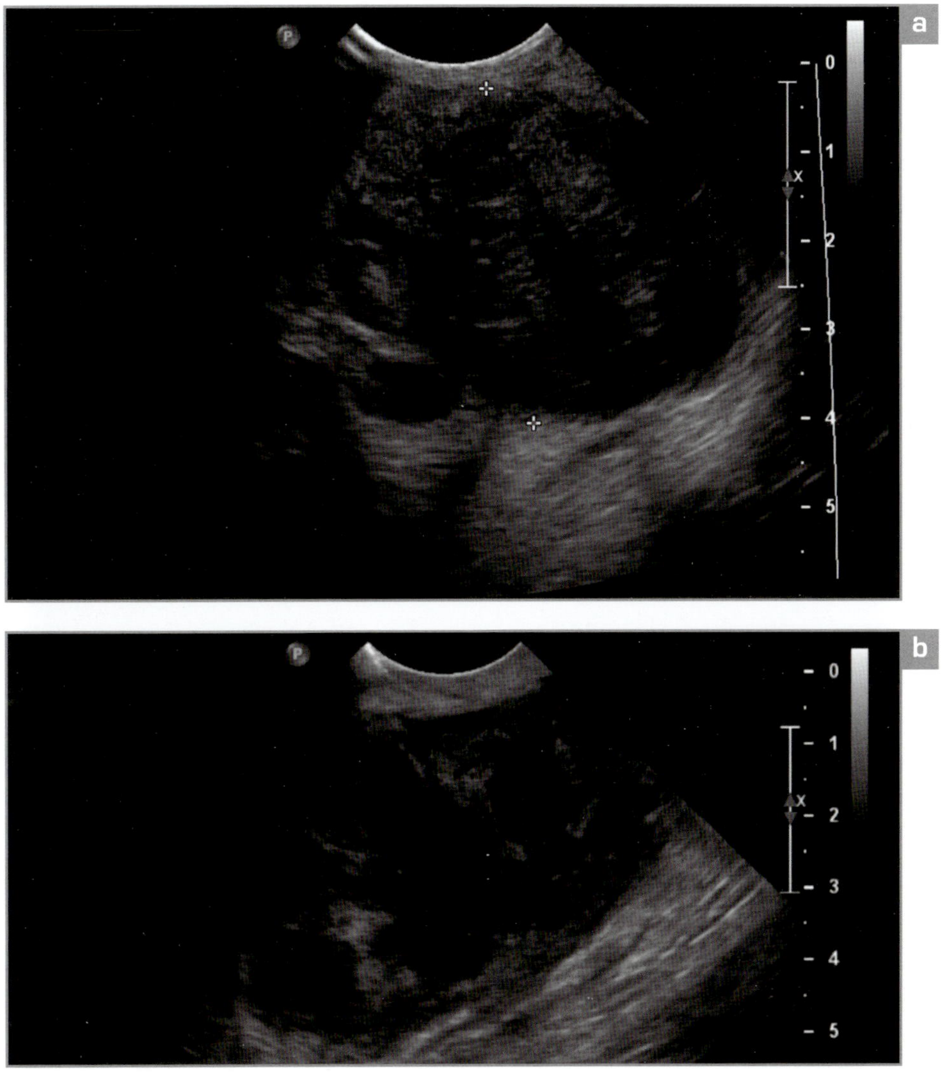

Figure 18. (a) Confirmed mammary gland carcinoma that appears as a mixed echogenicity mass in the right 5th mammary gland of a 10-year-old Labrador.
(b) Abscessed mammary gland carcinoma form from the 3rd mammary gland of the same animal. The mass content cavitary areas with small echogenic foci.

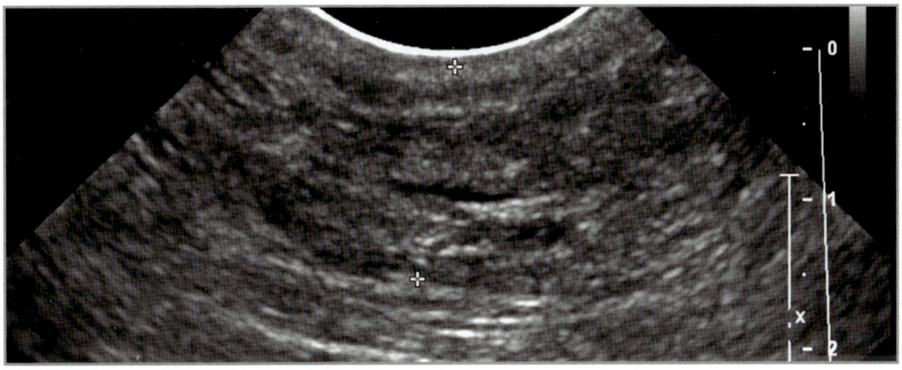

Figure 19. Thick mixed echogenicity mammary gland in a 4-year-old German Shepherd dog with mastitis.

14

CHAPTER

OVERVIEW OF ABDOMINAL ULTRASONOGRAPHY

The aim of an abdominal ultrasound examination is to evaluate every accessible abdominal organ or structure in a reasonable amount of time. The order in which the organs are examined is irrelevant, provided the examination is comprehensive. Ultrasonographers are encouraged to develop a systematic approach using a set protocol.

A 10–15 kg dog is ideal for beginners as this will allow the ultrasonographer to practice positioning and movements of the transducer without having to apply too much pressure.

Preparation of the examination

First of all, it is important to input the animal's data by creating a new patient card. This way, the animal's details as well as the date and time of examination will be saved and recorded with the stored images and clips.

It is best to start with a large organ, e.g. the liver, using a lower-frequency transducer. The frequency may be increased during the examination, particularly for the examination of more superficial structures. The depth, focal zone, and overall gain can be adjusted throughout the examination to optimise the image quality. The time gain compensation is usually adjusted at the beginning and is rarely modified during the examination.

You are now ready to start the examination. Although this chapter describes the technique in the order preferred by the author (see below), the organs may be examined in the order that best suits the veterinary surgeon.

> Beginners may find it difficult to locate and examine the left lobe and body of the pancreas and the right adrenal; however, with increased experience, this will become routine.

Recommended procedure for abdominal ultrasound examination

1. Position the patient in right lateral recumbency (dorsal recumbency can also be used) with the head pointing towards the ultrasound machine and the limbs towards the examiner. The transducer's marker should be displayed on the left side of the screen.

2. The liver is examined first. Place the transducer parallel to the tabletop with the marker pointing to the patient's head and orient it towards the shoulders. Rock the transducer in a craniocaudal direction until the liver "fills" the screen.

3. Fan the transducer towards the left and right side of the animal to examine the whole liver. Then, rotate the transducer 90° anticlockwise and fan it cranially and caudally along the whole length of the liver. The gallbladder should also be examined at the same time (Video 1). If the whole liver does not fit on the screen, you can examine the cranial half first, and then the caudal half.

If it is not possible to place the transducer caudal to the xiphoid due to the patient's conformation (e.g. deep-chested dogs), then the liver must be examined intercostally from both sides (see the Liver chapter).

Video 1. Liver and gallbladder technique

4. The stomach is the next organ to be assessed. With the transducer in the initial position (parallel to the tabletop and oriented towards the shoulders) and the marker pointing to the animal head, slide it caudally and to the left side to identify the stomach, located immediately caudal to the liver. Fan the transducer up and down to examine the whole stomach in transverse orientation. Then, rotate the transducer approximately 90° clockwise and rock it dorsally and ventrally to examine the fundus (dorsal rocking) and pylorus (ventral rocking) in a longitudinal orientation (Video 2).

Video 2. Stomach technique

5. The spleen is examined next. Starting from the liver, slide the transducer to the left, following the last rib (feeling the rib cranial to the transducer) until you identify the spleen. In some animals, the spleen will be found in a very dorsal location. At this point, you should be near the cranial splenic margin or just caudal to it. If the latter, slide the transducer cranially to identify the cranial margin of the spleen. Then, fan the transducer dorsally to examine the head of the spleen and then ventrally before returning to the starting position. Slide the transducer caudoventrally towards the tail of the spleen, repeating the fanning movement every couple of centimetres to assess the whole organ. Finally, rotate the transducer 90° clockwise and slide it cranially to examine the spleen in a transverse orientation (Video 3).

Video 3. Spleen technique

If the spleen cannot be identified, always remember to review the patient's history (e.g. has the animal undergone a splenectomy in the past?). If the spleen should be present and still cannot be identified, it is usually because it is located within the rib cage and/or is very small. In these cases, slide the transducer intercostally from the left side to identify it.

6. The next organ to be examined is the left lobe (limb) of the pancreas. This can be very challenging for a beginner and should be attempted once you are a little more experienced. To that end, identify the spleen and, just below it, the splenic vein on the screen. Slide the transducer dorsally towards the spine. Look carefully and identify the portal vein. You will find the left lobe of the pancreas between the splenic vein and the portal vein (Video 4).

Video 4. Left limb of the pancreas technique

7. The left kidney is imaged next. It can be identified by positioning the transducer caudal to the last rib, on the dorsal abdomen or, alternatively, sliding the transducer dorsally from the caudal edge of the spleen towards the spine. The examination of the kidney in its long axis is achieved by slight rotation of the transducer in a clockwise or anticlockwise direction. Once you have the maximum renal length on the screen, fan the transducer dorsally and ventrally, ensuring the whole kidney is examined. Finally, rotate the transducer 90° clockwise (short axis) and fan it cranially and caudally until you have examined the whole kidney (Video 5).

Video 5. Left kidney technique

8. The left adrenal follows in the examination. With the left kidney visible and the transducer oriented parallel to the spine, fan the transducer slowly until the aorta is visible across the screen. If you do not see the aorta crossing the screen (it may appear as an oval or rounded anechoic structure), it means that the transducer is oblique in position. To correct this, a slight rotation of the transducer is required. Once the aorta is visible across the screen, carefully identify the renal artery coming off the aorta near the kidney. Press, mildly to moderately, harder with the transducer and fan it slowly in a ventral direction until the left adrenal is identified next to the renal artery (cranial to the renal artery-aorta junction). Optimise the image by slightly rotating the transducer until both cranial and caudal poles of the left adrenal are visible on the screen (Video 6).

Video 6. Left adrenal technique

9. If the patient is an entire female, the left ovary can be found approximately up to 2 cm caudal to the left kidney.

10. The medial iliac lymph nodes can be examined next. They are found by following the aorta caudally from the left kidney to the aortic bifurcation (Video 7).

Video 7. Medial iliac lymph node technique

11. Ventral and caudal sliding of the transducer from the aortic bifurcation allows the identification of the urinary bladder. This organ is examined by fanning the transducer in sagittal and transverse orientation (Video 8).

Video 8. Urinary bladder technique

12. If the patient is a male dog, the prostate can be identified by sliding the transducer caudal to the urinary bladder (Video 9). If the prostate is intrapelvic and not visible, an assistant can help to make it more accessible by pushing it cranially (see the Prostate chapter for more details).

Video 9. Prostate technique

13. If the patient is a female, the uterus (or uterine stump if it is a neutered female) can be identified and examined. Place the transducer on the midline of the abdomen in a transverse orientation with the marker pointing up and parallel to the tabletop. Identify the urinary bladder and descending colon, and then slide the transducer caudally. The uterus (or uterine stump) is located between the urinary bladder and the descending colon. Finally, rotate the transducer 90° anticlockwise to examine the uterus in a longitudinal orientation (Video 10).

Video 10. Uterus technique

14. The small intestine is examined following a "castle" pattern (Video 11). The descending colon is located dorsal to the urinary bladder and can be followed to the ileocaecocolic junction. The descending duodenum may be examined during the evaluation of the right lobe of the pancreas. It is important to also examine the peritoneum and lymph nodes while examining the intestine.

Video 11. Intestines technique

15. In cats and small dogs, the right kidney (Video 12), right adrenal (Video 13) and right lobe of the pancreas (Video 14) can be examined by placing the transducer under the animal. The transducer is placed at the level of the umbilicus, parallel to the table and oriented towards the last rib. Press harder with the transducer to identify the right kidney, optimising the image with slight fanning and rotating movements.

Video 12. Right kidney technique (small dog)

16. The right adrenal can be examined next in cats and small dogs. Identify the kidney and keep the craneal pole in the middle, fan the transducer upwards to identify the caudal vena cava. Press harder and fan the transducer slowly ventrally to identify the right adrenal.

Video 13. Right adrenal technique (small dog)

17. Once the evaluation of the right kidney and right adrenal is complete, identify the right kidney release the pressure on the transducer. The descending duodenum then will "fall" into view with the right lobe of the pancreas visible just below. To confirm that the duodenum has been identified correctly, fan the transducer ventrally until it is pointing to the table, and then fan it slowly upwards. The first loop of intestine you encounter must be the descending duodenum.

Video 14. Right pancreas technique (small dog)

18. In large dogs, the examination of the right kidney is performed with the patient in left lateral recumbency with the head towards the ultrasound machine and the limbs away from the examiner. The right kidney is located near the spine, at the level of the last two intercostal spaces or just caudal to the last space. Once identified, optimise the image by rotating the transducer to lengthen the view of the kidney. The technique used to examine the right kidney is similar to that described for the examination of the left kidney (Video 15).

Video 15. Right kidney technique (large dog)

19. The right adrenal is examined next in large dogs. At the level of the right kidney, with the transducer parallel to the spine, fan the transducer dorsally to identify the aorta. Then, slide the transducer ventrally to identify the caudal vena cava (CVC). The CVC is the vessel located ventral to the aorta. Once it has been identified, fan the transducer slowly and carefully in a dorsal direction. The right adrenal is located between the right kidney and the CVC. The right adrenal is often identified just when the CVC disappears from the screen (Video 16).

Video 16. Right adrenal technique (large dog)

20. If the patient is an entire female, the right ovary should also be examined. It is usually located up to 2 cm caudal to the right kidney.

21. The duodenum and the pancreas are the next organs to be examined. In large dogs, identify the right kidney (as described in video 16) and slide the transducer ventrally until the first loop of small intestine is visible at the top of the screen; this is the descending duodenum. The right lobe of the pancreas is visible below the duodenum. Optimise the image by slightly fanning the transducer (Video 17).

Video 17. Right pancreas technique (large dog)

22. The body of the pancreas is located between the pylorus and the portal vein, and is commonly identified with the animal in right lateral recumbency for cats, small and large dogs (Video 18). It can also be identified with the animal in left lateral or dorsal recumbency.

Video 18. Body of the pancreas technique

23. The abdominal examination is complete.

RECOMMENDED FURTHER READING

Chapter 1. Machine set-up

Curry TS III, Dowdey JE, Murry RC. Ultrasound. In: *Christensen's Physics of Diagnostic Radiology*. 4th ed. Philadelphia. Lea and Febiger. 1990; 323-371.

Herring DS, Bjornton G. Physics, facts and artifacts of diagnostic ultrasound. *Vet Clin North Am Small Anim Pract*. 1985; 15:1107-1122.

Kremkau FW. Sonography *Principles and Instruments*. 8th ed. Philadelphia. Elsevier Saunders. 2011.

Mattoon JS, Berry CR. Fundamendals of Diagnostic Ultrasound. In: *Small Animal Diagnostic Ultrasound*. 4th ed. St Louis, Missouri. Elsevier Saunders. 2021; 1-48.

Chapter 3. Liver and gallbladder

Atalan G, Barr FJ, Holt PE. Estimation of the volume of the gall bladder of 32 dogs from linear ultrasonographic measurements. *Vet Rec.* 2007;160(4):118-122.

Bertolini G. Acquired portal collateral circulation in the dog and cat. *Vet Radiol Ultrasound*. 2010; 51:25-33.

Besso JG, Wrigley RH, Gliatto JM et al. Ultrasonographic appearance and clinical findings in 14 dogs with gallbladder mucocele. *Vet Radiol Ultrasound*. 2000; 41:261-271.

Biller DS, Kantrowitz B, Miyabayashi T. Ultrasonography of diffuse liver disease. A review. J *Vet Intern Med.* 1992; 6:71-76.

Book AP, Fidel J, Wills T et al. Correlation of ultrasound findings, liver and spleen cytology, and prognosis in the clinical staging of high metastatic risk canine mast cell tumors. *Vet Radiol Ultrasound*. 2011; 52:548-554.

Bromel C, Barthez PY, Leveille R et al. Prevalence of gallbladder sludge in dogs as assessed by ultrasonography. *Vet Radiol Ultrasound.* 1998; 39:206-210.

Crews LJ, Feeney DA, Jessen CR et al. Clinical, ultrasonographic, and laboratory findings associated with gallbladder disease and rupture in dogs: 45 cases (1997-2007). *J Am Vet Med Assoc.* 2009; 234:359-366.

D'Anjou MA, Penninck D, Cornejo L et al. Ultrasonographic diagnosis of portosystemic shunting in dogs and cats. *Vet Radiol Ultrasound.* 2004; 45:424-437.

D'Anjou MA. The sonographic search for portosystemic shunts. *Clin Tech Small Anim Pract*. 2007; 22:104-114.

D'Anjou MA. Liver. In: *Atlas of Small Animal Ultrasonography*. Iowa. Blackwell publishing. 2008; 217-262.

Dennis R, Kirberger RM, Wrigley RH, Barr FJ. Handbook of Small Animal Radiology and Ultrasound, Techniques and Differential Diagnoses. 2nd edition. Philadelphia, W.B. Saunders Co. 2010; 239-248.

Diana A, Guglielmini C, Specchi S, Di Tommaso M, Pietra M, Baron Toaldo M, Cipone M. Ultrasonographic evaluation of preprandial and postprandial gallbladder volume in healthy cats. *Am J Vet Res*. 2012, 73(10):1583-1588.

Faverzani S, Chinosi S, Valenti P, Caniatti M. Comparison between ultrasonography and cytology of liver focal lesions and parenchyma in the dog and cat. *Vet Res Comm.* 2006; 30 (Suppl. 1):293-296.

Hittmair KM, Vielgrader HD, Loupal G. Ultrasonographic evaluation of gallbladder wall thickness in cats. *Vet Radiol Ultrasound.* 2001; 42:149-155.

Ivancić M, Mai W. Qualitative and quantitative comparison of renal versus hepatic ultrasonographic intensity in healthy dogs. *Vet Radiol Ultrasound.* 2008; 49:368-373.

Lamb CR, Mahoney PN. Comparison of 3 methods for calculating portal blood flow velocity in dogs using duplex-Doppler ultrasonography. *Vet Radiol Ultrasound*. 1994; 35:190-194.

Leveille R, Biller DS, Shiroma JT. Sonographic evaluation of the common bile duct in cats. *J Vet Intern Med.* 1996; 10:296-299.

Moon Larson M, Mattoon JS, Lawrence Y, Sellon RK. Liver. In: *Small Animal Diagnostic Ultrasound*. 4th ed. St Louis, Missouri. Elsevier Saunders. 2021; 15: 355-421.

Penninck DG, Brisson JO, Webster CR. Sonographic assessment of gallbladder volume in normal cats. Vet Radiol Ultrasound. 2010;51(6):665-666

Pike FS, Berg J, King NW et al. Gallbladder mucocele in dogs: 30 cases (2000-2002). *J Am Vet Med Assoc.* 2004; 224:1615-1622.

Ramstedt KL, Center SA, Randolph JF, Yeager AE, Erb HN, Warner KL. Changes in gallbladder volume in healthy dogs after food was withheld for 12 hours followed by ingestion of a meal or a meal containing erythromycin. *Am J Vet Res*. 2008; 69(5):647-651.

Sonnenfield JM, Armbrust LJ, Radlinsky MA et al. Radiographic and ultrasonographic findings of liver lobe torsion in a dog. *Vet Radiol Ultrasound.* 2001; 42:344-346.

Spalding KA. Gallbladder wall thickness. *Vet Radiol Ultrasound*. 1993; 34:270-273.

Tivers M, Lipscomb V. Congenital portosystemic shunts in cats. Investigation, diagnosis and stabilisation. *J Feline Med Surg.* 2011; 13:173-184.

Warren-Smith CM, Andrew S, Mantis P, Lamb CR. Lack of associations between ultrasonographic appearance of parenchymal lesions of the canine liver and histological diagnosis. *J Small Anim Pract.* 2012; 53:168-173.

Chapter 4. Spleen

Crabtree AC, Spangler E, Beard D, Smith A. Diagnostic accuracy of gray-scale ultrasonography for the detection of hepatic and splenic lymphoma in dogs. *Vet Radiol Ultrasound. 2010; 51(6)*:661-664.

Cuccovillo A, Lamb CR. Cellular features of sonographic target lesions of the liver and spleen in 21 dogs and a cat. *Vet Radiol Ultrasound.* 2002; 43:275-278.

Dennis R, Kirberger RM, Wrigley RH, Barr FJ. Handbook of Small Animal Radiology and Ultrasound, Techniques and Differential Diagnoses. 2nd edition. Philadelphia, W.B. Saunders Co. 2010; 248-252.

Hanson JA, Papageorges M, Girard E, Menard, M, Hebert P. Ultrasonographic appearance of splenic disease in 101 cats. *Vet Radiol Ultrasound.* 2001; 42:441-445.

Hardie EM, Vaden SL, Spaulding K, Malarkey DE. Splenic infarction in 16 dogs: a retrospective study. *J Vet Intern Med.* 1995; 9:141-148.

Hecht S. Spleen. In*: Atlas of Small Animal Ultrasonography.* Iowa. Blackwell publishing. 2008. 263-280.

Mattoon JS, Duffy M. Spleen. In: *Small Animal Diagnostic Ultrasound*. 4th ed. St Louis, Missouri. Elsevier Saunders. 2021. 422-460.

O'Brien RT, Waller KR, Osgood TL. Sonography can features of drug-induced splenic congestion. *Vet Radiol Ultrasound.* 2004; 45:225-227.

SAUNDERS HM, NEATH PJ, BROCKMAN DJ. B-mode and Doppler ultrasound imaging of the spleen with canine splenic torsion: a retrospective evaluation. *Vet Radiol Ultrasound*. 1998; 39:349-353.

SCHWARZ LA, PENNINCK DG, GLIATTO J. Canine splenic myelolipomas. *Vet Radiol Ultrasound*. 2001; 42:347-348.

SPANGLER WL, CULBERTSON MR. Prevalence and type of splenic diseases in cats: 455 cases (1985-1991). *J Am Vet Med Assoc*. 1992; 201:773-776.

Chapter 5. Gastrointestinal tract

GOGGIN JM, BILLER DS, DEBEY BM, PICKAR JG, MASON D. Ultrasonographic measurement of gastrointestinal wall thickness and the ultrasonographic appearance of the ileocolic region in healthy cats. *J Am Anim Hosp Assoc*. 2000;36(3):224-228.

HOFFMANN KL. Sonographic signs of gastroduodenal linear foreign body in 3 dogs. *Vet Radiol Ultrasound*. 2003; 44:466-469.

LAMB CR, MANTIS P. Ultrasonographic features of intestinal intussusception in 10 dogs. *J Small Anim Pract*. 1998; 39:437-441.

MOON ML, BILLER DS, ARMBRUST LJ. Ultrasonographic appearance and etiology of corrugated small intestine. *Vet Radiol Ultrasound*. 2003; 44:199-203.

NEWELL SM, GRAHAM JP, ROBERTS GD, GINN PE, HARRISON JM. Sonography of the normal feline gastrointestinal tract. *Vet Radiol Ultrasound*. 1999; 40:40-43.

NEELIS DA, MATTOON JS, SLOVAK JE, SELLON RK. Gastrointestinal Tract. In: *Small Animal Diagnostic Ultrasound*. 4th ed. St Louis, Missouri. Elsevier Saunders. 2021; 491-525.

NYLAND TG, NEELIS DA, MATTOON JS. Gastrointestinal Tract. In: *Small Animal Diagnostic Ultrasound*. 3rd ed. St Louis, Missouri. Elsevier Saunders. 2015; 468-500.

PENNINCK D, SMYERS B, WEBSTER CRL, RAND W, MOORE AS. Diagnostic value of ultrasonography in differentiating enteritis from intestinal neoplasia in dogs. *Vet Radiol Ultrasound*. 2003; 44:570-575.

PENNINCK D, MATZ M, TIDWELL A. Ultrasonography of gastric ulceration in the dog. *Vet Radiol Ultrasound*. 1997; 38:308-312.

PENNINCK DG, NYLAND TG, KERR LY, FISHER PE. Ultrasonographic evaluation of gastrointestinal diseases in small animals. *Vet Radiol Ultrasound*. 1990; 31:134-141.

PENNINCK DG, NYLAND TG, FISHER PE, KERR LY. Ultrasonography of the normal canine gastrointestinal tract. *Vet Radiol Ultrasound*. 1989; 30:272-276.

STANDER N, WAGNER WM, GODDARD A, KIRBERGER RM. Ultrasonographic appearance of canine parvoviral enteritis in puppies. *Vet Radiol Ultrasound*. 2010; 51:69-74.

SUTHERLAND-SMITH J, PENNINCK DJ, KEATING JH, WEBSTER CRL. The morphological significance of ultrasonographic intestinal hyperechoic striations in dogs. *Vet Radiol Ultrasound*. 2007; 48:51-57.

SWIFT I. Ultrasonographic features of intestinal entrapment in dogs. *Vet Radiol Ultrasound*. 2009; 50:205-207.

TIDWELL AS, PENNINCK DG. Ultrasonography of gastrointestinal foreign bodies. *Vet Radiol Ultrasound*. 1992; 33:160-169.

YAM PS, JOHNSON VS, MARTINEAU HM, DICKIE A, SULLIVAN M. Multicentric lymphoma with intestinal involvement in a dog. *Vet Radiol Ultrasound*. 2002; 43:138-143.

Chapter 6. Pancreas

ETUE SM, PENNINCK DG, LABATO MA, PEARSIN S, TIDWELL A. Ultrasonography of the normal feline pancreas and associated anatomic landmarks: a prospective study of 20 cats. *Vet Radiol Ultrasound*. 2001; 42:330-336.

HECHT S, HENRY G. Sonographic evaluation of the normal and abnormal pancreas. *Clin Tech Small Anim Pract*. 2007; 22:115-121.

HECHT S, PENNINCK DG, MAHONY OM, KING R, RAND WM. Relationship of pancreatic duct dilation to age and clinical findings in cats. *Vet Radiol Ultrasound*. 2006; 47:287-294.

HESS RS, SAUNDERS HM, WINKLE TJ, SHOFER FS, WASHABAU RJ. Clinical, clinicopathologic, radiographic, and ultrasonographic abnormalities in dogs with fatal acute pancreatitis: 70 cases (1986-1995). *J Am Vet Med Assoc*. 1998; 213:665-670.

LARSON MM, PANCIERA DL, WARD DL, STEINER JM, WILLIAMS DA. Age-related changes in the ultrasound appearance of the normal feline pancreas. *Vet Radiol Ultrasound*. 2005; 46:238-242.

MANTIS P. Diagnostic imaging of the pancreas of the dog and cat. *European J Companion Animal Practice*. 2012; 22(4):15-22.

MATTOON JS, SLOVAK JE, SELLON RK. PANCREAS. In: *Small Animal Diagnostic Ultrasound*. 4th ed. St Louis, Missouri. Elsevier Saunders. 2021; 461-490.

NYLAND TG, MATTOON JS. Pancreas. In: *Small Animal Diagnostic Ultrasound*. 3rd ed. St Louis, Missouri. Elsevier Saunders. 2015; 438-467.

PENNINCK D. Pancreas. In PENNINCK D, D'ANJOU MA (eds): *Atlas of small animal ultrasonography*. Blackwell publishing. 2008; 317-337.

ROBBEN JH, POLLAK YWEA, KIRPENSTEIJN J, BOROFFKA SAEB, VAN DEN INGH TSGAM, TESKE E, VOORHOUT G. Comparison of Ultrasonography, Computed Tomography, and Single-Photon Emission Computed Tomography for the Detection and Localization of Canine Insulinoma. *J Vet Intern Med*. 2005; 19:15-22.

Chapter 7. Kidneys and ureters

ADAMS WH, TOAL RL, BREIDER MA. Ultrasonographic findings in dogs and cats with oxalate nephrosis attributed to ethylene glycol intoxication: 15 cases (1984-1988). *J Am Vet Med Assoc*. 1991; 199(4): 492-496.

ALLWORTH MS, HOFFMANN KL. Crossed renal ectopia with fusion in a cat. *Vet Radiol Ultrasound*. 1999; 40(4):357-360.

BARR FJ. Evaluation of ultrasound as a method for assessing renal size in the dog. *J Small Anim Pract*. 1990; 31:174-179.

BARR FJ, PATTESON MW, LUCKE VM, GIBBS C. Hypercalcemic nephropathy in 3 dogs: sonographic appearance. *Vet Radiol*. 1989; 30:169-173.

BILLER DS, SCHENKMAN DI, BORTNOWSKI H. Ultrasonic appearance of renal infarcts in a dog. *J Am Anim Hosp Assoc*. 1991; 27:370-372.

CHOI J, JANG J, CHOI H, KIM H, YOON J. Ultrasound features of pyonephrosis in dogs. *Vet Radiol Ultrasound*. 2010; 51:548-553.

D'ANJOU MA, BEDARD A, DUNN ME. Clinical significance of renal pelvic dilation in dogs and cats. *Vet Radiol Ultrasound*. 2001; 52:88-94.

D'ANJOU MA. Kidneys and ureters. In: Atlas of Small Animal Ultrasonography. Iowa. Blackwell publishing. 2008; 339-364.

ESSMAN SC, DROST WT, HOOVER JP, LEMIRE TD, CHALMAN JA. Imaging of a cat with perirenal pseudocysts. *Vet Radiol Ultrasound*. 2000; 41:329-334.

FORREST LJ, O'BRIEN RT, TREMELLING MS, STEINBERG H, COOLEY AJ, KERLIN RL. Sonographic renal findings in 20 dogs with leptospirosis. *Vet Radiol Ultrasound*. 1998; 39:337-340.

Jakovljevic S, Rivers WJ, Chun R, King VL, Han CM. Results of renal ultrasonography performed before and during administration of saline (0.9 % NaCl) solution to induce diuresis in dogs without evidence of renal disease. *Am J Vet Res.* 1999; 60:405-409.

Kyles AE, Hardie EM, Wooden BG, Adin CA, Stone EA, Gregory CR, Mathews KG, Cowgill LD, Vaden S, Nyland TG, Ling GV. Clinical, clinicopathologic, radiographic, and ultrasonographic abnormalities in cats with ureteral calculi: 163 cases (1984-2002). *J Am Vet Med Assoc.* 2005; 226:932-936.

Lamb CR. Ultrasonography of the ureters. *Vet Clin North Am Small Anim Pract.* 1998; 28:823-848.

Lamb CR, Gregory SP. Ultrasonographic findings in 14 dogs with ectopic ureter. *Vet Radiol Ultrasound.* 1998; 39:218-223.

Mantis P, Brockman D, Whatmough C, Gregory SP, Lamb CR, Mahoney P, Jakovljevic S. Sensitivity, specificity and accuracy of diagnostic imaging methods for the diagnosis of ectopic ureters in the dog. *Journal of the Hellenic Veterinary Medical Society.* 2006; 57(4):289-296.

Mantis P, Lamb CR. Most dogs with medullary rim sign on ultrasonography have no demonstrable renal dysfunction. *Vet Radiol Ultrasound*. 2000; 41:164-166.

Mareschal A, d'Anjou MA, Moreau M, Alexander K, Beauregard G. Ultrasonographic measurement of kidney-to-aorta ratio as a method of estimating renal size in dogs. *Vet Radiol Ultrasound.* 2007; 48:434-438.

Neuwirth L, Mahaffey M, Crowell W, Selcer B, Barsanti J, Cooper R, Brown J. Comparison of excretory urography and ultrasonography for detection of experimentally induced pyelonephritis in dogs. Am J Vet Res. 1993; 54(5):660-669.

Widmer WR, Mattoon JS. Urinary tract. In: *Small Animal Diagnostic Ultrasound*. 4th ed. St Louis, Missouri. Elsevier Saunders. 2021; 583-634.

Rivers BJ, Walter PA, Polzin DJ. Ultrasonographic-guided, percutaneous antegrade pyelography: technique and clinical application in the dog and cat. *J Am Anim Hosp Assoc*. 1997; 33:61-68.

Chapter 8. Adrenal glands

Barthez PY, Nyland TG, Feldman EC. Ultrasonographic evaluation of the adrenal glands in dogs. *J Am Vet Med Assoc.* 1995; 207(9):1180-1183.

Barthez PY, Nyland TG, Feldman EC. Ultrasonography of the adrenal glands in the dog, cat and ferret. *Vet Clin North Am Small Anim Pract.* 1998; 28:869-885.

Besso JG, Penninck DG, Gliatto GM. Retrospective ultrasonographic evaluation of adrenal lesions in 26 dogs. *Vet Radiol Ultrasound.* 1997; 38:448-455.

Douglas JP, Berry CR, James S. Ultrasonographic adrenal gland measurements in dogs without evidence of adrenal disease. *Vet Radiol Ultrasound.* 1997; 38:124-130.

Graham J. Adrenal Glands. In: Penninck D, d'Anjou MA (eds) *Atlas of Small Animal Ultrasonography*. Blackwell Publishing. 2008, pp. 385-396.

Grooters AM, Biller DS, Merryman J. Ultrasonographic parameters of normal canine adrenal glands: comparison to necropsy findings. *Vet Radiol Ultrasound.* 1995; 36:126-130.

Hoerauf A, Reusch C. Ultrasonographic examination of the adrenal glands in six dogs with hypoadrenocorticism. *J Am Anim Hosp Assoc.* 1999; 35:214-218.

NeelIS Da, Matton JS, Sellon RK. Adrenal Glands. In: *Small Animal Diagnostic Ultrasound*. 4th ed. St Louis, Missouri. Elsevier Saunders. 2021; 566-582.

Wenger M, Mueller C, Kook PH, Reusch CE. Ultrasonographic evaluation of adrenal glands in dogs with primary hypoadrenocorticism or mimicking diseases. *Vet Rec.* 2010; 167(6):207-210.

Zimmer C, Hörauf A, Reusch C. Ultrasonographic examination of the adrenal gland and evaluation of the hypophyseal-adrenal axis in 20 cats. *J Small Anim Pract*. 2000; 41(4):156-160.

Chapter 9. Urinary bladder and urethra

Benigni L, Lamb CR, Corzo-Menendez N, Holloway A, Eastwood JM. Lymphoma affecting the urinary bladder in three dogs and a cat. *Vet Radiol Ultrasound*. 2006; 47:592-596.

Cherbinsky O, Westropp J, Tinga S, Jones B, Pollard R. Ultrasonographic features of grass awns in the urinary bladder. *Vet Radio Ultrasound.* 2010; 51:462-465.

Geisse AL, Lowry JE, Schaeffer DJ, Smith CW. Sonographic evaluation of urinary bladder wall thickness in normal dogs. *Vet Radiol Ultrasound.* 1997; 38:132-137.

Lamb CR, Gregory SP. Ultrasonography of the ureterovesicular junction in the dog: a preliminary report. *Vet Rec.* 1994; 134: 6-8.

Leveille R. Ultrasonography of urinary bladder disorders. *Vet Clin North Am Small Anim Pract*. 1998; 28:799-821.

Lobetti RG, Goldin JP. Emphysematous cystitis and bladder trigone diverticulum in a dog. *J Small Anim Pract.* 1998; 39:144-147.

Martinez I, Mattoon JS, Eaton KA, Chew DJ, DiBartola SP. Polypoid cystitis in 17 dogs (1978-2001). *J Vet Intern Med*. 2003; 17:499-509.

Nyland TG, Wallack ST, Wisner ER. Needle-tract implantation following us-guided fine-needle aspiration biopsy of transitional cell carcinoma of the bladder, urethra, and prostate. *Vet Radiol Ultrasound*. 2002; 43:50-53.

Nyland TG, Widmer WR, Mattoon JS. Urinary tract. In: *Small Animal Diagnostic Ultrasound*. 3rd ed. St Louis, Missouri. Elsevier Saunders. 2015; 557-607.

Petite A, Busoni V, Heinen MP, et al. Radiographic and ultrasonographic findings of emphysematous cystitis in four nondiabetic female dogs. *Vet Radiol Ultrasound*. 2006; 47:90-93.

Sutherland-Smith J. Bladder and Urethra. In: *Atlas of Small Animal Ultrasonography*. Iowa. Blackwell publishing. 2008; 365-396.

Takiguchi M, Inaba M. Diagnostic ultrasound of polypoid cystitis in dogs. *J Vet Med Sci.* 2005; 67: 57-61.

Tipisca V, Murino C, Cortese L, Mennonna G, Auletta L, Vulpe V, Meomartino L. Resistive index for kidney evaluation in normal and diseased cats. *J Feline Med Surg*. 2016;18(6):471-475.

Chapter 10. Peritoneal cavity, lymph nodes and major abdominal vessels

Agthe P, Caine AR, Posch B, Herrtage ME. Ultrasonographic appearance of jejunal lymph nodes in dogs without clinical signs of gastrointestinal disease. *Vet Radiol Ultrasound.* 2009; 50:195-200.

De Swarte M, Alexander K, Rannou B, D'Anjou MA, Blond L, Beauchamp G. Comparison of sonographic features of benign and neoplastic deep lymph nodes in dogs. *Vet Radiol Ultrasound*. 2011; 52:451-456.

Finn-Bodner ST, Hudson JA. Abdominal vascular sonography. *Vet Clin North Am Small Anim Pract*. 1998; 28:887-942.

Merlo M, Lamb CR. Radiographic and ultrasonographic features of retained surgical sponge in eight dogs. *Vet Radiol Ultrasound.* 2000; 41:279-283.

Nyman HT, Lee MH, McEvoy FJ, Nielsen OL, Martinussen T, Kristensen AT. Comparison of B-mode and Doppler ultrasonographic findings with histologic features of benign and malignant superficial lymph nodes in dogs. *Am J Vet Res.* 2006; 67:978-984.

Mayer MN, Lawson JA, Silver TI. Sonographic characteristics of presumptively normal canine medial iliac and superficial inguinal lymph nodes. *Vet Radiol Ultrasound.* 2010; 51:638-641.

Pugh CR. Ultrasonographic examination of abdominal lymph nodes in the dog. *Vet Radiol Ultrasound.* 1994; 35:110-115.

Schreurs E, Vermote K, Barberet V, Daminet S, Rudolf H, Saunders J. Ultrasonographic anatomy of abdominal lymph nodes in the normal cat. *Vet Radiol Ultrasound*. 2008; 49:68-72.

Volta A, Bonazzi M, Gnudi G, Gazzola M, Bertoni G. Ultrasonographic features of canine lipomas. *Vet Radiol Ultrasound.* 2006; 47:589-591.

Widmer WR, MatToon JS, Sellon RK. Peritoneal fluid, Lymph nodes, Masses, Peritoneal Cavity, and Great vessel Thrombosis. In: *Small Animal Diagnostic Ultrasound*. 4th ed. St Louis, Missouri. Elsevier Saunders. 2021; 526-543.

Chapter 11. Prostate gland and testes

Bigliardi E, Ferrari L. Contrast-enhanced ultrasound of the normal canine prostate gland. *Vet Radiol Ultrasound.* 2011; 52:107-110.

England GCW. Ultrasonographic diagnosis of non-palpable Sertoli cell tumours in infertile dogs. *J Small Anim Pract*. 1995; 36:476-489.

Feeney DA, Johnston GR, Klausner JS. Two-dimensional gray-scale ultrasonography: applications in canine prostatic disease. *Vet Clin North Am Small Anim Pract* .1985; 15:1159-1176.

Johnston GR, Feeney DA, Johnston SD, O'Brien TD. Ultrasonographic features of testicular neoplasia in dogs: 16 cases (1980-1988). *J Am Vet Med Assoc*. 1991; 198:1779-1184.

Johnston GR, Feeney DA, River B, Walter PA. Diagnostic Imaging of the male canine reproductive organs: Methods and limitations. *Vet Clin North Am Small Anim Pract*. 1991; 21:553-589.

Newell SM, Neuwirth L, Ginn PE, Roberts GD, Prime LS, Harrison JM. Doppler ultra-sound of the prostate in normal dogs and in dogs with chronic lymphocytic lymphoplasmacytic prostatitis. *Vet Radiol Ultrasound*. 1998; 39:332-336.

Mattoon JS, Davidson A. Prostate and Testes. In: Small Animal Diagnostic Ultrasound. 4th ed. St Louis, Missouri. Elsevier Saunders. 2021; 635-664.

Ober CP, Spaulding K, Breitschwerdt EB, Malarkey DE, Hegarty BC. Orchitis in two dogs with Rocky Mountain spotted fever. *Vet Radiol Ultrasound*. 2004; 45(5):458-465.

Ruel Y, Barthez PY, Mailles A, Begon, D. Ultrasonographic evaluation of the prostate in healthy intact dogs. *Vet Radiol Ultrasound*. 1998; 39:212-216.

Stowater JL, Lamb CR. Ultrasonographic features of paraprostatic cysts in dogs. *Vet Radiol*. 1989; 30:232-239.

Chapter 12. Ovaries, uterus and mammary glands

Barr FJ. Pregnancy diagnosis and assessment of foetal viability in the dog: a review. *J Small Anim Pract*. 1988; 29: 647-656.

Beccaglia M, Luvoni GC. Comparison of the accuracy of two ultrasonographic measurements in predicting the parturition date in the bitch. *J Small Anim Pract.* 2006;47:670-673.

Beck KA, Baldwin CJ, Bosu WTK. Ultrasound prediction of parturition in the queen. *Vet Radiol*. 1990; 31:32-35.

Bigliardi E, Parmigiani E, Cavirani S, Luppi A, Bonati L, Corradi A. Ultrasonography and cystic hyperplasia-pyometra complex in the bitch. *Reprod Domest Anim*. 2004; 39:136-140.

Diez-Bru N, Garcia-Real I, Martinez EM, Rollan E, Mayenco A, Llorens P. Ultrasonographic appearance of ovarian tumors in 10 dogs. *Vet Radiol Ultrasound*. 1998; 39:226-233.

England GCW, Allen WE. Ultrasonography and histological appearance of the canine ovary. *Vet Rec*. 1989; 125:555-556.

England GCW, Allen WE, Porter DJ. Studies on canine pregnancy using B-mode ultrasound: Development of the conceptus and determination of gestational age. *J Small Anim Pract.* 1990; 31:324-329.

England GCW, Yeager AE. Ultrasonographic appearance of the ovary and uterus of the bitch during oestrus, ovulation and early pregnancy. *J Reprod Fertil Suppl*. 1993; 47:107-117.

England GCW. Ultrasonographic assessment of abnormal pregnancy. *Vet Clin North Am Small Anim Pract.* 1998; 28:849-868.

England GC, Russo M. Ultrasonographic characteristics of early pregnancy failure in bitches. *Theriogenology*. 2006; 66:1694-1698.

Hecht S. Female reproductive tract. In: *Atlas of Small Animal Ultrasonography*. Iowa. Blackwell publishing. 2008; 397-416.

Kim Y, Travis AJ, Meyers-Wallen VN. Parturition prediction and timing of canine pregnancy. *Theriogenology*. 2007; 68:1177-1182.

Kutzler MA, Yeager AE, Mohammed HO, Meyers-Wallen VN. Accuracy of canine parturition date prediction using foetal measurements obtained by ultrasonography. *Theriogenology*. 2003; 60:1309-1317.

Lopate C. Estimation of gestational age and assessment of canine foetal maturation using radiology and ultrasonography: a review. *Theriogenology*. 2008; 70:397-402.

Luvoni GC, Beccaglia M. The prediction of parturition date in canine pregnancy. *Reprod Domest Anim.* 2006; 41:27-32.

Luvoni GC. Ultrasonographic study of gestation in dogs and cats. *Rev. Bras. Reprod. Anim., Belo Horizonte.* 2013; 37:172-173.

MATTOON JS, DAVISON A. Ultrasonography of the genital system. In: *Veterinary Diagnostic Ultrasound*. Philadelphia, Pennsylvania, WB Saunders. 1995; 141-164.

MATTOON JS , NYLAND TG, SELLON RK. Ovaries and Uterus. In: *Small Animal Diagnostic Ultrasound*. 4th ed. St Louis, Missouri. Elsevier Saunders. 2021; 665- 688.

PHARR JW, POST K. Ultrasonography and radiography of the canine postpartum uterus. *Vet Radiol Ultrasound*. 1992; 33:35-40.

SRIDEVI P. Ultrasonographic diagnosis and monitoring of pregnancy in the bitch – a review. *J Vet Anim Sci*. 2013; 44:1-7.

STÖCKLIN-GAUTSCHI NM, GUSCETTI F, REICHLER IM, GEISSBÜHLER U, BRAUN SA, ARNOLD S. Identification of focal adenomyosis as a uterine lesion in two dogs. *J Small Anim Pract*. 2001; 42:413-416.

TOPIE E, BENCHARIF D, BRIAND L, TAINTURIER D. Early pregnancy diagnosis and monitoring in the queen using ultrasonography with a 12.5 MHz probe. *J Fel Med and Surg. 2015*; 17(2): 87-93.

YEAGER AE, CONCANNON PW. Serial ultrasonographic appearance of postpartum uterine involution in beagle dogs. *Theriogenology*. 1990; 34:523-33.

YEAGER AE, MOHAMMED HO, MEYERS-WALLEN V, VANNERSON L, CONCANNON PW. Ultrasonographic appearance of the uterus, placenta, fetus, and foetal membranes throughout accurately timed pregnancy in beagles. *Am J Vet Res*. 1992; 53:342-351.

ZAMBELLI D, CASTAGNETTI C, BELLUZZI S, BASSI S. Correlation between the age of the conceptus and various ultrasonographic measurements during the first 30 days of pregnancy in domestic cats (*Felis catus*). *Theriogenology.* 2002; 57:1981-1987.

Chapter 13. Artifacts.

KIRBERGER RM. Imaging artifacts in diagnostic ultrasound: a review. *Vet Radiol Ultrasound*. 1995; 36:297-306.

KREMKAU FW. Artifacts. In: *Sonography Principles and Instruments*. 9th ed. Philadelphia. Elsevier Saunders. 2016; 183-216.

MATTOON JS , BERRY CR. Fundamentals of diagnosic ultarsond. In: *Small Animal Diagnostic Ultrasound*. 4th ed. St Louis, Missouri. Elsevier Saunders. 2021; 26-32.